THE PRIMACY OF CARING

The *Primacy of Caring* presents the reader with a way to view the practice of nursing at the bedside. . . . finally someone has organized ideas that nurses have always known but didn't quite know how to classify. . . . Benner and Wrubel have not only captured the true essence of nursing but have provided a much needed coupling of the science with the art of nursing . . . [they have] taken some of the most controversial issues currently addressed by the profession and provided new and understandable insights.

Sheila Packard, RN, PhD
University of Connecticut

The content is unique. It is where nursing is and what nursing is all about . . . a very powerful project which holds promise for becoming one of the best approaches to patient care.

Jean P. Gilbert, RN, EdD
Northeastern University

The Primacy of Caring

Stress and Coping
in Health and Illness

PATRICIA BENNER, RN, PhD, FAAN
JUDITH WRUBEL, PhD

ADDISON-WESLEY PUBLISHING COMPANY

Health Sciences Division, Menlo Park, California
Reading, Massachusetts • New York • Don Mills, Ontario
Wokingham, England • Amsterdam • Bonn • Sydney
Singapore • Tokyo • Madrid • San Juan

Sponsoring editor: Nancy Evans
Production supervisor: Judith Johnstone
Book designer: Paul Quin
Copyeditor: Antonio Padial
Proofreader: Steven Sorensen

Library of Congress Cataloging in Publication Data

Benner, Patricia E.
    The primacy of caring : stress and coping in health and illness /
Patricia Benner, Judith Wrubel.
        p.   cm.
    Includes bibliographies and index.
    ISBN 0-201-12002-X
    1. Nursing—Psychological aspects.   2. Nursing—Philosophy.
3. Caring.   4. Sick—Psychology.   I. Wrubel, Judith.   II. Title.
    [DNLM: 1. Nursing Care—psychology.   2. Philosophy, Nursing.
3. Stress. Psychological.   WY 87 B469p]
RT86.B395 1988
610'.73'019—dc19
DNLM/DLC
for Library of Congress   88-14489
                                                                           CIP

      10 11 -MA- 97

ISBN   0-201-12002-X

Addison-Wesley Publishing Company
Health Sciences Division
2725 Sand Hill Road
Menlo Park, California 94025

To Carol Carr and to the memory of Terry Carr. Carol, your instantiation of caring reminded us once again of the possibilities.

To the memory of Irene O. Duke.

To Jane and John Culbertson who kept us honest by showing how courage is doing what you have to do.

To the many expert nurses who know more than they can tell and who taught us in their expert caring.

PUBLISHER'S FOREWORD

It is rare that Addison-Wesley adds a prefatory statement to a book we have published. Each book that bears our imprint implies our assessment of its inherent worth and importance.

However, certain books merit more than the endorsement implicit in our imprint because of their significance to the intended audience. We believe that, for nurses, *The Primacy of Caring* is such a book.

The Primacy of Caring is unique and remarkable, not only because it eludes classification within the curricular and practice arenas of professional nursing, but also because it offers a totally new view of stress, coping, and caring. The authors define and describe the essence of nursing practice, and make visible and powerful the hidden expertise of that practice.

In a sense, this work could be called a book on nursing theory. It is more than that, however, because its unique premise is that theory derives from practice, and it demonstrates how theory is applied to practice in various clinical areas.

Like Patricia Benner's earlier work, *From Novice to Expert,* this book is enriched by many clinical exemplars from expert nurses whose caring made a critical difference for their patients and their families. Vivid and moving, these first-person accounts help articulate the uniqueness of nursing practice and the profound impact of expert caring.

We believe this book will have enduring value and appeal for nurses in research, education, and practice. Nurse scholars and theorists will respect the quality of the research, the theory, and its presentation. Nurse educators will welcome the insights this book offers into the context of nursing practice. Nurses in practice will be empowered by this reminder of what nursing is and what nurses do.

Nursing has been called the science of caring. We believe this book represents a landmark contribution to the literature of that science and to the ultimate health of all of us whom that caring touches.

Nancy Evans
Senior Editor, Health Sciences
Addison-Wesley Publishing Company

FOREWORD

This thoughtful and thought-provoking book needs little introduction to prospective readers already familiar with Patricia Benner's highly valued study, *From Novice to Expert.* I believe the nursing world recognized in it a report of clinically focused research that, because of its nature and scope, might materially affect practice and the preparation of nurses for practice.

While the theoretical base of *The Primacy of Caring* is even broader than that of *From Novice to Expert,* it also is clinically focused. Its most instructive and memorable aspect is the application of theory to the care of particular patients, whose stories, told here by practicing nurses, engage the interest and sympathy of readers.

The very title of the book tells us that the authors see a person's sense of being cared for as therapeutic. The "wisdom of the body" is stressed, as is the fallacy of considering mind and body as separate entities. What they have to say about psychosomatic illness and differentiation of objective and subjective symptoms is significant for those who have not studied the meaning of "holistic" care.

It is tempting to quote many passages of this remarkable book, but the following may suffice to suggest its particular value in an age often referred to as "depersonalized" and its medical care as dominated by technology.

> The enabling condition of connection and concern is also what we mean by the primacy of caring. Caring (about someone or something) places the person in the situation in such a way that certain aspects show up as relevant. . . . For example, parenting "techniques" will not work unless a basic level of attachment and caring are in place. . . . Similarly, in studying what makes expert nurses effective, we conclude that mere techniques and knowledge are not enough. . . . In fact caring (a certain level of involvement) is required for expert human practice. *Dreyfus and Dreyfus, 1986*

Speaking parenthetically, while the authors cite H.L. and S.E. Dreyfus frequently and M. Heidegger as, or more, often, attributing considerable weight to the latter's influence, this is a wide-ranging and scholarly work that demonstrates familiarity with an impressive body of literature, dating back to ancient Greece, that bears on the argument underlying their central themes of caring, stress and coping.

To borrow from the authors themselves:

The phenomenological view of stress and coping presented here grew out of a desire to develop a language that more adequately captured the possibilities lived out by actual people coping with events as divergent as birth, childhood illnesses, aging, and death. . . . The languages of positivistic social science and the natural sciences were too impoverished to give an adequate account of what actually occurs in everyday life. This work stems from dissatisfaction with atomic mechanistic and strictly utilitarian views of life.

The more theoretical philosophical chapters include frequent references to clinical practice, but the second half of the book is devoted to coping with coronary illness, with cancer, and with stroke. The final chapter, "Coping with Caregiving," is an understanding view of what it means to nurse as nursing is described in this book. It persuades the reader that in spite of its scholarly nature it is based equally on the reality of caring in today's world.

Virginia Henderson, RN, MA
Senior Research Associate, Emeritus
Yale University School of Nursing

PREFACE

This book examines the relationships between caring, stress and coping, and health, and claims that caring is primary. Caring is a basic way of being in the world—caring sets up what counts as stressful and what coping options are available. This work extends the thesis begun in *From Novice to Expert: Excellence and Power in Clinical Nursing Practice* (Benner, 1984), the thesis that caring is central to human expertise, to curing, and to healing. Nursing is viewed as a caring practice whose science is guided by the moral art and ethics of care and responsibility. It is argued that caring as a moral art is primary for any health care practice.

Nurses provide care for people in the midst of health, pain, loss, fear, disfigurement, death, grieving, challenge, growth, birth, and transition on an intimate front-line basis. Expert nurses call this *the privileged place of nursing.* Clinical nursing practice offers a perspective on stress and coping in health and illness that is distinctly different from a purely psychological, physiological, or biomedical view, and even different from behavioral medicine, though nurses draw on these disciplines. In expert nursing practice, nurses focus on the lived experience in health and in stressful situations. One of the aims of the book is to distinguish the nursing perspective from purely psychological, physiological, or biomedical views. The nursing perspective offered is based upon the notion of good inherent in the practice and the knowledge embedded in the expert practice of nursing. *Herein lies the premise of the book: An articulation of alternative approaches to health promotion, restoration, and even curing practices based upon the primacy of caring.*

This book shares the phenomenological and feminist goal of making visible the hidden, significant work of nursing as a caring practice. Phenomenology and feminism have influenced the work, but expert nursing practice illuminates all the theoretical points. The theoretical perspective taken in this book is based on the phenomenology of Martin Heidegger, Maurice Merleau-Ponty, and the teachings of Hubert L. Dreyfus and Richard S. Lazarus at the University of California, where both authors studied. Practice is viewed as theory in the tradition of Heidegger (1962, 1982), Taylor (1985), and MacIntyre (1981). As this work is read, the critical question of how this perspective would affect health care practice, caring, and curing should never be far from the reader's mind.

ILLNESS AS HUMAN EXPERIENCE

Since nurses deal with health and illness, growth and loss, as they are lived, a distinction is made between illness and disease (Cassel, 1976; Kleinman, Eisenberg, and Good 1978). Illness is the human experience of loss or dysfunction, whereas disease is the manifestation of aberration at the tissue, cellular, or organ levels. Nurses attend to the patient's story of the illness in the formal or informal nursing history. Understanding how symptoms are noticed, or what they interrupt, nurses know that the patient's interpretation of the symptoms is essential to providing adequate nursing and medical care (see Chapter 4). In this view, symptoms are laden with meaning. Understanding the context and meaning of the symptoms is central to curing and healing.

The direction of influence between illness and disease goes both ways. Illness, the human experience, affects disease through a meaningful climate of hopefulness, fear, despair, and denial, and the disease can alter the illness experience through direct impact of neuroendocrine and other bodily changes and states (e.g., hunger, fatigue, thirst, muscle weakness, paralysis). This can never be a simple story of one direction (mind over matter), or a physical determinism (body over mind), because the mind and body are not dual realities as the Cartesian tradition of a mind/body (subject/object) split portrays. We will call this a transactional relationship between the embodied person and the situation. The mind is both constituted by, and constitutes, the body. The influence between mind and body is synergistic and mutual.

Most people agree that the mind and body are inseparable; however, the language of Cartesianism abounds, as evidenced by distinctions between "subjective" and "objective" symptoms. A major task of this book is to offer a view of the person that is an alternative to Cartesianism. This is the view of stress and coping; growth and development across the lifespan; health and health promotion; stress and coping related to chronic illness; and coping with caregiving itself. While holism is firmly established in nursing theory and practice, it will remain an abstract ideal as long as the dominant explanatory systems and methods explicitly or implicitly present a dualistic view of the person. Holism cannot be "layered on" or placed external to mechanistic models of the person; it must shape the view of the person and consequently shape the science of studying human beings.

SEPARATING POPULAR AND SCIENTIFIC NOTIONS OF STRESS AND COPING

Stress and coping as a systematic scientific field is plagued with a confusion between the popularized versions of "stress" and "stress management" that have been taken up as a part of the technological self-understanding and the whole range of stressful transactions people may experience. As a consciousness-raising exercise, students in our classes on stress and coping are asked to differentiate the meanings of "stress" and "suffering." They are asked to say all the words that come to mind when thinking of stress and suffering. The words most often associated with suffering relate to meaningful losses, whereas associations with stress have to do with loss of control, poor management, overload, sense of time urgency—all the exigencies of bureaucratic individualism and modern living. This exercise is used to show that the word *stress* has become popularized to exclude the normal meaningful losses that are "stressful" in the scientific sense. Indeed, the popularized definition of stress can be called a modern folk disease, the scientific findings have become so enmeshed in the popular self-understanding and interpretation of illness. The popularized view of stress and coping is *not* the one presented in this book. Instead, we provide a critique of this popular ideology and an alternative explanation. Stress includes growth and challenge and is defined as threats to significance as well as to goal achievement. Stress management or coping includes strategies for engagement and involvement as well as strategies for increased control and distance. The goal is to avoid a simplistic problem-oriented approach to human suffering, because human beings cope not only with "problems" that can be solved, but also with dilemmas and tragedies. Sometimes there are no solutions, and endurance while maintaining one's concerns and meanings is the most that can be accomplished.

Stress management as popularly viewed could be considered the appropriate technology to manage an autonomous self that develops troubled relationships with a chaotic, capricious environment (a technological self-understanding). Such a technology of self-management logically follows as almost necessary equipment for private, autonomous, individual selves who must create a meaningful order from the ground up and who must manage their own responses. While this is indeed a pervasive view of the modern Cartesian self, and while it is legitimate to claim that the popularity of stress and coping may be laid to this modern technological self-understanding, this is *not* an accurate portrayal of stress and coping in health and illness as they are experienced. Therefore, this book calls into question the major ideological and popularized versions of stress and coping and health promotion, and offers an alternative perspective that can explain and go beyond the current theoretical perspectives.

The scientific discourse on stress and coping presented in this book relates directly to the everyday experience of health and illness. The stress management strategies promote involvement and appropriation of meaning in the midst of pain, suffering, loss, growth, and change. Popularized stress-management strategies that offer increased distance and control are frequently useful—for example, for the person dealing with an untenable commitment to a lost limb. Still, increased distance and control are insufficient for the kinds of human suffering that nurses often help patients confront. Even in the lost-limb example, the person must be able to appropriate meanings that foster reintegration and engagement; a positive phantom of the lost limb (a positive memory of past skilled capacities) assists in extending a sense of embodiment into the artificial limb (Sacks 1984).

The premise that there is a "right" way to cope with human dilemmas as divergent as birth and death is untenable from a nursing-practice perspective and will not be presented in this book. Such a diagnostic, normative view takes a "pathological" or "deficit" approach to human practices and concerns related to health, illness, disease, and suffering, and arrogantly recommends "appropriate" responses in the process. A strictly pathological view cuts off the clinician from the possibilities inherent in the person's own history, skill, practices, and concerns. This work presents an alternative to the current nursing diagnostic label of *ineffective coping*, and encourages the traditional nursing questions: "Coping with what? To what end? With what skills and resources?"

Stress and coping are viewed as historical through and through, meaning that one's stressful experiences and coping options are constituted by the way one is involved in the situation, the skills and concerns, the meanings, and the particular history, including the way one anticipates or projects oneself into the future. Likewise, emotions are viewed as meaningful integral aspects of practical knowledge and embodied intelligence, not as a block to "rationality" or disruptions that must always be coped with.

VALUING CARING IN A TECHNOLOGICAL, INDIVIDUALISTIC CULTURE

This book was written in the context of the societal devaluation of nursing and an acute nursing shortage that is predicted to be permanent. It addresses the cultural and ideological background that lies at the root of the nursing shortage—the devaluation of nursing care and other caring practices. In a highly technical society that values autonomy, individualism, and competitiveness, caring practices have always been fragile, but this societal blindness causes those who value technological advances to overlook the ways these advances are rendered dangerous and unfeasible without a context of skillful, compassionate care.

The dominant view of knowledge in the Western tradition emphasizes abstract, general, theoretical knowledge while overlooking and devaluing local, specific, practical knowledge and expert skillful clinical judgments about particular clinical situations. The way involvement is central to expert knowledge is overlooked, reinforcing the myth that the expert must stand outside the situation, aloof and detached, in order to pronounce expert judgment.

Nursing and other caring practices have become paradoxical in a highly technical culture that seeks sweeping technological breakthroughs to provide liberation and disburdenment. For example, American health care emphasizes the heroics of trauma centers, while overlooking and under-funding programs for nutrition and prenatal care. Heart transplants receive tremendous funding and attention while preventive measures are less exciting and fundable because they are less culturally appealing. In the case of heart transplantation, people typically focus on the dramatic stitching in of a transplanted heart as the "breakthrough." Few notice that the intensive medical and nursing followup—solving the day-to-day problems of living with a transplanted organ, treating sores in the mouth due to immunosuppression, coping with a new hormonal milieu, promptly recognizing and responding to infection and rejection—were all caring "breakthroughs" that led to the eventual success of heart transplantation. These essential day-to-day nursing-care issues had to be solved in order to make heart transplantation a viable therapy. Yet they are all but overlooked in the scientific and popular media coverage of the transplant story.

The theoretical perspective presented here provides an alternative basis for legitimizing and valuing the caring practices and expert knowledge embedded in nursing practice. Caring practices and clinical knowledge development that encompass the particular as well as the general, contextual, and relational knowledge as well as rule-governed abstract principles, cannot rely on seventeenth century notions of science, nor on an oppositional, highly individualistic, technological view of the person. The goal is to set up a basis for a nursing science that examines the lived experience of human illness and the relationships among health, illness, and disease. Such a science can include relevant human concerns and the ways in which human-concern meanings shape health, illness, and disease.

ACKNOWLEDGMENTS

To be true to the thesis of this book we must acknowledge many people who have made the work possible. The expert practice of many nurse clinicians has inspired this work and, indeed, has shaped it. If we have accomplished what we intended, we have captured a portion of the knowledge, wisdom, and ways of being in the best of nursing practice. Hubert L. Dreyfus' lectures, coaching, and writings show up on almost every page. We value beyond words his mentorship and enthusiasm for this work. The teaching, coaching, and writings of Richard S. Lazarus are also central to this work, as will be amply evident. We thank him for his sponsorship and for starting us down this path. The work of Dr. Jane Rubin, who is currently a lecturer at the University of California, San Francisco, School of Nursing, has had a pervasive and profound influence on this work. We have drawn heavily on her teaching and her unpublished manuscript, which provides a new interpretation of the work of Sören Kierkegaard. Charles Taylor's writings, and his visiting professorship at Berkeley, came at the right times to help us see more clearly how an alternative understanding of the person could and should reshape the study of human beings.

Virginia Henderson inspired the direction and content of Patricia Benner's understanding of nursing from her early texts and from more recent conversations and letters. We fervently hope that this work is in the Henderson tradition and are grateful to Virginia Henderson for writing the foreword to this work. Helen Nahm sponsored, recognized, and affirmed the early directions in *From Novice to Expert*, and we hope that we have been true to the insights she values.

Lucille Petry Leone, has been an inspirational coach and prod. We cannot recall a conversation with her over the past seven years in which she has not recommended at least one important book relevant to the work. Her affirmation and confidence in nursing practice is central to the work, and we trust that we have done justice to it.

Many other colleagues have supported and encouraged the work. Nancy Diekelmann, at the University of Wisconsin at Madison, and Christine Tanner deserve special mention for their advice, critiques, and enthusiasm early and late in the work. Jeanne Quint Benoliel's teaching and dialogue have been influential. Mary Mallison, Senior Editor of the American Journal of Nursing, has sponsored, questioned, and affirmed at crucial points. Dr. Deborah Gordon participated early and late in insightful conversations about this work. Our colleagues at the University of California, San Francisco, have provided stimulating conversations and scholarly background for the work.

Many doctoral students have participated in this work. A few must be mentioned because of their critiques, thoughtful questions, and enthusiasm. Karen Brykcynski, Catherine Chesla, Nancy Doolittle, Margaret Dunlop, Mary Hartfield, Annemarie Kesselring, Vickie Leonard, Harriet Lionberger, Linda McKeever, Catherine Popell, Erne Schilder, Lee Smith, Colleen Stainton, Cynthia Stuhlmiller, and Larry Wornian have all participated in strengthening the work. All are conducting research relevant to the theory and tenets of this work.

This work is the culmination of a twelve-year conversation between the authors. The conversation has been ongoing during the births of children and the illness and death of ones close to us, always in the context of the love and support of our husbands, Richard V. Benner and Bob Wrubel, and our children, John and Lindsay Benner, and Rob, Bradley, Benjamin, Joel, and Luke Wrubel. Patricia Benner's parents, Shirley and Charles Lindsay, and Judith Wrubel's parents, John and Jane Culbertson, introduced us to caring practices and provided loving support during the work. Harry Duke provided coaching, proof reading, and encouragement throughout the project.

While the themes in this work have been explored in teaching and conversations over a twelve-year period, this book has been written during the last three. Chapter Six was written first and was jointly written in our favorite form of exchange and dialogue. The rest of the work was divided into major responsibility for writing first and final drafts as follows: Chapters One, Three, Five, Seven, Eight, and Ten were written primarily by Patricia Benner. Chapters Two, Four, and Nine were primarily written by Judith Wrubel.

We owe a large measure of gratitude to Nancy Evans, Senior Editor at Addison-Wesley. Nancy understood the work before it was written and coached, encouraged, stimulated, and improved it. Thank you, Nancy! We are also indebted to Judith Johnstone at Addison-Wesley for her design and production expertise. Antonio Padial, copy editor, suffered through our need to be precise and to defy the usual subject/object splits embedded in English grammar.

Finally, we would like to thank the reviewers who contributed many valuable comments and suggestions during the development of the manuscript. We are indebted to them for helping us see the work through new eyes. They are: Jean P. Gilbert, Northeastern University; Edith (Pat) Lewis, noted editor and writing consultant; Brenda Lyon, Indiana University; and Sheila Packard, University of Connecticut.

Patricia Benner
Judith Wrubel

ABOUT THE AUTHORS

PATRICIA BENNER, RN, PhD, FAAN is an Associate Professor in the Department of Physiological Nursing in the School of Nursing at the University of California, San Francisco. She is author of the widely acclaimed *From Novice to Expert,* named an *American Journal of Nursing* Book of the Year for nursing education and nursing research in 1984. She is an internationally noted researcher and lecturer on health, stress and coping, and clinical skill acquisition. She is currently conducting a research study on expert nursing practice in intensive-care units that is sponsored by the Helene Fuld Foundation. She is co-investigator on a research project on coping with asthma, funded by the Center for Nursing Research, National Institutes of Health.

JUDITH WRUBEL, PhD, is an Assistant Clinical Professor in the School of Nursing at the University of California, San Francisco. She has published in the areas of stress and coping, social competence, and clinical knowledge. She is a research consultant specializing in interpretive methodology, as well as a sought-after guest lecturer. Her current research projects focus on coping with infertility and on the role of personal concerns in seeking and receiving social support.

NURSE CONTRIBUTORS

Lisa Chickadonz, RN, MS

Mary Cucci, RN, BS

Mary Culnane, RN, MS

Judith DeChristopher, RN, BS

Margret Fenton, RN

Susan Hager, RN

Clare Hastings, RN, MS

Nancy Karthas, RN, BSN

Robin Fireman Kramer, RN, MS

Gail L. Marculescu, RN, MS

Michelle Marin, RN, BS

Dorothy Merner, RN

Pamela Minarik, RN, MS

Sharon Olsen, RN, MS

Barbara Ridley, RN

Laura Ryan, RN, MS

CONTENTS

CHAPTER ONE

The Primacy of Caring

I went into his room and he yelled at me, "Are you listening?" I said yes pretty calmly, and he began crying softly and talking. He knew I was listening. *Mary Culnane, RN, MS*

Why Caring Comes First

Caring as it is used in this book means that persons, events, projects, and things matter to people. Caring is essential if the person is to live in a differentiated world where some things really matter, while others are less important or not important at all. "Caring" as a word for being connected and having things matter works well because it fuses thought, feeling, and action—knowing and being. And the term *caring* is used appropriately to describe a wide range of involvements, from romantic love to parental love to friendship, from caring for one's garden to caring about one's work to caring for and about one's patients.

Because caring sets up what matters to a person, it also sets up what counts as stressful, and what options are available for coping. Caring creates possibility. This is the first way in which caring is primary. It determines both what will be stressful and what will count as coping. Caring (having things matter) puts the person in a place of risk and vulnerability. Relationships, things, events, and projects do not show up as stressful unless they matter. If the person does not care, an event cannot be stressful. But the nature of caring is such that it also sets up what coping options are available and acceptable to the person.

Caring sets up the condition that something or someone outside the person matters and creates personal concerns. Without care, the person would be without projects and concerns. Care sets up a world and creates meaningful distinctions, and it is these concerns that provide motivation and direction for people. This book departs from theories of motivation based purely on need satisfaction, or drives, and

1

asserts that motivation is based on concern and caring about specific people, projects, things, and events. Meaninglessness (a place of not caring) and *anomie* (the loss of a feeling of belonging) are the positions most bereft of coping options, because all things appear equal—nothing stands out as relatively more or relatively less important or inviting. Nothing really matters. In the modern sense, the person is free from care and attachments. But this is a negative freedom that makes all options look equally plausible and provides no direction for choosing one over another.

In our modern era, when care and caring are devalued, it can seem that caring is a problem—or *the* problem. From a place of care, the person can neither claim complete autonomy nor be the absolute source of all meaning. This runs counter to the dominant quest in our culture for extreme individualism, the quest to be in charge of one's own life and control all options, including feelings and responses to events. Embracing this version of negative freedom, in which one finally loses all bonds and is free from every care, deprives one of the positive freedom to choose and to act. Of course, such utter disconnectedness is a practical impossibility, and the quest for negative freedom frustrates as it impoverishes.

The risks and vulnerability inherent in caring lead to the temptation to create safe places of "controlled caring" where the person dictates fully what matters and exercises the freedom to stop caring when the person or project is threatened. Many stress-management strategies are designed to increase distance and control. However, if such strategies are inappropriately used and understood to mean that detachment is always preferable and least "stressful," they effectively rob the person of the possibilities and meanings inherent in caring. Worse yet, "preferred coping strategies" for stress management that offer the illusion of distance, control, and equanimity in the midst of suffering can trivialize distress and cut people off from expressing their pain and fear.

A premise of this book is that caring is the essential requisite for all coping. For this reason, the coping strategies discussed here do not usually focus on the mainstays of stress management—strategies for relaxation, distraction, distance, and increased sense of control. More often, we offer descriptions of how nurses help patients to recover caring, to appropriate meaning, and to maintain or reestablish connection. The three paradigm cases[1] presented later in this chapter illustrate this.

Because caring is always specific and relational, the reader will find no context-free lists of advice on "how to cope," nor will the stock-in-trade of stress management techniques be offered as the "solution" to all stress. Instead, we celebrate the possibilities inherent in involvement and caring. Involvement and caring may lead one to experience loss and pain, but they also make joy and fulfillment possible. In our view, coping cannot cure or abolish loss and pain. Coping can help one manage those experiences, but coping based on caring also allows for the possibility of joy, the satisfactions of attachment. Coping "prescriptions" all too often overlook the importance of maintaining the caring relationship, because the caring relationship appears to be the source of the stressful experience.

Thus, we acknowledge that detachment and distancing strategies are useful for gaining perspective and respite, but we disagree that detachment and control are always the preferred modes of coping. In many situations, detachment and control are possible only if one does *not* care, and not caring has its own negative consequences when one cannot exit from the situation. For example, nurses who have dealt with abused children know firsthand the havoc that detachment and disengagement bring to families. The tasks involved in child care are countless, and the work it entails is demoralizing if the parent does not care for the child and is not engaged by the child's laughter, smiles, language, and cries. But when there is caring and concern, parents find ways to manage, even in extreme conditions of multiple births or chronic illness.

Likewise, athletes endure great deprivations and make extraordinary demands of themselves because they care about their sport, care about being the best they can be, and care about winning. They accomplish great feats with little sense of deprivation because caring about the event or accomplishment is the focus. Caring allows the person to focus on the event or the one cared for rather than on personal threat. For example, people may be quite heroic in caring for a

---

1. The three exemplars in this chapter were originally presented at the National Institutes of Health in celebration of Nurses' Week, October 17, 1984. Clare Hastings, Mary Culnane, and Laura Ryan each prepared narrative accounts of clinical situations in which they made a difference. These were presented with interpretive commentary by Patricia Benner.

loved one with a serious illness. To someone not in the situation, this kind of caregiving often appears courageous. The caregiver, however, does not feel "courageous" because the person is doing the only thing that he or she can do. There is no other option compatible with being who this person is, that is, a person who cares for a loved one. When people are praised for their courage or devotion in caring for a seriously ill loved one, they typically respond, "I just did what I had to do." Walking away or not caring simply does not occur to the person.

This enabling condition of connection and concern is another way in which caring is primary. Caring (about someone or something) places the person in the situation in such a way that certain aspects show up as relevant. This is what enables people to discern problems, to recognize possible solutions, and to implement those solutions. For example, parenting "techniques" do not work unless a basic level of attachment and caring exists. In fact, parenting techniques are not even useful or possible unless the parent is already engaged in the parenting situation through caring. But for those already involved in caring for and about particular children with particular concerns, some techniques will show up as more desirable and workable than others.

Similarly, in studying what makes expert nurses effective, we conclude that mere technique and scientific knowledge are not enough. Although the nurse-patient relationship is not on the same level as the parent-child relationship, caring is nonetheless central to effective nursing practice. Caring makes the nurse notice which interventions help, and this concern guides subsequent caregiving. Caring causes the nurse to notice subtle signs of improvement or deterioration in the patient. In fact, caring (a certain kind of involvement) is required for expert human practice (Dreyfus and Dreyfus 1986).

Finally, caring is primary because it sets up the possibility of giving help and receiving help. The same act done in a caring and noncaring way may have quite different consequences. A caring relationiship sets up the conditions of trust that enable the one cared for to appropriate the help offered and to *feel* cared for. This is why nursing can never be reduced to mere technique because humor, anger, "tough love," administering medications, and even patient teaching have different effects in a caring context than a noncaring one. When analyzing the practice of expert nurses, we cannot generalize by isolating effective actions and transferring the same interventions to another situation. We must consider the caring context because the nature of the caring relationship is central to most nursing interventions. The flexibility and diversity of expert practice depend on the nurse's involvement in the situation. In this book, we view caring as a concept that is central not only to our theory of stress and coping but also to our theory of nursing practice.

Caring, Nursing Practice, and Nursing Theory

It is self-evident that theory must be informed by real-world experience and experiments, which are in turn subject to theoretical interpretation. Nursing theories are currently under-investigated and have been developed for curriculum building rather than for or from practice (Meleis 1985). Consequently, nursing theory has not been adequately shaped by the practice of nurses. A theory is needed that describes, interprets, and explains not an imagined ideal of nursing, but actual expert nursing as it is practiced day to day. This type of theory could be used to develop curricula in which practice informs nursing education in a way that nursing education has always influenced practice.

This view is consistent with the recent interest in the nature and qualities of caring practices (Larson 1987, Drew 1986, Mayer 1986, Reiman 1986, Swanson-Kauffman 1986, Brown 1986, Wolf 1986). Rieman (1986), for example, asked patients to identify non-caring interactions with nurses. Non-caring amounted to *not* being present with the patient, but rather being there "only to get the job done." Patients reported feeling dehumanized, devalued, angry, and fearful when nursing care was hurried and distant. Of note is the fact that clumsily performed technical procedures were not raised as instances of non-caring.

Swanson-Kauffman (1986) found five kinds of caring wanted by women who had suffered miscarriages. Caring involved "knowing" that the woman's loss is unique to her as a person, "being with" the woman in an engaged manner, "doing for" the woman by providing comforting and supportive measures, "enabling" the woman to grieve for the loss, and finally "maintaining the belief" that the woman could bear a child. All of these caring practices are central to our understanding of the way caring is always related to issues of concern and significance.

Brown's (1986) study of patients' perceptions of caring demonstrates another central aspect of caring: *Caring is always understood in a context.* In other words, when the situation calls for technical proficiency, then technical proficiency (swift, accurate ac-tions) is experienced as caring. When the patient situation does not require technical actions, expressive actions such as recognition of the patient's uniqueness are identified as caring.

Nursing theorists have been overly constrained by the stringent requirements of the received view of formal theories and have found it difficult to capture the embodied, relational, configurational, skillful, meaningful, and contextual human issues that are central to expert nursing care (Benner 1984). Formal theories that are in the tradition of classical seventeenth-century science embody an atomistic, mechanis-tic view of the person. That is, they either support the view that all processes are irregular, random motions of unchangeable particles or elements, or they maintain that a human being, like the universe, can be considered machinelike, orderly, predictable, observable, and measur-able (Dijksterhuis 1961, 1986).

Nursing theorists typically take exception to atomistic and mechanistic views of the person. At least three other nursing theorists place caring at the center of their views of nursing (Diekelmann in press, Leininger 1981, Roach 1984, Watson 1979). However, in most other nursing theories this exception is stated in the assumptions of the theories but is not integrated into the model or may even conflict with the model. This is understandable, since by its nature a model is atomistic and explicit, with measurable constructs that can be causally related. In short, because of their givens, models are mechanistic.

In addition to being mechanistic, models come to be viewed as templates to be placed over practice. Thus, knowledge comes to be viewed as a product to be utilized, and the role of the clinician in developing knowledge is overlooked. Virginia Henderson has provided an alternative view that the clinical nurse develops knowledge through the practice of nursing [see especially her landmark text with Gladys Nite, *Principles and Practice of Nursing* (6th edition 1968)]. David Evans (1980) asserts that Henderson and Nite's text contains the revo-lutionary view that:

> The habits of mind which inform the everyday tasks of the nurse are exactly the same as those which undergird the very finest published research; in this way Everynurse ought not just to *do* simple research tasks as part of her work, but she ought also *always* to *be* a researcher, whether or not she writes or speaks a word in print or public. Nurses are given lots of token encouragement to participate in research or to be

aware of the need for research-based nursing care, but not enough emphasis has been placed on those qualities of mind that essentially make the
publishing scholar *identical,* in a way, to Everynurse, when she is truly
being a nurse as she should (1980, pp. 338–339).

This book is both an endorsement and extension of this view. Exemplars included in this work show how knowledge is extended and
developed in practice.

This book is devoted to an interpretive theory of nursing practice
as it is concerned with helping people cope with the stress of illness. In
their practice, nurses deal with health and illness, and growth and loss
as they are lived or experienced. This seemingly simple statement is
what this book is about, and the rest of the book will be devoted to
amplifying it and explaining what it means. The goal here is threefold:
to demonstrate (a) the primacy of caring as the producer of both stress
and coping in the lived experience of health and illness, (b) the primacy of caring as the enabling condition of nursing practice (indeed, of
any practice), and (c) the ways that nursing practice based in such
caring can positively affect the outcome of an illness.

This book takes a phenomenological stance based on the work of
Martin Heidegger (1962, 1982) and Maurice Merleau-Ponty (1962)
and focuses on the lived experiences of being healthy and being ill.
Being healthy and being ill are understood as distinct ways of being in
the world. These phenomenologists consider the person's way of being
in the world as prior to reflective thought; and that way of being sets up
the conditions under which treatments will be sought or help will be
appropriated. Kestenbaum (1982) points out that phenomenology is a
style of thought:

> [Phenomenology] advances not only our knowledge of human nature but
> also our understanding of the awareness that a health professional needs if
> his or her practice is to convey more than simply an adequate technical
> comprehension of bodies and persons. To grasp the meaning of illness for
> humanity, the patient, and the humanity of the patient is more than simply
> to "identify" with the patient or to feel compassion. It is to appropriate at
> least one of the conditions necessary for professional judgment inspired
> by human wisdom (p. viii).

In this book, human wisdom is taken to be more than rational calculation. Although problem solving and goal attainment are important
functions, the understanding of what it is to be human also includes

issues of significance. Therefore, human studies can be reduced neither to mathematical accounts nor to causal statements about the relationships between isolated elements.

The rest of this chapter describes a nursing perspective on health and illness, first by distinguishing illness from disease and then by describing how nursing is concerned with the relationships between disease and the lived experience of health and illness. Understanding nursing practice as the care and study of the lived experience of health, illness, and disease gives us a new perspective on several important areas. The old mind-body duality gives way to an integrated view of the person. Likewise the opposed roles of instrumental and expressive are redefined when they are viewed in the context of their function. Thus, nursing care may be both instrumental and expressive, just as medical care may be both. This shift in perspective uncovers the primacy of care in bringing about cure. Cure cannot be understood or accomplished without a background of care and caring practices.

HEALTH, ILLNESS AND DISEASE

Health is not the absence of illness, and illness is not identical with disease (Kleinman, Eisenberg, and Good 1978). *Illness* is the human experience of loss or dysfunction, whereas *disease* is the manifestation of aberration at the cellular, tissue, or organ level. As Oliver Sacks notes, "animals get diseases,but only man falls radically into sickness" (1985, p. xiii).

A person may have a disease, and yet not experience himself or herself as being ill. And so, except for routine checkups that may uncover pathologic conditions, people do not seek health care unless they experience a disruption, loss, or concern. Furthermore, patients do not experience illness as symptoms that can be mapped empirically onto a medically diagnosed syndrome (unless they are medically over-socialized or hypochondriacal). The patient experiences the symptom as an interruption, an inconvenience, or a health worry. Typically, he or she seeks to have troubling aspects of the symptom removed or ex-plained in ways that minimize the disruption or allay the health worry. A disease that matches the symptom may or may not be found, but curing of the disease does not automatically cure the illness (that is, the human response to the symptom).

Since illness and disease are not mirror images of one another, illness cannot be reduced to merely a nonscientific account of disease. Illness as the human experience of loss or dysfunction has a reality all its own. In the end, all treatment must make sense in terms of the human experience; the efficacy of the treatment will be hindered and suffering will increase when the treatment does not match the patient's understanding of the illness.

NURSING PRACTICE AND THE LIVED EXPERIENCE OF ILLNESS

The best nursing practitioners understand the differences and relationships among health, illness and disease. This understanding leads nurses to seek the patient's story in formal and informal nursing histories, because they know that every illness has a story—plans are threatened or thwarted, relationships are disturbed, and symptoms become laden with meaning depending on what else is happening in the person's life. Understanding the meaning of the illness can facilitate treatment and cure. Even when no treatment is available and no cure is possible, understanding the meaning of the illness for the person and for that person's life is a form of healing, in that such understanding can overcome the sense of alienation, loss of self-understanding, and loss of social integration that accompany illness.

A paradigm case written by Clare Hastings illustrates the worth of understanding the lived experience of the illness regardless of what other medical or nursing therapies may be available.

PARADIGM

The Lived Experience of the Illness: Making Contact with the Patient

Clare Hastings, RN, MS
Clinical Nurse Specialist
National Institutes of Health

I had a powerful clinical experience when I was working in the Rheumatology Screening Clinic. It changed my understanding of how nurses can affect patients even during brief encounters. This event took place in the screening clinic, where we see patients who are referred for evaluation and consideration for entry into research protocols. The clinic was set up so that patients spent a fair amount of time with one of the nurses, who went over why they had been referred to the clinic and orienting them to the National Institutes of Health. The setting was what is now the "chemo room" on one of the clinics. It had several beds and a desk. It was a crowded space with not a lot of privacy.

An older woman in a wheelchair came with her daughter. I remember that she had *terrible* rheumatoid arthritis. When we say "terrible rheumatoid arthritis," we mean someone who might be presented in a textbook—one with a lot of deformities, who can't walk and is all twisted up and in pain. We talked about this patient later as a "medical disaster." She came to us after having been treated by a lot of physicians and really not having had what we would have recommended as appropriate medical therapy. She had gone through many years of what I considered almost useless suffering.

When I see patients in this kind of situation, I usually begin by asking them some background questions about why they're here, what their history is, how long they've been ill, and so on. The first thing I asked her was whether she usually used a wheelchair. Was that the way she usually got around? And that question brought a flood of expression from her. Apparently, even though I thought her extremely disabled and deformed, this was the first time she had needed to use a wheelchair. She had somehow managed to cope with all the things that arthritis means, get around her house, take care of her family, and do her job, without having to resort to the symbolic state of "being in a wheel chair." Right away, that put us in touch with each other, and the encounter shifted to an emotional level. We were talking about feelings right from the beginning, before I had found out much about her.

It's hard to express, but there is a sense when you feel that you are making contact with the patient—and again I don't know whether it is the way you talk about the illness, the way you approach the patient, the kinds of questions you ask, or the language you use—but somehow, patients know that you know what they are talking about, that you have seen these kinds of things before. You understand *what they are*. You have dealt with the disease and the consequences of the illness daily, and you have a thorough knowledge of it. The illness is horrible to most people, and they never talk about it to the patient, but it is an everyday thing to you, something you have dealt with, something you know about, and therefore not horrendous or awful. I could feel that between us—that contact.

I then moved into doing a physical assessment and looking at her various joints. Thinking about this later, I realized one of the ways I was able to communicate with her, really get to some of the things she felt, was just by the *way* I looked at her joints. I made distinctions about swelling, the level of inflammation, and so on. It is possible to touch a person and move the person's hand or wrist, and say: "I can tell that this must be really painful right now," or "It looks like you haven't been able to use this hand for a long time," or "What is this finger doing way out here? This must be really difficult when you take a bath." I asked her to move her arms, and I saw that she couldn't even get them up past her shoulders.

10

I asked: "Does anyone help you get dressed in the morning?" Actually these are the kinds of questions I typically ask.

As we were methodically looking at her whole body, she was getting more emotional; probably she had never discussed these personal things before. Maybe the fact that her daughter was there had something to do with it. She had never really discussed anything with anyone beyond: "This knee hurts" and "This finger is swollen." She had never talked about what the symptoms meant to her. She had never said: "This means that I can't go to the bathroom by myself, put my clothes on, even get out of bed without calling for help."

When we finished I said something like: "Rheumatoid arthritis really has not been nice to you." She burst into tears, and her daughter did also, and I sat there, very close to losing it myself.

She said: "You know, no one has ever talked about it as a personal thing before, no one's ever talked to me as if this were a thing that mattered, a personal event."

That was the significant thing about the encounter. I didn't really have much else to offer her. She ended up not being eligible for what we were doing at NIH. She had what we call "old disease," or "burned out rheumatoid arthritis." The disease had wrecked her joints years ago. What she really needed was for someone to put a lot of new hardware inside her, and maybe some physical therapy, but it wasn't the kind of thing we were offering. I knew at the end of the interview that we would probably not be following her, and I had to tell her that. I gave some advice about ways she could go about getting help in the community, but that was clearly not what was significant about the event. Something really significant had happened between us, something that she valued and would carry away with her.

This was a paradigm case (see Benner 1984a) for Clare Hastings because it made her recognize the significance of understanding the lived experience of the illness. No one had ever *understood* what the illness meant to this woman before, and the understanding alone was a great gift, because it moved back the walls of isolation and suffering created by the disease. In our strategic, instrumentally oriented culture, we overlook the human importance of understanding. Understanding can be therapeutic or healing even when there are no possible instrumental interventions, because illness can cut the person off from self-understanding and familiar relationships and ground with others. Scheper-Hughes and Lock (1987) point out:

Sickness is not just an isolated event, nor an unfortunate brush with nature. It is a form of communication—the language of the organs—

through which nature, society, and culture speak simultaneously. The individual body should be seen as the most immediate, the proximate terrain where social truths and social contradictions are played out, as well as a locus of personal and social resistance, creativity and struggle (p. 31).

Clare Hastings called this incident "making contact with the patient," that peculiar ground where the nurse's understanding of the illness builds a bridge to the patient's lived experience of the illness. "Making contact," as Clare Hastings defines it, is based on a deep understanding of the illness and a personal coming-to-terms with the implications of the illness so that the nurse is comfortable talking about the daily consequences. The nurse has, in some sense, personally come to terms with the reality of the illness and is able to convey acceptance and understanding to the patient.

Clare Hastings demonstrates a deep knowledge of the disease and the illness and the relationship between the two. For example, in her detailed physical assessment she not only accounted for pain, inflammation, and swelling but also took into account their personal consequences. The deft examination revealed her knowledge and understanding of the disease. Her attentiveness and thoroughness was received as an acknowledgement of concern and understanding.

Jean Johnson's (1973) research demonstrates that information given to help people prepare for procedures should be as close to the actual sounds and sensations as possible. Howard Leventhal (1975) points out that attentiveness to the lived experience of the illness would transform the usual mode of giving medical information:

> Even if patients are fully aware of the medical implications of their diagnoses, they may not connect the diagnoses to their personal experiences. There are several things physicians can do to connect their statements to the patient's world. The first is to make clear how medical tests and therapeutic procedures will feel. "Feel" subsumes the full range of sensory experiences elicited by a test or treatment procedure: coldness, numbness, tingling, sharpness, and so forth. The second concerns how the procedure will change one's body and its ability to do things. The third concerns the full range of implications of these changes for one's future life. These three types of statement (sensory feeling, bodily changes, future self) form a dimension of information about the self which ranges from concrete sensory experience to abstract issues of self-definition. The usual process of informing patients, for example, naming a medical procedure, or describing how it is performed, does not tell patients how the procedure will affect their experiences and their lives (p. 142).

By connecting with the meaning of the illness and with the way her patient lived out the illness, Clare Hastings addressed all the dimensions outlined by Leventhal.

Clare Hastings's paradigm case is a good example of expert coaching (Benner 1984a). The nurse makes that which is generally abhorrent and unapproachable into something interpretable and approachable. This kind of coaching is exemplified by the nurse in a clinical-knowledge development seminar who commented that a patient had asked her at the end of her preoperative teaching on mastectomy if she, the nurse, also had had a mastectomy. The nurse had not, but she considered this comment a compliment to her teaching. She had not stood outside the patient's realm of experience in her teaching. Instead, she had truly stood alongside the patient, and in her teaching she had conveyed that this could happen to her, too. She was not the aloof health care professional standing outside the patient's community and realm of possibility.

This ability to presence[2] oneself, to be with a patient in a way that acknowledges your shared humanity, is the base of much of nursing as a caring practice. Simons (1987) has captured this sense of presencing in her review of research on caring.

> The presence of the nurse who pays attention was interpreted as caring by patients. Such attention includes more than mere physical presence. It reflects a being "in tune" with each other, an awareness of unique person-hood. Specific actions such as eye contact, body language, and tone of voice are indications of caring as perceived by patients. These actions take no additional time and yet may make a difference in patient well-being (p. 2).

Clare Hastings demonstrates this ability to presence herself with the patient. This ability is a part of the gift of understanding and is illustrated well by Mary Culnane, who describes a paradigm case that

---

2. The phrase "to presence oneself" comes from Martin Heidegger's *Being and Time,* translated from German to English by John Macquarrie and Edward Robinson (Heidegger 1962). The German words *Anwesenheit* and *Zugegensein* were translated "presencing oneself" as the closest English equivalent to the German meanings which include "to enjoin" or "to be accessible." To presence oneself with another means that you are available to understand and be with someone. Presencing oneself contrasts with standing aloof and outside the situation, or being preoccupied with other thoughts while being physically present with the person.

taught her how to presence herself. A second case demonstrates how this learning opened up new avenues of helping for her.

PARADIGM

Presencing

Mary Culnane, RN, MS
Clinical Nurse Specialist
National Institutes of Health

I want to present two examples that are complementary. They reflect the changes I have experienced during these years as an oncology nurse. In the first clinical experience, the patient taught me; in the second, I was able to translate my previous experiences to make a difference for the patient.

Jim Smith was forty-five years old when I met him. He was happily married for a second time, had no children, worked in a bar, and was busy on weekends playing banjo in a country band. He was admitted to the cardiopulmonary unit where I was working (I had not yet become an oncology clinical nurse specialist). The patient had an eight-hour history of slurred speech and blurred vision. The symptoms had cleared up prior to his admission and he was now admitted for a diagnostic workup.

He and his wife had a lot of questions about the diagnostic test he was going through. We would visit the procedural laboratories, or I would introduce him to patients who had recently completed that particular test. He was worked up for transitory ischemic arterial spasms. Four days later he went home with a negative workup. Two days after that he was readmitted after having a seizure at home. I was on holiday at the time, and by the time I returned he had a diagnosis of metastatic lung cancer.

I do not know how he responded to the initial diagnosis—when I returned, I didn't go in to see him for a couple of days. I was really frightened about seeing him because I did not know what to say or do. He made it easy for me, and I did begin working with him again, concentrating on teaching him about his chemotherapy and radiotherapy. I felt that I was teaching him a lot, but actually he taught me. One day he said to me (probably after I had "delivered" some well-meaning technical information about his leukopenia), "You are doing an OK job Mary, but I can tell that every time you walk in that door you are walking out."

He was right. He had developed so much meaning in his illness and life that I was not relating to. This man had really expanded the context of his life into areas where I could have been effective, had I had some understanding. He gave me that understanding.

Because of this, future clinical experiences were different. One Sunday when I was returning from lunch I heard some angry screaming. I recognized the voice. It was a man named Dave (also in his early forties, with a diagnosis of lung cancer). I can't remember the treatment modalities he had been through, but at the time he was going to receive a Phase I agent.

He was yelling that he wanted everything packed up. I felt a panic among the staff. It was a very disruptive outburst, and sometimes it is hard to say what is really going on. It was apparent to me that he wanted to communicate. I went into his room and he yelled at me: "Are you listening?" I said yes pretty calmly, and he began crying softly and talking. He knew I was listening.

For about an hour he told me about the first time he went to the oncologist, his biopsy, waiting for results, the first time he had chemotherapy, what it was like to have "recurrence." He reviewed with me at that time his relationships with family and friends. Ironically, he said what Jim Smith had said: "They are walking out when they come through that door." It was great that he wasn't saying that to me. I knew that I did not relate like that anymore.

Our conversation ended that day, but during the following weeks we spent some intensive time going over what needed to be accomplished. He realized for himself that things were going to be OK for his family, friends, and associates. We began concentrating on his issues: chemotherapy at home, volunteers coming into his house, pain management. It was great, because with support he made the most of his time.

In the second clinical example that Mary Culnane gives, it is evident that she is now able to, in Clare Hastings words, "make contact" with the patient. She is also able to be present. She no longer needs to run away. This paradigm case also points up the importance of understanding the lived experience of the illness. Mary Culnane demonstrates the capacity to develop clinical knowledge, the ability to learn from patients. Her elaborate and technically correct teaching was transformed into expert coaching so that the patient learned what he needed to know when he needed to know it, and the information was presented in the light of the patient's own goals and agendas.

Mary Culnane's paradigm case also illustrates the common meaning pervasive in nursing that Benner (1984a) has called *situated meaning*. Patients who experience extreme deprivations do not respond as an outsider looking in might expect. They do not respond to the situation solely in terms of what they have lost. Instead, they continue to be engaged by concerns, meanings, and even a limited future. Their goals and pleasures are circumscribed by what is possible. Their responses come from their understanding of the situation, and they respond as the situation demands and as it unfolds in time (Dreyfus 1979). Both of Mary Culnane's patients experienced *situated* possibility, and Mary learned to respond to this uniquely human capacity.

Benner remembers the patient who initiated her into this meaning commonly understood by experienced nurses: Mr. Baker was dying. Medicine had nothing left to offer. She entered his room with a sense of despair, wondering what she could offer in what seemed to be a hopeless situation. Mr. Baker taught her that life continues even for the dying. Mr. Baker still liked his coffee hot, he loved to be positioned so that he could see the sunrise and sunset. He relished his visits with his wife. A rather elaborate management strategy helped him cope with his colostomy. He wore brilliant green socks, and he made jokes about leprechauns and the touch of the Irish. All of his efforts were aimed toward returning home one more time before he died.

Like Jim Smith and Dave, Mr. Baker experienced situated possibility and taught his nurses to appropriate this meaning. Indeed, experienced nurses know that nothing is sadder than when those close to the dying person cease to notice that the person is still alive, still has a world, still has concerns. Social death that precedes actual death is particularly sad.

Getting the patient's story is often just a beginning in nursing practice. Knowing what the illness interrupted and how the patient understands the symptoms helps the nurse see the patient in the patient's context, but as the illness progresses and a treatment program is initiated, that context changes. Here the nurse can become not just someone who understands but an interpreter of the situation for the client. This is illustrated in an excerpt from an interview with Mary Cucci, who is a coronary care nurse:

> I look at people. I think anyone else might have noticed if they had looked. I notice people. I am looking at the physical. I am reading demeanor, body language, facial expression, what they have on, whether they have combed their hair. It is not the cosmetic things, it is the other things. I can remember a patient who had ventricular tachycardia. He was not my patient, but for some reason I went into his room. I spoke to him because he appeared in his physical presentation as either sad or needy; he was physically still and very tense. When people are very still they are needy.
>
> I: "You are reading . . ."
>
> I am reading his body and his tones, and I am reading his exhausted-looking face, and I comment to him about that: "You look as if you need a

16

friend. You look as if something is wrong." It opened up a whole problem for him. Someone had defibrillated him while he was conscious.

I: "Describe that for me."

Well, he remembered being defibrillated, and that is something that people do remember (someone anticipates that the person may not be revivable, and gets in there too quickly). People remember it as something almost more unbearable than the fear of the arrythmia—that kicking, jolting thump—a painful memory, and he was sort of paralyzed by it. It is the type of thing that makes people fear going to sleep. They are afraid that it is going to happen again. They have to be protective of themselves, watchful. This had happened in another hospital. When patients arrive, there is at first no trust established, and sometimes it takes a while to reassure them. "Yes, it has happened, but we are aware how painful that can be and what a trauma it can be." In this particular case, the patient said that just my empathy relieved him; that telling him, "Oh no, we do not do that here," relieved him. He turned to me and said, "You should be a psychiatrist."

Mary Cucci's deep understanding of the situation and her ability to read the patient's body language allowed her to understand his fear, give an interpretation, and provide realistic reassurance that he would not suffer the same pain again. This understanding was sufficient to restore his trust in his body and his situation.

Interpretive skills are at the heart of any expert clinical nursing practice because nursing practice is always concerned with the human world. Mary Cucci rightly understood the man's posture as indicating deep worry. She was able to find out what was worrying him, interpret his current situation, and allay that anxiety. With other patients, it is not the situation that requires interpretation, but the patient's personal *meanings*. This is illustrated by Laura Ryan's paradigm case from a psychiatric setting.

PARADIGM
The Delicate Use of Humor as a Means of Relating
Laura Ryan, RN, MS
Clinical Nurse Specialist
Mental Health and Alcohol Nursing Services
Clinical Center
National Institutes of Health

A nineteen-year-old art student (I'll call her Jane) was admitted for a study on a psychiatric research ward because of a serious suicide attempt, chronic depression, and an inability to cope in her first year of college.

She was the only child of a professional couple, both of whom were involved in the behavioral sciences. In fact, her psychologist father had performed many psychological experiments on her when she was a baby in her crib. Her suicide attempts had a chilling seriousness about them, and she came to NIH directly from an intensive care unit following ingestion of rat poison. One of the first things that struck me about Jane was her use of symbolic communication; in fact, this became the core of our work together. For instance, I felt that the choice of rat poison for her suicide attempt was not insignificant but rather a reflection of how she viewed herself as less than human. I thought it was also pertinent to her care that she was in a research setting which might evoke feelings about her early participation in her father's experiments.

The initial challenge for nursing was to establish sufficient trust to open channels of communication and, of course, to carefully assess her suicide potential and provide a secure environment. Long-range goals were designed to assist her in completing the tasks of adolescence that she had failed to do. My initial work with Jane required finely tuned observations of her appearance, her gestures, her interests, and her non-verbal communications as well as her words. I discovered that she was much better able to communicate her mood and inner discomfort through her art than through verbal communications. Inferences had to be shared with her for confirmation, but art provided the groundwork for our relationship, and it seemed that she was testing the waters of trust during these interactions. Intuitively, I felt that a light touch might be more effective than a serious approach in relating to her. The judicious use of humor seemed to defuse some of the tension, and she began sharing a series of codes she had developed to maintain her secrecy.

These word codes were quite elaborate, and I had the feeling that she used them to cover up the ugliness she felt inside, which was also depicted by the many monsters she drew. These figures were always done in black and white, and when she was suicidal, red dots appeared— certainly not very subtle clues.

She often wrapped herself up in her green blanket and refused to let anyone, including her frustrated therapist, know what was going on with her. One idea dawned on me as I sat with Jane during a time when she was bundled up in her green blanket. She was on strict suicidal precautions since her suicidal ideation continued to be quite lethal. We were never sure what she was thinking, and her potential for self-harm was quite high. As I observed the many objects in her room, my eyes landed on a bowl with two pet turtles. I thought how much she reminded me of a turtle— covered in green, with a very hard shell into which she retreated.

During our next session, I brought up the turtles, and it seemed like the door of a vault was opened. She began to talk about the turtles as if they were human, focusing on the one turtle whom she described as depressed. She went on to to talk about how that felt, how afraid the turtle must be. For her, it was the beginning of true self-disclosure and the start of some good work that she was able to do on her low self-esteem. She eventually asked for what she called "grounds therapy," which meant continuing the discussions during walks outside on the grounds. Eventually, the basis for trust was established. As she learned to trust me and the other nurses, a "mutual regulation" developed whereby we could trust her, and she, in turn, learned to trust and depend on herself. Little by little, the wholeness of her being emerged, and she was perceived as an endearing individual whose needs went far beyond the limits of the research.

Laura Ryan appropriately leaves out the humorous exchanges between herself and Jane because they are not easily understood out of context. Her use of humor was effective in establishing rapport and slightly altering this situation of grave seriousness and despair. Expert nurses frequently use humor as an avenue of communication. However, they are hesitant to talk about their use of humor because it is so specific to the situation and so easily misunderstood. Humor can help reframe a situation; however, effective use of humor requires a deep background understanding of the situation and at least a modicum of trust and respect.

In Laura Ryan's example, the skills required to understand the lived experience of the illness are extensive, and understanding is won only through very detailed observation and attentiveness. Laura Ryan talks about finely tuned observations of Jane's appearance, her gestures, and her nonverbal communication. The observations are enriched by education and experience. There are no blueprints with detailed instructions for this clinical interaction. In expert nursing, as in any expert practice, the actual practical situation is more complicated than can be captured by any formal theory or causal modeling. The practice itself is a form of inquiry.

FROM PRACTICE TO THEORY AND BACK AGAIN

The view of practice presented here is based on two premises:

1. Nursing practice is a systematic whole with a notion of excellence inherent in the practice itself (MacIntyre 1981).

2. Theory is derived from practice.

The first premise asserts that excellence is embodied in practice itself, therefore the practice is a moral art and not merely an applied science or technology.[3] Though nursing practice depends on science, nursing care requires more than science for its legitimacy and direction. While the ethos and procedures of science are value-neutral with regard to application and human implications, the practice of nursing cannot be. Curtin (1982) has also taken the stance that the moral art of nursing must guide its science and technology.

The second premise that theory is derived from practice is based upon the Heideggerian view that practical engaged activity is more basic than, and is prior to, reflective theoretical thinking (Dreyfus in press, Heidegger 1982). The practical human world is more complicated and dynamic than can be captured by any formal theory. Theory is necessarily a skeletal, simplified version of reality. The power of theory lies in its ability to simplify and demonstrate relationships and patterns in the world. We take the stance that theory about human action and concerns cannot be mechanistic and causal in the formal sense. Theory about human issues and concerns must be descriptive and interpretive. Understanding is the goal.

Theory in the human sciences frames the questions, and tells the practitioner where to look for legitimate concerns and what constitutes legitimacy. Advanced clinical practice may go beyond any current theoretical account; therefore, expert practice may demonstrate new knowledge and new understanding (Benner 1984a). For this reason, it is important to study the practice of experts to determine new areas of knowledge, new lines of inquiry, and new puzzles or confusion that may exist in advanced levels of practice. The nurse is a knowledge worker and a developer of clinical knowledge.

One might ask, why teach or have theories at all if the expert practitioner's knowledge goes beyond current formal knowledge? This is easily answered because, of course, the expert practitioner has not always been an expert. The nurse entering practice, like the person learning to fly an airplane, requires all the guidance possible to avoid mistakes so that patients and nurses alike survive long enough to develop advanced skills (see Benner 1984a; Dreyfus and Dreyfus 1986). Interpretive accounts of advanced practice create public discourse and the basis for developing knowledge from practice. Also, in

---

3. For a similar view of medicine see: Haurerwas S: *The Suffering Presence*. Notre Dame, Indiana: University of Notre Dame Press, 1986, pp. 39–62. For a similar view of the limits of science see: Schwartz, B: *The Battle for Human Nature*. New York: W.W. Norton, 1986.

novel situations experts must rely on analytical thinking and available formal knowledge.

A second question from a persistent inquirer might be, why should anyone even read this book, since the nurse may come to the same conclusions directly in her or his own practice? After all, did not the nurses held up as examples here perform without the benefit of this particular book? The exemplars taken from expert practice demonstrate the notion of good and the knowledge embedded in advanced levels of practice. By articulating them and holding them up as examples, we can extend them, confirm them, and use them as the basis for new visions of practice. Indeed, the expert nurses themselves extended their understanding by examining and refining areas of knowledge and lines of inquiry directly from their practice. In most cases, an exemplar is presented as a singular outstanding clinical situation. By examining them, we hope to make them more accessible to nurses in comparable situations.

Theory frames the issues and guides the practitioner in where to look and what to ask. Clinical situations are always more varied and complicated than theoretical accounts, and therefore clinical practice is an arena of inquiry and knowledge development. Expert practice embodies the notion of excellence; by studying it we uncover new knowledge. Thus, theory shapes practice, and practice shapes theory. In the best of worlds, practice and theory set up a dialogue that creates new possibilities.

INTEGRATED MIND AND BODY

More than any other helping professionals, nurses attend to the relationship between illness and disease (Benner 1984a, 1985). The human experience of illness affects disease through a meaningful climate of hope, fear, despair, or denial. The disease, in turn, can alter the illness experience through the direct impact of neuroendocrine and other bodily changes and states (e.g., hunger, fatigue, thirst, muscle weakness, paralysis). This relationship can never be a simple one of mind over matter or of body over mind because the mind and body are not dual realities.

Today, most people agree that the mind and body are interrelated and that the influence between them is synergistic and mutual; however, the language of mind-body dualism still abounds, as, for example, when distinctions are made between "subjective" and "objective" symptoms. As long as this legacy from the seventeenth-century scientific

21

revolution continues to pervade nursing theory, it will be impossible to interpret expert nursing practice that acts on an understanding of the relationship and the difference between illness and disease. That is, we believe that the notion of a mind-body dualism prevents people from seeing how nursing practice uses its access to, and grasp of, the meaning of illness to help and, when possible, to heal. The clinical examples cited earlier illustrate this point. From the perspective of mind-body dualism, Clare Hastings should have assessed the arthritic woman as not having "realistically" accepted the limitations of her disease. And Mary Culnane should have sent for a psychiatric intern to deal with her cancer patient's "anger" and "denial." Cassell (1982) describes this problem for medicine:

> If the mind-body dichotomy results in assigning the body to medicine, and the person is not in that category, then the only remaining place for the person is in the category of the mind. Where the mind is problematic (not identifiable in objective terms), its reality diminishes for science, and so, too, does that of the person. Therefore, so long as the mind-body dichotomy is accepted, suffering is either subjective and not truly "real"— not within medicine's domain—or identified exclusively with bodily pain. Not only is such an identification misleading and distorting, for it depersonalizes the sick patient, but it is itself a source of suffering (p. 640).

Suffering is a part of the illness experience, a part of the human world of meaning. In this book, meaning is understood to be *constitutive* as well as descriptive. In other words, a person is created by some meanings that define what it is to be a person and thus govern *what* can be an issue or a concern. Participation in a meaningful world enables, or creates, possibility. Meanings do not just refer to or designate objects and events; they also create new options, new ways to think, feel, and relate (Taylor, 1985).

When mind and body are viewed as distinct and separate entities, stress is defined as a private and subjective experience. In this view, the same damaging event could be considered as opportune by one person and threatening by another, the only difference being their "thinking." Common meanings are overlooked, and the private subject is left with the private responsibility and understanding that "thinking makes it so." Freedom comes to mean a private, subjective freedom of mind over matter. Therefore anyone who is "stressed" can be accused of not having the right mental attitude or not possessing the appropriate coping repertoire (see for example, Weisman 1979). This is the common "blame-the-victim" pitfall in the stress and coping literature.

In this book, we counter mind-body dualism with the phenomeno-logical view (Heidegger 1982, Dreyfus in press). From this perspective, the person is viewed as a participant in common meanings. It is this participation in a world along with the commonalities of embodiment (Merleau-Ponty 1962) that make perceptions common, shared, and mutually accessible. Once the mind and body are understood as unified being, then the person can been seen as participating in a meaningful world. We describe this participation as *situated freedom* (Taylor 1979). (See discussion of radical freedom in Chapter 2, pp. 53–54.) This is the stance that freedom in the fullest sense of human agency comes only when the person is situated in a web of social relations, meanings, concerns, and equipment. The situation offers both what the person may want to be free from and what the person may want to be free to be or to accomplish, because the situation offers alternatives that show up as relatively more or relatively less desirable. This is the definition of participating in a meaningful world.

This view contrasts sharply with a currently popular idea of the self, which we trace back to mind-body dualism. In this utilitarian view, the self is seen as purely instrumental and disengaged, one who sets goals and achieves them. Pleasure in this view, is one of the most rational and powerful goals. People are seen as fundamentally free to abandon any commitment or membership simply because it is "stress-ful" and because it interferes with pleasant feelings. Likewise, they are free to choose and to engage in any stress-management strategies, even those that create untenable distance and control over constituting or self-defining relationships.

The notion of situated freedom has important clinical implications in that people are not viewed as freely choosing all their actions all the time. In this view persons are neither fundamentally free nor unfree. They enter into situations, with their own sets of meanings, habits, and perspectives. And the particular ways of being in the situation set up particular lines of action and possibilities. New possibilities can be learned, but they are encountered or introduced only in the context of the old habits, skills, practices, and expectations. This is what it means to live in a meaningful world.

For example, when people cope with a chronic illness over time, they develop a set of habits, practices, and expectations; that is, they develop a practical knowledge about how to live with the illness. As the disease or health state changes, some patterns become obsolete. However, coping strategies are seldom developed in a purely deliberative and conscious manner. People may have very little access to or understanding of their coping practices. The practices they evolved to manage systems may have become their way of being in the world and understanding themselves. What the nurse sees as an obviously obsolete coping pattern the patient may take for granted as a way of being in the world.

Because people have situated freedom, they also have situated possibility based upon their self-understanding, their history, and their projected future (see Benner 1984a and b, Wrubel 1985). Effective interventions must relate to situated possibilities that include meanings, practices, and personal concerns. Simple homeostatic adaptation models do not adequately capture situated possibility because they systematically ignore meaning and history (a feat that human beings cannot perform!). From a stance of situated freedom and situated possibility, people are viewed as constituted by their meanings, practices, social relationships, and memberships. In contrast to the modern version of the self, they do not stand outside their concerns and interests and decide from scratch what their interests and affinities are, and then select issues, concerns, and relationships that match those isolated interests and talents. It is the concrete, specific relationships that *create* or *constitute* what counts as an interest or a concern. Consequently, caring is our starting point for understanding stress and coping and for understanding which helping strategies actually help.

REFERENCES

Benner P: *From Novice to Expert: Excellence and Power in Clinical Nursing Practice.* Menlo Park, Calif.: Addison-Wesley, 1984a.

Benner P: Quality of Life: Explanation prediction and understanding in nursing science. Adv Nurs Sci 1:1–14, 1985.

Benner P: *Stress and Satisfaction on the Job: Work Meanings and Coping of Mid-Career Men.* New York: Praeger Scientific Press, 1984b.

Brown L: The experience of care: Patient perspectives. Top Clin Nurs 8:56–62, 1986.

Cassell EJ: The nature of suffering and the goals of medicine. N Engl J Med 30:639, 1982.

Curtin L: The nurse patient relationship: Foundation, purposes, responsibilities, and rights. In L Curtin, MJ Flaherty (eds). *Nursing Ethics: Theories and Pragmatics.* Bowie, Maryland: Brady Publications, 1982.

Diekelmann N: *The Curriculum as Dialogue and Meaning—An Alternative for Professional Nursing Education.* Madison: University of Wisconsin Press, in press.

Dijksterhuis EJ: *The Mechanization of World Picture,* Dikshoorn C (trans.). Princeton, N.J.: Princeton University Press, 1961, 1986.

Drew N: Exclusion and confirmation: A phenomenology of patients' experiences with caregivers. *Image* 18:39–43, 1986.

Dreyfus HL: *Being-in-the-World: A Commentary on Being and Time Division I.* Cambridge: Cambridge University Press, in press.

Dreyfus HL: *What Computers Can't Do: The Limits of Artificial Intelligence,* rev ed. New York: Harper & Row, 1979.

Dreyfus HL, Dreyfus SE, with Athanasiou T: *Mind over Machine: The Power of Human Intuition and Expertise in the Era of the Computer.* New York: The Free Press, 1986.

Evans D: Everynurse as researcher: an argumentative critique of principles and practice of nursing. Nurs For 19:337–349.

Heidegger M: *Being and Time.* Macquarrie J, Robinson E (trans). New York: Harper & Row, 1962.

Heidegger M: *The Basic Problems of Phenomenology.* Hofstadter A (trans.) Bloomington: Indiana University Press, 1982.

Henderson V, Nite G: *Principles and Practice of Nursing.* New York: Macmillan Co., 1978.

Johnson J: Effects of accurate expectations about sensations on the sensory and distress components of pain. J Pers Soc Psych 27:261–275.

Kestenbaum V (ed): *The Humanity of the Ill: Phenomenological Perspective.* Knoxville: The University of Tennessee Press, 1982.

Kleinman A, Eisenberg L, Good B: Culture, illness, and care: Clinical lessons from anthropologic and cross-cultural research. Ann Intern Med 88: 251, 1978.

Larson P: Comparison of cancer patients' and professional nurses' perceptions of important nurse caring behaviors. Heart Lung 16:187–192, 1987.

Leininger MM: *Caring: An Essential Human Need.* Thorofare, N.J.: Charles B. Slack, 1981.

Leventhal H: The consequences of depersonalization during illness and treatment: An information-processing model, p. 120. In *Humanizing Health Care,* Howard J, Strauss, A (eds). New York: Wiley, 1975.

MacIntyre A: *After Virtue.* Notre Dame, Indiana: University of Notre Dame Press, 1981.

Mayer D: Cancer patients' and families' perceptions of nurse caring behaviors. Top Clin Nurs 8:63–69, 1986.

Meleis AI: *Theoretical Nursing: Development and Progress.* New York: Lippincott, 1985.

Merleau-Ponty, M: *The Phenomenology of Perception.* London: Routledge & Kegan Paul, 1962.

Reiman D: Noncaring and caring in the clinical setting: Patients' descriptions. Top Clin Nurs 8:30–36, 1986.

Roach S: *Caring: The Human Mode of Being: Implications for Nursing—Perspectives in Caring.* Monograph 1. Toronto: Faculty of Nursing, University of Toronto, 1984.

Sacks O: *The Man Who Mistook His Wife for a Hat and Other Clinical Tales.* New York: Simon & Schuster, 1985.

Scheper-Hughes N, Lock MM: The mindful body: A prolegomenon to future work in medical anthropology. Med Anthropol Q 1: 6, 1987.

Simons JE: Science update: Patients' and nurses' perception of caring. *The Research Review: Practice Studies for Nursing* 4:2, 1987.

Swanson-Kauffman K: Caring in the instance of unexpected early pregnancy loss. Top Clin Nurs 8:37–46, 1986.

Taylor C: *Hegel and Modern Society.* Cambridge: Cambridge University Press, 1979.

Taylor C: Theories of meaning. In *Human Agency and Language: Philosophical Papers*, vol 1, pp. 248–292. Cambridge: Cambridge University Press, 1985.

Watson J: *Nursing: The Philosophy and Science of Caring.* Boston: Little, Brown, 1979.

Weisman AD: *Coping with Cancer.* New York: McGraw-Hill, 1979.

Wolf Z: The caring concept and nurse identified caring behaviors. Top Clin Nurs 8:84–93, 1986.

Wrubel J: Personal meanings and coping processes. Unpublished doctoral dissertation, University of California at San Francisco, 1985.

CHAPTER TWO

On What It Is
To Be a Person

Eventually the basis for trust was established. As she learned to trust me and the other nurses, a "mutual regulation" developed whereby we could trust her, and she in turn learned to trust and depend on herself. Little by little, the wholeness of her being emerged, and she was perceived as an endearing individual whose needs went far beyond the limits of the research. *Laura Ryan, RN, MS*

Introduction: Why Philosophy?

Socrates reportedly said that the unexamined life was not worth living. We believe that, in matters of theory, the unexamined assumption is not worth having. We intend to examine some of the assumptions underlying our current popular and scientific notions of what it is to be a person. We have some fairly well worked out notions of what it is to be a person that are at the base of the theory of stress and coping presented in Chapter Three. These notions differ in major ways from the usual view. To describe this different idea of what it is to be a person completely and fairly, we need to examine the usual notion. This means examining it in terms of its origins as well as its assumptions. And this means sketching very roughly some history of philosophy and entering into some philosophical considerations.

Why philosophy? There are several answers to that question. The first answer is our belief that we are formed by (and we also reciprocally form) both our personal and our cultural history. Our cultural history as it occurs in the present connects us to the past because it contains meanings that have been passed down. Indeed, the term *philosophy* goes back as far as Socrates. It comes from the Greek (as do a number of terms used in this chapter) and means "love of wisdom." And our prevailing notion of what human wisdom is also goes back to Socrates.

Socrates was always trying to find out what people knew and how they could know anything. So he questioned different experts about such things as justice, piety, and the good and concluded that they knew very little. But in these questionings or "dialogues," as they are known, Socrates always explicitly left out anyone with skilled knowledge, like the shoemaker or the cook. Skilled knowledge was not concerned with such abstract ideals as the beautiful and the good, and skilled knowledge could not be abstracted from its concrete, situational expression.

How Greek philosophy, particularly that of Socrates' student Plato, has shaped our idea of what it is to be a person is discussed further below. The point here is to indicate that our very understanding of ourselves has been shaped by a long cultural history, for example, our idea that abstract knowing is the highest and most desirable form of knowledge, and that skilled activity is of a lower order and is not true knowledge. And so, if we are ever to be in a position to affirm or deny that notion of the person, we must examine it from its beginnings.

Why else philosophy? Why digress from the topic of the role of caring in nursing practice and stress and coping to entertain philosophical considerations of what it is to be a person? Because theories of nursing practice, of stress and coping, and of health and illness, whether they are formal or informal theories, are all based on assumptions about what it is to be a person, that is, on assumptions about being, knowing, and knowledge.

This brings us to our final reason for explicitly stating the philosophical basis of our approach. If our work and our approach are to be useful to anyone in his or her practice, it has to be fully understood. What we are offering here is neither a template that can be placed over a situation nor a set of rules for improving patient coping. Rather, it is an approach, a way of thinking, a method. We are not ourselves philosophers, but we have found that philosophy has provided us tools for understanding within the frameworks of our respective disciplines. We wish all of our readers to be so equipped. Although it will be clear (if it is not already) that we have considerable enthusiasm, even passion, for our topic, we know that not everyone will agree with our premises or with our conclusions. The important aspect is not that readers agree or disagree but that they understand why they do.

This chapter falls into five somewhat uneven segments. First comes a discussion of the mechanistic model of the person, which includes both a brief historical review of how this model came about and a critique of the position. Then come two sections, one on the cognitivist and the other on the structural/organismic view of the person. Both views, we will argue, are based on mechanistic assumptions. The fourth section presents our (Heideggerian) phenomenological account of what it is to be a person. The fifth and last section is, in a sense, mechanism revisited. Instead of examining mechanistic notions of what it is to be a person in formal theory, however, we turn to an examination of our culture and of the way mechanistic assumptions influence how we think of ourselves and others in our everyday lives. This section comes after the phenomenological theory of what it is to be a person because only once the alternative view is clear can the deeply embedded cultural meanings be interpreted.

The Mechanistic Model of the Person

The notion of what is involved in being a person, that is, the notion of human being that is most often used in theories about human activity, is rooted in the mechanistic "model."[1] It has become so familiar that often its basic assumptions are taken for granted and not expressed explicitly. As a result, even theories that aim to present an alternative approach can be based in essentially mechanistic assumptions. Because of this hidden or unexplicit factor, we point out mechanistic assumptions throughout the book when addressing approaches to stress and coping and health care. It may at times appear an annoying quirk of ours, but we do so deliberately to jog the reader's thinking. We believe that the mechanistic model is inadequate for explaining human activity, and we have also found that its assumptions as expressed in health theories can lead to a noncaring stance in health care givers (see the discussion of psychosomatic symptoms in Chapter Five for an example of this). So, our pointing out mechanistic assumptions wherever they occur is a deliberate act of "consciousness raising" on our part.

The mechanistic model of the person was born out of the causal-

---

1. The word *model* has been placed in quotation marks because it is the term commonly used by social scientists trying to describe what it is to be a person. We avoid the term because it is explicitly mechanistic. Our view of what it is to be a person cannot be modeled because the term presupposes an objective assessment, that is, a notion of the person as object with definable parts, rather than a being, agent, or actor situated in a meaningful context.

mechanistic framework of seventeenth- and eighteenth-century English empiricists, and articulated as a psychological view by early twentieth-century American behaviorists. When the limits of behaviorism as a useful theory for understanding human beings became apparent, another "model" sprang up, that of cognitivism. The cognitivists' notion of the person was aimed at correcting the worst extremes of behaviorism, but, as it will be shown below, it, too, is based on mechanistic assumptions. The rest of this section is devoted to describing and critiquing the four overlapping assumptions that underlie the mechanistic model:

1. The primacy of efficient causality in scientific inquiry
2. The person as reactive organism
3. The necessity for reductionism
4. Knowing as representation.

They will be presented as they appeared historically to give some sense of their cultural roots.

EFFICIENT CAUSALITY

The seventeenth and eighteenth centuries were the occasion of a major revolution in thought in Western Europe. This revolution gave birth to ways of thinking that have provided the basis for the technological advances of our era and particularly for the great strides of the natural sciences. Before that time, natural, visible objects and occurrences were interpreted in terms of their relation to supernatural (that is, spiritual) meanings. The natural world was a manuscript wherein Divine intentions could be read.

We owe to the Greek philosopher Aristotle (384–322 B.C.) the definition of the four causes of change. He thought that distinctions among the causes were necessary because "knowledge is the object of our inquiry, and men do not think they know a thing till they have grasped the 'why' of it (which is to grasp its primary cause)" (1941, p. 240). He labeled them the material, the efficient, the formal, and the final cause. And he described them in terms something like these:

The *material cause* of an object is what it is made up of, as, for instance, a house is composed of bricks. The *efficient cause* is the force or agent that moves the object. If we continue the example of the house, this could be the bricklayer. The *formal cause* is the pattern or form of an object, such as bungalow, split-level, or igloo. The *final*

30

cause is the end or purpose of the object, as, for instance, the purpose of a house is to provide shelter.

When these terms are applied to people instead of things, a psychologist could say that the material cause is the physiological base, that is, the body and its organic capacities. The efficient cause could be the indepedent variable, or the antecedent condition. The formal cause would be the genetic substrate (e.g., DNA), and the final cause could be some developmental endpoint.

British philosopher Francis Bacon (1561–1626) was influential in rejecting formal and final causes to explain natural phenomena. Formal causes did not provide explanations but rather different ways of classifying objects and events. And, Bacon saw final causes as involving "that for the sake of which" a thing exists; an inappropriate form of explanation for natural science because it attributes intentions, goals, or purposes to things.

Eliminating formal and final causes from the study of natural science freed that area of investigation from the then current anthropomorphic vision and allowed for a stunningly rapid advance of knowledge. The power of the natural science approach in advancing understanding is very attractive, and the human sciences have strived during this century to be equally "scientific" in the pursuit of understanding human beings. There is one central problem with this adaptation of the form of inquiry used in the natural sciences. With people, formal and final causes are very much to the point, because people are everywhere engaged in purposeful activity.

If final causes are excluded as a legitimate form of explanation in the study of human activity, then agency can be viewed and understood only in strategic terms, that is, in terms of the success in achieving certain ends (Taylor 1985b). And the person as an agent of significance, that is, a being who has concerns and issues, cannot be considered. Taylor (1985b) states that if we understand

> . . . an agent essentially as a subject of significance, then what will appear evident is that there are matters of significance for human beings which are peculiarly human, and have no analogue with animals . . . matters of pride, shame, moral goodness, evil, dignity, the sense of worth, the various human forms of love, and so on. If we look at goals like survival and reproduction, we can perhaps convince ourselves that the difference between men and animals lies in a strategic superiority of the former: we can pursue the same ends much more effectively than our dumb cousins.

31

But when we consider these human emotions, we can see that the ends which make up a human life are *sui generis*. And then even the ends of survival and reproduction will appear in a new light. What it is to maintain and hand on a human form of life, that is, a given culture, is also a peculiarly human affair (p. 102).

Stress and coping are impoverished if we can consider only strategic superiority and cannot address the significance issues that are at the heart of human emotion. Taylor (1985b) is clear that the view of the human being in purely strategic terms is the result of trying to rid the human sciences of all anthropocentric properties (final causes) and results in a hopelessly reductive human science, in which goals such as survival and reproduction are the ultimate explanatory factors, and issues of significance are ignored altogether.

THE PERSON AS REACTIVE ORGANISM

John Locke (1632–1704) was the most important progenitor of British empiricism, and his thinking has been clearly adopted by American behaviorists. From Locke we get the notion of the person as a passive receptor of stimuli from the external environment. Locke proposed that the mind at birth is a blank slate (*tabula rasa*). Ideas are mental copies of reality. (Some copies may be relatively more or relatively less accurate than others.) These ideas are impressed upon the mind and constitute its total contents. Locke called the basic, irreducible unit of information a "simple idea." The mind passively receives and responds to sensory experiences and cannot create knowledge; however, the mind can put the simple ideas together in various combinations to form complex ideas.

REDUCTIONISM

Reduction is the principle that empiricists see as guiding the process of science. For reductionists, the complex can be best understood in terms of its basic, atomic components, components that bear no intrinsic relation to one another.

The first two assumptions of the mechanistic model combine to pave the way for how reductionism applies to the study of people. If social scientists must look to efficient causality in their explanations, (that is, the external force, antecedent condition, or independent variable) and if all complex ideas can be seen as combinations of simple ideas originating in the external world, then, to understand people, researchers need to discover the basic, atomic terms (the "simple ideas") that precede behavior. Taylor's (1985b) description of the problem with this atomistic view is brief and to the point:

> The actions we are inclined to take are identified by their purposes, and frequently these are only intelligible against the background of significance. For instance, we understand the inclination to hide what is humiliating only through understanding the humiliating. Someone who had no grasp of a culture's sense of shame would never know what constituted a successful case of hiding (p. 108).

Human actions, human concerns, or even complex physiological systems cannot adequately be captured by combining atomic elements because the contents of elements make qualitative differences and the relationship between the elements changes their nature and functioning.

KNOWING AS REPRESENTATION

Representation describes one way of conceptualizing how the person relates to and understands his or her world. This notion can be traced to the theories of the French philosopher René Descartes (1596–1650), who held that the mind and the body are distinct entities. In his view, the mind exists in time only, whereas the body, unlike the mind, is physical and has extension in space. Since the mind cannot come into direct contact with the external world, it has to operate with representations of the world that are more or less correct approximations of reality. The contents of the mind are private, accessible only to the individual. Behavior, by contrast, is public and available for all to see.

Internal, that is, mental, experience is causally related to events in the external world by means of the body. The body, through sense organs, becomes the vehicle for external events to become impressed on the mind. In this way, the body becomes part of the external environment as far as the mind is concerned. Since the body is the only vehicle by which the mind can express the internalizations garnered from experience, behavior is the only information available for a person to understand another's mental experience, which is otherwise inaccessible.

In sum, in the Cartesian view, representation describes the person-context relation. The world as currently experienced through the sense organs is represented in the mind. The world as understood and remembered is stored in memory and represented through recall. Because the world is not apprehended directly but is represented mentally by the person, personal meanings are private and idiosyncratic. Personal meanings cannot be understood as expressing commonalities between people because, first, they are individual creations, and second, they are not directly accessible to another person. Only the person's behavior is accessible to another.

In psychology this assumption of the privacy of meaning has for decades created controversy about how to study people and has resulted in a number of different tactics for research. Strict behaviorists believe that only behavior is accessible for study. Nonbehaviorist personality and social psychologists believe that meaning cannot be studied directly, it must be inferred, but with many protections against the skewness of individual perceptions. Thus, data are often mistrusted or questioned if based on "self-report," that is, the person just saying what he or she thought or did. In a great deal of the research in clinical psychology, but especially in psychoanalytically influenced clinical psychology, what people say about what they think or do is the basic information used. But it is treated with suspicion and analyzed in terms of what the person is trying to hide or cover up, either consciously or "unconsciously."

All these approaches in psychology have one thing in common: Meaning is understood to be idiosyncratic. In itself, meaning is not the object of study because idiosyncratic meaning reveals only aspects of a particular person but nothing about people in general. Thus, researchers devise ways of conceptualizing, organizing, and describing personal meanings not in terms of specific content of a life over time but in abstract or generalized categories to which groups of people might belong.

If we accept the notion of representation as how people are in the world, then personal meanings are not only private but also a less-than-perfect apprehension of what is really out there in the world. In short, personal meanings are subjective and reality is objective. This assumption has had major implications both for how some social scientists conceive the health or illness of human functioning should be assessed and for how most conceive of their method of study in the first place. The degree of skewness among the researcher's assessment of behavior, the researcher's inferences concerning personal meanings, and objective reality forms the basis for assessing health and level of adaptation for some psychologists. (For an example, see the discusion of Haan in

Chapter Three.) Also, because of the assumption of an objective world versus subjective meanings, many social scientists tend toward methods of study that permit the study of the person as an object. For this reason, their conclusions will be judged objective and communicable, giving other social scientists a basis for judging the truth or accuracy of the findings.

Thus, in this approach, people must always be viewed as objects, and methods for studying them must fit certain criteria of objectivity. As a result, the person cannot be seen as a creative, generating being who lives embedded in a context of meaning, a being whose actions and understandings form a comprehensible whole.

Cognitivism

The clearest expression of enlightenment views in social science was found in the behavioristic stimulus-response (S-R) model, which predominated in American psychology for several decades. In its strict interpretation of the tenets sketched above, behaviorists limited the study of people to their behavior, that is, to their objectively viewable actions. This meant that the study of people could not be concerned with internal mental activity, which, in the view of behaviorists, is private and subjective. That is, mental activity can never be studied objectively. Of course, this creates a rather barren field of study, since people could not be studied in terms of their reported emotions, goals, or purposes. And yet, it seems obvious that people's actions can be understood only in terms of their emotions, goals, and purposes.

Behaviorism has fallen out of favor these days as a theoretical explanation of human activity. But elements of mechanism remain in the belief in the need for objectivity, in the distrust of subjectivity, and the continued belief in the rules of natural science as the appropriate rules for the study of people—indeed, in the belief that nothing true about people can be discovered unless the rules for natural science are followed.

Aspects of behaviorism have been borrowed for use in different areas. For example, clinical interventions using behavior modification techniques have been widely popularized. Further, in moving away from behaviorism, many theoretical psychologists have nonetheless retained elements of the mechanistic concept of the person and tried to find other explanations than the now seemingly simplistic notion of S-R

35

psychology. Cognitive psychologists have now taken over the reins from the behaviorists (Bolles 1974, Dember 1974). And yet cognitive psychologists still retain the Cartesian notion of representation and its corollary of the mind-body split. Some cognitivists have even borrowed the idea of the mechanism, and the modern mechanism of the computer has become their model of a person.

The most thorough critique of the computer-based concept of the person has been offered by Hubert Dreyfus (1972) in his critique of the field of artificial intelligence, which strives to model the human mind on a computer. He argues that the computer model of the person cannot account for some of the most important human activities, such as emotions, embodied knowledge, and skilled behavior. Furthermore, the computer model cannot account for shared meanings, the role of the situation in shaping meaning, or the way people use context to grasp meaning.

If the mind is to be seen as like a computer, it must be understood to function by taking in data in bits. What is taken in is meaningless, that is, the information taken in is neutral and uninterpreted until the mind "processes" it and decides what it means. The mind contains what is variously called a cognitive map, psychological structures, or formal rules that make the information interpretable. In the computer analogy in its crudest sense, the brain is the hardware, the "mind" is the software, and human experience is neutral bits of data. Thus, the model retains the Cartesian dualism between mind and body and the assumption that meanings are subjective.

Because the person is understood to take in neutral information and assign it meaning, meanings (that is, the organizing capacity that makes sense of incoming information) must necessarily exist in the mind. Because the model requires that information be received in this neutral way, it cannot account for the role of the situation in shaping people's understanding. For example, someone with a chronic symptom with known causes will react differently from someone who is experiencing a similar symptom for the first time. The situation sets up expectations so that some interpretations and options will just appear obvious, while others will not even be considered.

Not only does the computer model of the mind require that information be neutral until taken in and interpreted, it also requires that information be received in bits. This requirement cannot allow for (or account for) the role of context. We propose that context plays a continuous role in people's lives. Especially important is the capacity of context to shift between background and foreground. The Gestaltists discovered how this works visually and have demonstrated it with pictures. One picture shows either a vase or two profiles, depending on how one looks at it. It is not possible to see both the vase and the profiles at the same time, because each is background for the other. In daily life, things can be in the background and move into the foreground. For example, in a time of grieving, routine events that were formerly taken for granted and formed the background of the relationship may be a signal of loss and change. The routine may then move into the foreground of the grieving person's attention.

Situations set up a context for feelings. But just as the computer model cannot account for the situation, so also it cannot adequately deal with feelings. Miller and Johnson-Laird (1976) describe how awkwardly feelings are handled in the information-processing model of the mind:

> The information-processing system that emerges from these remarks is fearfully cognitive and dispassionate. It can collect information, remember it, and work toward objectives, but it would have no emotional reaction to what is collected, remembered, or achieved. Since in this respect it is a poor model of a person, we should add at least one more predicate to this list of those that take "person" as their first argument. We will use *Feel* (person, x) to indicate that people have feelings as well as perceptions, memories, and intentions. It might be possible to subsume *Feel* under *Perceive* on the grounds that our feelings are a special class of perception of inner states. Or we might discuss feelings under *Remember*; the recognition that some word or object is familiar, is after all, a matter of feeling a certain way about it. Or, since we have already recognized that there is a strong affective component to our intentions, we might link *Feel* to *Intend*. . . . All these considerations testify to the sytematic importance of this psychological predicate. Nevertheless, we will have little to say about *Feel* in the following pages (pp. 111–112).

The quotation illustrates the difficulty at the heart of the matter. Because incoming information is neutral until processed, emotion, if it is to have any place in this model, has to exist in the system of formal rules that conducts the processing business. And no one knows how a system of formal rules could have feelings and concerns at all. *Feel* does not have "systematic importance," as Miller and Johnson-Laird assert, it has human importance.

Essentially, any cognitive model of the person, whether it uses the computer analogy or not, cannot account for the role of the situation in shaping emotions, the experience of stress, or the possibilities available for coping. A cognitive view of the person necessarily sees the mind as the originator of meaning. The situation in this view becomes at best a mitigating factor.

The extreme end of this view, but one that is becoming all too common, is the "thinking-makes-it-so" idea of human involvement in a situation. The person's way of thinking is seen as the reason for his or her own illness. It is but a brief step from this position to the "blame-the-victim" stance, the judgmental position that the illness is the person's own fault. For example, before it was discovered that Parkinson's disease had a neurologic cause, it was proposed that the disease was the result of excessive suppressed hostility (Booth 1948, Jelliffe 1940).

The computer analogy of the person is particularly inadequate for explaining salience, that is, the person's immediate grasp of a situation in terms of meaning for the self. Or, if we use the language of the computer model itself, how is it that people distinguish between hot and cold information? Zajonc (1980, 1984) and Lazarus (1982, 1984) have publicly debated about which comes first, emotion or cognition. Zajonc argues for the separation of emotion and cognition and cites empirical evidence for emotion being primary and distinctly separate from cognition.

Lazarus (1984), by contrast, argues that there can be no emotion without cognitive appraisal. He denies that this cognitive appraisal must consist of clear, explicit conceptual thinking. Their debate points up the crisis in the Cartesian view of the person because neither position can adequately account for the meaningful way in which the person relates to the situation or the way in which the skilled body responds to meaningful situations.

The Structural View

Although most cognitivists have adopted the computer model of the mind, not all psychological theories are so "mechanically minded." There has been a strong movement in psychology, especially among developmentalists, toward a theory of the person that would reflect both the organic aspect of the person and the role of the environment. Thus, "organismic" theories of human development came into vogue (see Overton and Reese 1973). At the center of this movement was a reaction against the view of the person as a passive receiver of stimuli from the environment who is not active in shaping his or her world but can only respond to what is presented. Researchers such as Piaget, Langer, and Werner noted a movement for growth and development that they believed could best be accounted for as having an internal and physiological ("organismic") origin.

First, human development seemed too orderly to be accounted for by the bombardment of the person by random external stimuli. It seemed to these theorists that there were too many commonalities among children of the same ages and also among adults who had experienced very different "stimuli" from their environments. They reasoned that some other factor must be involved in shaping lives.

Second, it was clear to those involved in actual observation of children (e.g., Piaget 1950, 1954, 1968) and clinical work with them (e.g., White 1963) that the children were not passive receivers of the environmental stimuli but were active in their exchanges with the environment: active not only in that they sought out certain kinds of exchanges but active also in how they shaped and took in what came from the environment.

Third, the developmental changes that took place were not continuous. Development, according to S-R psychology, should occur on a continuum because development is the result of an accretion over time of a stimulus history. But Piaget discovered major discontinuities in children's cognitive development. The most familiar is conservation of number. Piaget gave children two groups of six small objects, one group bunched up and the other spread out. Before the child reaches a certain cognitive level, if one asks which group has more, the child will say that the group that is spread out has more. After reaching the cognitive level, the child will say that both groups are the same and might give the interviewer a funny look for asking such a silly question. Apparently, the conservation of number is not a concept that is grasped slowly, with the child sometimes making mistakes and going back and forth between getting it and not getting it. Thus, this cognitive stage is discontinuous with the preceding one in that it represents a qualitative change in a way of thinking. Piaget proposed that the discontinuity was not total, however, because the old mode of thinking is incorporated into the new. In this incorporation, however, there is a transformation that gives the appearance of discontinuity. The important point is that the changes are qualitative and cannot be accounted for by accretions of experience.

Piaget is used here simply as an example of a structural/organismic developmentalist. Much more could be said about his theory of cognitive development. However, the issue at hand is that, at base, his theory is a structural one. It concerns cognitive structures. Other developmental approaches emphasize personality structures (e.g., Block 1971). Cognitive or personality structures are mental frameworks that determine how the world is to be understood as well as what behavioral response is to be given. A mental structure is essentially just the same notion as the computer model's cognitive map, and thus all the difficulties inherent to cognitivism are also inherent to structural theories of personality or cognitive development.

A mental structure is a generalization, an abstraction devoid of situational content. If a mental or personality structure is to work, it has to be generalizable (and as far as researchers are concerned, recognizable) across situations. Structures cannot be thought of in terms of the specific content of personal meanings because such content is too situation specific. The point of a structure is that it is applicable to different contents. For example, according to a structural approach, a person who exhibits the trait of dominance to a high degree will respond to an examination, a marriage proposal, and the death of a parent in ways that reflect that characteristic, and the responses will be similar to those given by others who exhibit that trait to a similar degree.

Thus, a mental structure is like a set of rules for how to act. An understanding of the structure can be gained by observing it in actual situations, but the structure itself is understood as applying across situations. Because mental structures are ideas, forms, or organizers, they cannot themselves be conceived of or understood in terms of contextually relevant particulars. And because they apply across individuals and are used as a way of grouping individuals, they cannot be thought of in terms of individual life experience.

To sum up, although originally intended to counter the mechanistic model, the organismic model, by positing mental structures, retains the central element of mechanism. That central element is representational thought as the only way of encountering the world. In our critique thus far, we have brought up a number of concepts that we believe are important and must be accounted for in any discussion of what human being is. These include embodied ways of knowing, personal meanings that are neither private nor subjective, and an inhabited world that is a context, not an environment, and that is organized according to human purposes. We give a fuller account of these aspects of the person in the following section, and also in Chapter Three.

A Phenomenological View of the Person: The Self-Interpreting Being

As noted at the beginning of the chapter, we do not use the term *model* for our description of a person because, in the phenomenological view proposed here, the person cannot be modeled. That is, the person cannot be understood if treated as an object.

When we talk about a phenomenological view of the person, we are not even beginning from the same point as the Cartesian-based mechanistic view. Descartes began by asking the question, "How do I know?" His solution resulted in the mind-body dualism that has dominated scientific thought for several centuries. Descartes believed that by answering the epistemological question, he had answered the ontological one. In other words, he believed that by answering the question of how a person knew things, he had answered the question of how a person was or existed. He summed up his solution in the sentence, "Cogito, ergo sum" ("I think, therefore I am").

In the phenomenological view of the person proposed by Heidegger (1962), which is the view drawn on here, the ontological question takes precedence over the epistemological one. For Heidegger, the question of being is prior to the question of knowing, and the answer to the question of knowing arises out of the answer to the question of being.

According to Heidegger, a person is a self-interpreting being, that is, the person does not come into the world predefined but becomes defined in the course of living a life. A person also has, Heidegger proposes, an effortless and nonreflective understanding of the self in the world. People can have this understanding because they are always situated in a meaningful context and because they grasp meaning directly. This is not to say that people are not capable of thinking reflectively or conceptually. But deliberative, abstract thought is not the only way in which people encounter the world. In fact, one would not know what to do with such abstract, conceptual thinking if one were not situated in a meaningful context. But it is easy to see how one could believe that all knowledge was reflective knowledge, because whenever one stands outside of a situation, one is in a reflective position. Heidegger's concern was to illuminate what kind of knowing occurs when one does not stand outside of the situation, but is involved in it. This concern was preeminent because it seemed to him that most of a person's being was engaged in particular situations.

This is a different understanding of the term *phenomenology* than is widely used in nursing (Oiler 1982, Omery 1983), psychology (e.g., Kohler 1966, MacLeod 1964), and sociology (e.g., Berger and Luckman 1966). Those conceptions of phenomenology are based on Husserl's work. Edmund Husserl (1859–1938) was another German philosopher and a teacher of Heidegger. But Heidegger's phenomenological view of the person differs radically from Husserl's (1964). Husserl's view still contains the Cartesian elements we discussed above. First, Husserl's *noema* (an abstract mental structure that accounts for the mind's directedness toward objects) is a cognitive, representational view of the mind. Second, Husserl believed that the individual assigns meanings to the situation. This individual assignment of meanings results in an intersubjectivity that is based on a consensus of private meanings (see Dreyfus 1982 for a fuller discussion). In Heidegger's formulation, however, the person grasps the situation directly in terms of its meaning for the self. The person does not assign meanings to the situation once it is apprehended because the very act of apprehension is based on taken-for-granted meanings embedded in skills, practices, and language.

This immediate grasp of a situation in terms of its meaning for the self is made possible by several aspects of our humanness. One is the fact that our bodies as well as our minds are knowers, and this embodied knowledge enables us to move through situations and encounter situations in terms of meaning and in rapid, nonreflective ways. Another is the fact that we are brought up in meanings and understand the world in terms of these meanings, which Heidegger calls "the meaning of being." Yet a third aspect of our humanness is that things matter to us. We have the capacity to care, and our caring causes us to be involved in and defined by our concerns. And finally, because we are able to encounter situations in a nonreflective way (that is, not as subjects reflecting on objects but as involved participants), and because care involves us in the world, situations have the capacity to engage us and to constitute us. We discuss each one of these aspects in turn below to explain what they are, how they work, and how they all together describe a phenomenological view of the person.

EMBODIED INTELLIGENCE

It should be clear by this point that the assumption of a mind-body split in the Cartesian view of the person left no room for an embodied intelligence. This is one reason why the concept of an embodied intelligence has not been very widely investigated. There are two other reasons why the intelligence of the body has been so neglected. One is in the nature of our cultural heritage, and the other is in the nature of emodied intelligence itself.

Skilled activity, which is made possible by our embodied intelligence, has been long regarded as "lower" than intellectual, reflective activity. This prejudice goes back as far as Plato, who lived in Greece in the fifth century B.C. He explicitly stated that true knowledge was of abstract notions, such as the good and the beautiful, and that the understanding of skilled craftsmen was not really knowledge. This distinction persists today throughout our culture. However, this hierarchical ordering of skilled action versus abstract reasoning misses the point that skilled action is a way of knowing and that the skilled body may be essential even for the application of the so-called higher levels of human intelligence (Dreyfus 1979).

The other reason for the neglect of embodied intelligence is that it works best when it is not noticed, and it is usually brought to a person's attention only when it is not working well. When embodied intelligence works well, it is rapid, nonconscious, and nonreflective. When embodied intelligence does not work well or when it breaks down altogether, it loses its essential embodied, taken-for-granted quality and becomes something one reflects on consciously. Indeed, reflection tends to cause a breakdown. Thus, smoothly functioning intelligence is difficult to notice, much less study.

Understanding embodied intelligence means understanding the various rapid, nonexplicit, and nonconscious ways of grasping the significance of a situation for the self that are available for human beings. Embodied intelligence is involved in a wide range of activities, from recognition of familiar faces and objects and integrated recollection of our past experiences to maintaining posture and moving our bodies without conscious attending (Sacks 1985). It is an integral part of the highly complex skills of the jazz pianist (Sudnow 1978) or of the expert nurse (Benner 1984a). All of these are part and parcel of the kind of beings we are. That is, we are the kind of beings who have an ontological capacity to respond to meaningful situations (Dreyfus 1979; Merleau-Ponty 1962, 1968).

That we have this embodied intelligence, then, means not only that we are beings with a mind-body unity but also that we have the capacity to be in a situation in meaningful ways. When we speak of meaning here, we speak of meaning as it is lived out by the person. A simple example is the ready recognition of fleeting facial expressions. Our notions that meaning begins with the abstract and general and then becomes personal and that the greatest power for understanding comes from mastery of the abstract reflect a cultural, intellectual bias. The vacuity of the abstract is recognized only when the completely taken-for-granted capacity for personal meaning is lost. Sacks (1985) provides such an example in his case study of a man with visual agnosia.

> "What is this?" I asked, holding up a glove.
> "May I examine it?" he asked, and, taking it from me, he proceeded to examine it as he had examined the geometrical shapes.
> "A continuous surface," he announced at last, "infolded on itself. It appears to have"—he hesitated—"five outpouchings, if this is the word."
> "Yes," I said cautiously. "You have given me a description. Now tell me what it is."
> "A container of some sort?"
> "Yes," I said, "and what would it contain?"
> "It would contain its contents!" said Dr. P., with a laugh. "There are many possibilities. It could be a change purse, for example, for coins of five sizes. It could . . ."
> I interrupted the flow. "Does it not look familiar? Do you think it might contain, might fit, a part of your body?"
> No light of recognition dawned on his face. [. . .]
> Visually, he was lost in a world of lifeless abstractions (p. 13).

Only in the absence of the embodied capacity to recognize the familiar and its relation to the self is it possible to see how dehumanizing it would be to live in a world of abstractions. What a deprived existence it would be, what impoverishment of life, if one were unable to recognize a glove, a rose, the faces of one's spouse, children, or friends.

People as embodied intelligences are able to live in the world and recognize it as their world, a world of meaning. Also, as embodied intelligences, people are able to live in this world easily, comfortably. They are "at home" here. Developmentally, we begin with the body's innate capacity to be in the world and go on to the ways that the body learns cultural meanings, the use of tools, and skilled behavior.

Over time people acquire a culturally skilled habitual body. For example, people learn culturally appropriate distances for standing in different social situations (Hall 1959). It is all right to stand very close in a crowded bus, but the same distance is not acceptable when one stands in line in the supermarket. We never learn these distances conceptually in terms of feet and inches. Indeed, having to think consciously of one's cultural habitual body is an exhausting experience. Imagine, for example, moving to Japan as an adult and having to think consciously of bowing. In Japan the act of bowing is part of the cultural habitual body. It would be a strain to have to think reflectively and decide each time one bowed that this was the appropriate situation in which to bow, and then to decide how many times to bow and how deeply. It would be similarly straining to decide reflectively to stand 28 inches behind the person in front of you at the checkout stand.

The habitual cultural body is so taken for granted that it is most often completely invisible to reflexive awareness. It is easier to understand the value and necessity of an embodied intelligence when thinking of the skilled use of tools. We can often remember the first times we used a tool in a skilled activity, e.g., giving an injection or suctioning a patient, using a typewriter, or looking through a microscope. The awkwardness and crudeness of accomplishment in spite of completely focused attention are striking to us. Then gradually the body takes over. The needle and syringe move quickly and smoothly as a unit, and the injection is accomplished without jerking and slipping. The suction tube finds its mark without curling. The fingers know themselves where to find the letters on the keyboard with no conscious messages from the eyes via the brain, and the hand brings the slide into focus rapidly while the eye scans the slide as readily as it might read a page. Tools used in this skilled way become like extensions of the body (Polanyi 1966).

To sum up, the innate capacities that humans start out with make it possible for them to experience an embodied self and to inhabit a world that has meaning for that self. The cultural, habitual body allows the person to perceive a context organized according to human purposes and past concrete experiences, complete with their significances (Dreyfus and Dreyfus 1986). And the use of tools as extensions of the body organizes context-meanings in terms of practical behavior (Dreyfus 1972, Merleau-Ponty 1962). All of these aspects of embodied intelligence make possible a nonreflective grasp of a situation in terms of its meaning for the self. What those meanings might be is described in the next two sections, "Background Meaning" and "Concern."

BACKGROUND MEANING

We are used to thinking of meaning in subject-object terms. In these terms, subjective meaning is private and accessible only to the individual. When reflected upon, subjective meaning becomes objective and can be made explicit. The stated task of psychoanalysis, for example, is to take subjective—that is, private, unconscious meanings—and through reflection make them conscious and explicit.

It is also common to think of meanings as propositional knowledge. Psychological and sociological studies of "values" and beliefs follow this pattern. Even when researchers are seeking commonly held, culturally derived meanings, they see them as beliefs that such-and-such an explicitly statable thing is so.

Background meaning, according to Heidegger (1962), is neither subjective nor propositional. Rather, background meaning is what a culture gives a person from birth; it is that which determines what counts as real for that person. It is a shared, public understanding of what is. Background meaning is not itself a thing, it is rather a way of understanding the world. Although it does not exist as a thing itself, it is what allows for the perception of the factual world. Merleau-Ponty (1962) has offered the analogy of background meaning to a light. You do not see the light, you see what it illuminates, and without it, you would see nothing.

Because people are embodied intelligences, they can take in cultural background meanings from birth, even before they have reflective consciousness. Caudill and Weinstein (1969) give an example of how this works. They observed and carefully recorded mother-child interactions in both Japan and the United States. They found that the babies became thoroughly Japanese or American by the age of three or four months. The Japanese babies were physically passive and content to be watchful of things and people around them. The American babies were physically active and constantly engaging vocally as well as physically with their mothers. They traced these culturally recognizable ways of being to the culturally distinct interactive patterns of mother and child. The researchers understood the different cultural meanings in the following way: The Japanese understand the newborn to be a separate, uncivilized being who needs to be brought into the family and made civilized; the Americans understand the newborn to be a helpless, dependent being who needs to be encouraged to become autonomous.

For an individual, background meaning is provided by the culture, subculture, and family to which that person belongs. Background meaning is taken up in individual ways from the cultural background meaning, but only within the range of what is possible within a culture. For example, in the United States personal control is a cultural background meaning that has borne the scrutiny of social scientists for several decades. Rotter's (1966) work is probably the most well known. His Internal-External Locus of Control Scale has been widely used because so many other measures correlate with it.

More recently, Wrubel (1985) has shown that the relation between scores on the Rotter Scale and individual coping in actual situations can be understood only in the light of an individual's personal background meanings. But even though, in these cases, the background meaning of personal control is uncovered and interpreted, the full meaning of personal control can never be made totally explicit because in its deepest form it is tied to what it means to be a person in our culture. It is not limited to attitudes or belief systems but is embedded in cultural practices and skilled activity. Moreover, personal control is known in bodily ways that enable people to navigate through life, and bodily understanding is not fully amenable to conscious reflection. Finally, personal control, or any other aspect of background meaning, is not complete or finished. As people in a culture live out the background meaning over time, it is modified and takes on new forms.

CONCERN

The last two sections have described two aspects of a phenomenological view of the person. We have illustrated how background meaning and embodied intelligence help life go smoothly without effortful conscious attending. Embodiment allows people to live in the world and understand it in relation to themselves, and background meaning provides the content of what is understood. But there is yet another facet of what it is to be a person, and that is that things matter to us. And because things (including other people) matter to us, we become involved in the world. Heidegger (1962) calls this way of being involved "concern."

Although the term *commitment* is commonly used by social scientists describing (or measuring) what is important to people, the term *concern* is used here because it is more qualitative and more descriptive of meaning than *commitment* is. In its use in social science, commitment is quantitative; it is a continuous variable that is always analyzed in terms of its strength or weakness (Kelley 1977). At the positive end of the continuum, a strong commitment is defined by the researcher, usually in ideal terms. For example, a strong commitment in marriage could be characterized by how likely the person is to stay in the marriage. All couples studied would be rated on the strength of their intent to stay married in order to measure strength of commitment. Couples who did not possess strong intent would be rated as low on commitment. By contrast, in the phenomenological view of the person, concern, like the concern for a spouse, is described in its own terms, in its meaning for the person. This perspective makes it possible to describe the content of the concern and the likely intents.

Concern describes the peculiarly human way of being in the world. Heidegger (1962) clarifies what this means by contrasting the different ways one can use the word *in* to describe an object and to describe a being who has concern. Both an object and a person can be described as being "in" in a spatial sense. For example, the chair and the woman are in the house. But only the person can be "in" in the sense of being involved, for example, being in love. This existential rather than spatial sense of the preposition "in" is concern. It is an essential part of human existence (see Dreyfus in press).

Concern is a key characteristic of the phenomenological view of the person. Although embodied understanding and background meaning can account for *how* the person can be in the world and grasp meaning directly, concern accounts for *why*. Traditionally, the queston of why people do things, make the choices they make, has been answered by mechanistic theories of motivation. If people are seen as separate from their world, and the world as an object to be taken in and reflected upon, then what motivates people has to be either people's own internal drives, needs, or structural traits or external prods or rewards in the environment.

By seeing people as involved in a context, or as Dreyfus (in press) interpreting Heidegger puts it, as inhabiting their world, the issue of motivation becomes a nonquestion. The motivational question is "What moves people?" *Move* in this sense means literal motion. That is, what gets people going toward or away from some thing or person or goal? In the phenomenological view, the person does not move toward or away as subject to object; the person, through concern, is involved with the other. This involvement means that the world is understood in the light of the concern (e.g., what threatens the concern, threatens the person). Furthermore, rather than having a subject-to-object relation—or owner-to-possession relationship, as Sandel (1982) describes it—the person is defined by his or her concerns.

Because concern is qualitative (i.e., a meaning term) we can talk about how the concern is lived out. For example, Heidegger (1962) talks about two types of concern: (a) the kind of solicitude that leaps in and "takes over for the Other that with which he is to concern himself" and (b) the kind of solicitude that "leaps ahead" of the Other, "not in order to take away his (or her) 'care' but rather to give it back to him (or her) authentically. . . ." In the first kind of concern, the Other is thrown out of his or her own position, and he or she can either be disemburdened completely or take it up again "as something finished and at his disposal" (pp. 158–159). When patients are extremely ill and dependent, there is no choice but to "leap in" and take over, but the problem is that this kind of "taking over" can extend past the point of necessity either on the part of the one caring or the one cared for. That is, the one cared for may find it difficult to take up his or her care again. The first kind of solicitude, the kind that "leaps in" for the Other, can easily slip into domination and dependency or even oppression, even if this domination is subtle and not apparent to those involved. The second kind of solicitude is a form of advocacy and facilitation. It empowers the Other to be what he or she wants to be, and this is the ultimate goal in nursing care relationships.

THE SITUATION

Because of concern, people are involved in a context. They inhabit their world, rather than live in an environment. Because of embodied intelligence, background meaning, and concern, people grasp a situation directly in terms of its meaning for the self. This is what is meant by phenomenology. Furthermore, because of this direct apprehension of meaning, and because people do inhabit their worlds in an involved rather than subject-object way, people are constituted by their worlds and solicited by them. This point is often missed. Our understanding of situation or context is influenced by the ingrained Cartesian notions of the separate subject who touches the world only indirectly through representation, who is the source of all meaning, and so who can only be self-constituted (Taylor 1985c).

But sometimes smooth functioning breaks down. In all this discussion of embodied selves, personal/cultural background meaning, and concern, it is easy to forget that embodied, self-interpreting people live in a real world and that over time real-world contexts change. Marriage, divorce, widowhood, promotion, and unemployment—to name but five of the more common such changes out of the many that occur—all place the person in a situation in which the old self-understandings are no longer comepletely relevant. No amount of mental rehearsal can prepare one fully for such changes, because people cannot reflectively encounter all the taken-for-granted aspects of their being. It is only in the changed context that the hitherto unnoticed background meanings, habitual body understanding, and concern are seen to no longer allow for smooth functioning. People become aware of them and reflect on them.

This breakdown in smooth functioning is what we mean by stress. It is clear from the above discussion that such breakdown, even on a small scale, involves the person as a whole. One of the situations that almost always involves the breakdown of smooth functioning is illness. Many taken-for-granted aspects of one's being can no longer work smoothly for one during a serious or a chronic illness. Background meanings, concerns, and bodily understanding all go by the boards. And if the person is hospitalized, the context itself can be foreign, causing the person to feel desituated. Or, conversely, if the person is used to the institutional context, the situation could be laden with cues for a sense of dependence, unwellness, security, and so on.

Influence of the Mechanistic Model on Current Views of What It Is To Be a Person

Our culture is steeped in the assumptions of the mechanistic model. Both our ordinary ways of thinking and talking about ourselves and our formalized, theoretical approaches to knowledge have been profoundly influenced by mechanistic thinking. Now that a phenomenological view of the person has been presented, the implications of the mechanistic model and the pervasiveness of the concept in our culture can be more easily understood. We shall describe how mechanism has influenced our cultural understanding of three central aspects of personhood. We call them the technological view of the self, the disembodied view of the self, and the radically free self.

TECHNOLOGICAL SELF-UNDERSTANDING

The Cartesian notion that the mind and body are separate and that the subject is private and knows an objective world through observation that is more or less veridical is a representational theory of knowledge and truth. Truth is a correct representation, or at least has a high correspondence with objective reality. This model holds that intelligibility is rooted in rationality.

This assumption of Cartesianism has deeply influenced our modern sense of what it is to be a person. It has led to the belief that rationality and the ability to represent things clearly are the path to all understanding. The question of agency—freedom to plan and decide one's course—is determined by strategic abilities. In this view, what makes human beings "superior" to animals and computers is their strategic superiority in achieving goals. Instrumental reasoning becomes crucial because the best kind of planning is that done when options have been clearly delineated and evaluated in terms of the probability of attaining known goals (Taylor 1985b).

Thus, the person is viewed as an agent who engages in rational calculation to determine what goals to set and how to attain them, and the journey through the life course is conducted on the basis of a cost-benefit analysis. The person is enabled in this task by the objectivity afforded by analytical, strategic thinking about the world. Indeed, the only relationship the person has to the world (and for *person,* read here *mind*) is a representational one. The body, which unlike the mind is material, also becomes part of the world as far as the mind is concerned. This person, then, is an agent who sees the world and the body objectively, that is, as objects that are essentially the raw material used by the agent to gain desired goals.

The technological view that grew out of the Enlightenment accounts for the huge strides made in modern times in science and technology. Without the impetus of this approach, the understanding of the physiology of the body and the processes of disease would have remained cloaked in the prohibitions and superstitions of the Dark Ages. And twentieth-century health care providers would have a much poorer armamentarium with which to fight disease. When the technological view is turned on the nonhuman world, that is, on objects that really are objects, the result can be an increase in understanding of diseases and in the ability to combat or cure them. When the technological view is used as the basis for studying people (i.e., human action) or as the basis for one's own sense of self, the result is confusion, impoverished understanding, and alienation.

When people are studied objectively in the Cartesian sense of the term, then one thing that must be left out is the person's connection to and embeddedness in a situation. Researchers who have tried to acknowledge this relationship but who still approach the study "objectively" have been forced into the position of proliferating variables, each variable representing another aspect of the situation. The result of this kind of approach can only be confusion.

An alternative view of the person, one not based on a strategic or instrumental view of the person, is offered by Taylor (1985b). Here the distinguishing characteristics of the person cannot be judged on strategic powers and performance criteria alone. Being a human agent means that things and people matter in essential ways. The person is a creature of significance constituted by relationships, meanings, and memberships, in short, a creature of culture. And so what matters to people—what enables them to take up human concerns—must also be considered. When we consider human concerns, we encounter human forms of love, pride, shame, moral goodness, evil, dignity, suffering, and so on. Furthermore, these very concerns or human issues determine the worth of and approach to our strategic efforts toward reproduction, health maintenance, self-care, and other health issues. Outcome is no longer the only issue. Saving a life and prolonging dying become issues. Here, instrumental or means-ends strategic thinking can no longer be the only consideration. Maintaining ties, human connectedness, and human concerns become not just ends but are understood as constituting what it means to be a person. The self is understood as a member/participant in part constituted by relationships with others. Nurses promote healing by helping the patient maintain the human ties and concerns. And it is this human connection that gives people the courage to weather illness.

DISEMBODIED VIEW OF THE SELF

Since, under the Cartesian view, the body is separate from the mind and is represented in the mind like any other object, it is not possible to understand the body itself as a knower or as having skilled capacities and embodied intelligence. As noted earlier, this disregard of embodied knowing and skilled knowledge goes back to Plato, who proposed that knowledge of abstract ideas—e.g., "the good"—was the highest kind of knowledge and specific, skilled knowledge—e.g., how to make good soup or good shoes—was of a lower order and not really knowledge at all. This assumption from our Greek philosophical tradition has shaped much of our thinking for centuries. If we add to that the Cartesian assumption that all knowledge is the result of mental representation and reflection on that representation, it is not surprising that bodily knowledge has been neglected.

Understanding the body as an active capacity to act and as a ground for knowledge has major implications for caring for people with bodily breakdown or alterations. Old habits, sets to action, and capacities to act may no longer be relevant, yet the patient may still continue to exhibit these habits, bodily expectations, and sets to action. Such bodily expectations occur in amputees who report phantom limbs, and such sets to action appear in partially paralyzed stroke victims who describe leaping up as if they still had the capacity to walk.

The notion of the body as a way of knowing and as integrated with the mind can have profound implications for the care of the body during extreme breakdown. In this view, the body is not ever an object, the body is continuous with the person. This should have a profound impact on our treatment of the body, as in the use of physical restraints (see Schilder 1986), in the care of mothers and infants (see Stainton 1985), and in providing messages of comfort and activity through care of the body (Dunlap 1986).

Understanding embodied intelligence also has major implications for comprehending skilled nursing practice. Expert performance of complex skills (e.g., making decisions and clinical judgments or administering medications to maintain a patient within specified physiological parameters) depends on a bodily takeover of the skill to some degree so that the body's set to action becomes appropriate to a range of typical actions in the complex skill. Even seeing patterns in a complex array of clinical information is an example of embodied intelligence. Patterns can be recognized without prespecification. It is the unique, remarkable capacity of the body to cope with vague, "fuzzy" information and regions of influence and tension that makes possible the human capacity to function in ambiguous, underdetermined situations (Benner and Tanner 1987). This provides a sharp contrast to a mentalistic view of intelligence modeled on the information-processing paradigm, which requires that everything understood be equally clear and specifiable, that the situation be built element by element, and that relations be analytically connected.

Much of skilled performance requires a bodily takeover of a probe or tool so that perceptually it acts like an extension of the body (Merleau-Ponty 1962, Polanyi 1966). For example, an intravenous intracatheter becomes a sensitive probe that allows the experienced nurse to feel the venous walls and the surrounding tissue.

PURE INTENTIONALITY AND RADICAL FREEDOM

The Cartesian mental representation theory of the mind has only one form of intentionality, a pure conceptual or cognitive form that takes the cognitivist stance of internal mental judgments about external events as a way of describing the person in the situation (describing how the internal relates to the external). Even the Freudian unconscious, which is based upon a representational theory of the mind, has this kind of representational intentionality. Although human beings clearly do possess pure forms of intentionality, they can and do make clear plans to achieve certain ends and even succeed. However, this view of intentionality is too narrow. It leaves out the precognitive forms of intentionality: meaningful, purposive behavior that is based on skilled practices, habits, and language. This alternative form of intentionality is more basic and pervasive than pure forms of intentionality and makes possible smooth functioning and behavior without elaborate conscious deliberation.

This notion of precognitive intentionality has major implications for stress and coping. The person is no longer viewed as freely choosing all actions all the time. People are neither radically free nor radically unfree. They have situated freedom (Taylor 1979). Radical freedom is the modern view that people can choose *all* their meanings *all* the time. But this view ignores that the choice of meanings is predicated on the meanings available in the person's own background, culture, and language. Situated freedom is the view that persons come to situations with their own meanings, habits, and perspectives and that this history actually sets up the possibilities in the situation. We propose that the person has situated freedom and situated possibility (see Benner 1984a, 1984b; Wrubel 1985). Effective interventions must relate to this situated possibility, a possibility that includes meanings, practices, and personal concerns. Simple homeostatic adaptation models do not adequately capture situated possibility because they systematically ignore meaning and history, a feat that human beings cannot perform.

The view of the self is not limited to a purely instrumental and disengaged self-seeking to achieve prespecified ends. In this view, persons are not radically free to abandon any commitment or membership simply because it is "stressful." Nor are they free to engage in stress-management strategies that create untenable distance and control from self-constituting relationships. Clearly stress-management strategies need to include the positive strategies of appropriating meanings and fulfilling commitments, as well as the currently usual ones of allowing for disengagement and tension reduction.

REFERENCES

Aristotle: *Physics*. Hardie RP, Gaye, RK (trans). In McKeon R (ed): *The Basic Works of Aristotle*. New York: Plenum, 1941.

Benner P: *From Novice to Expert: Excellence and Power in Clinical Nursing Practice*. Menlo Park, Calif.: Addison-Wesley, 1984a.

Benner P: *Stress and Satisfaction on the Job: Work Meanings and Coping of Mid-Career Men*. New York: Praeger Scientific Press, 1984b.

Benner P, Tanner C: Clinical judgment: How expert nurses use intuition. Am J Nurs 87:23, 1987.

Berger PL, Luckman T: *The Social Construction of Reality*. Garden City, N.Y.: Doubleday, 1966.

Block J with Haan N: *Lives through Time*. Berkeley, Calif.: Bancroft Book, 1971.

Bolles RC: Cognition and motivation: Some historical trends. In Weiner B (ed): *Cognitive Views of Human Motivation,* pp. 1–20. New York: Academic Press, 1974.

Booth G: Psychodynamics in parkinsonism. Psychosom Med 10(1): 1, 1948.

Caudill W, Weinstein H: Maternal care and infant behavior in Japan and America. Psychiatry 32:12, 1969.

Dember WN: Motivation and the cognitive revolution. Am Psychol 29:161, 1974.

Dreyfus HL: *Being-in-the-World: A Commentary on Heidegger's Being and Time, Division I*. Cambridge, Mass.: MIT Press, in press.

Dreyfus HL: (ed) with Hall H: *Husserl, Intentionality and Cognitive Science*. Cambridge, Mass.: MIT Press, 1982.

Dreyfus HL: *What Computers Can't Do: The Limits of Artificial Intellgence.* Rev ed, New York: Harper & Row, 1979.

Dreyfus S, Dreyfus HL: *Mind over Machine*. New York: The Free Press, 1986.

Dunlop MJ: Is a science of caring possible? J Adv Nurs 11:661, 1986.

Hall ET: *The Silent Language.* Greenwich, Conn.: Fawcett Publications, 1959.

Heidegger M: *Being and Time*. Macquarrie J, Robinson E (trans). New York: Harper & Brothers, 1962.

Husserl E: *The Idea of Phenomenology.* Alston W, Nakhikan G (trans). The Hague: Nijhoff, 1964.

Jelliffe SE: The parkinsonian body posture: Some considerations on unconscious hostility. Psychoanal Rev 27:467, 1940.

Kelley HH: An application of attribution theory to research methodology for close relationships. In Levinger G, Rausch HL (eds): *Close Relationships,* pp. 87–113. Amherst: University of Massachusetts Press, 1977

Kohler W: *The Place of Value in a World of Fact.* New York: Liveright, 1966.

Lazarus RS: On the primacy of cognition. Am Psychol 39:124, 1984.

Lazarus RS: Thoughts on the relations between emotion and cognition. Am Psychol 37:1019, 1982.

MacLeod RB: Phenomenology: A challenge to experimental psychology. In Wann TW (ed): *Behaviorism and Phenomenology: Contrasting Bases for Modern Psychology*, pp. 47–73. Chicago: University of Chicago Press, 1964.

Merleau-Ponty M: *Phenomenology of Perception*. Smith C (trans). London: Routledge & Kegan Paul, 1962.

Merleau-Ponty M: *The Visible and the Invisible*. Lingis A (trans) Evanston, Ill: Northwestern University Press, 1968.

Miller GA, Johnson-Laird DA: *Language and Perception.* Cambridge, England: Cambridge University Press. Cambridge, Mass.: Harvard University Press, 1976.

Oiler C: The phenomenological approach in nursing research. Nurs Res 31:178, 1982.

Omery A: Phenomenology: A method for nursing research. Adv Nurs Sci 5:49, 1983.

Overton WF, Reese HW: Models of development: Methodological implications. In Nesselroade JR, Reese HW (eds): *Life Span Developmental Psychology: Methodological Issues*. New York: Academic Press, 1973.

Piaget J: *The Construction of Reality in the Child*. Cook M (trans). New York: Basic Books, 1954.

Piaget J: *The Psychology of Intelligence.* Piercy M, Berlyne DE (trans). London: Routledge & Kegan Paul, 1950.

Piaget J: *Structuralism.* Maschler C (trans). New York: Harper & Row, 1968.

Polanyi M: *The Tacit Dimension.* Garden City, N.Y.: Doubleday, 1966.

Rotter JB: Generalized expectations for internal versus external control of reinforcement. Psychological Monographs: General and Applied 80 (609): entire issue, 1966.

Sacks O: *The Man Who Mistook His Wife for a Hat and Other Clinical Tales.* New York: Simon & Schuster, 1985.

Sandel M: *Liberalism and the Limits of Justice.* London: Oxford University Press, 1982.

Schilder E: The use of physical restraints in an acute care medical ward. Unpublished doctoral dissertation, University of California at San Francisco, School of Nursing, 1986.

Stainton C: Culture and cue sensitivity: A phenomenological study of mothering. Unpublished doctoral dissertation, University of California at San Francisco, School of Nursing, 1985.

Sudnow D: *Ways of the Hand: The Organization of Improvised Conduct.* Cambridge, Mass.: Harvard University Press, 1978.

Taylor C: *Hegel and Modern Society.* Cambridge, England: Cambridge University Press, 1979.

Taylor C: *Philosophical Papers,* vols. 1 & 2. Cambridge, England: Cambridge University Press, 1985a.

Taylor C: The concept of a person. In *Human Agency and Language. Philosophical Papers,* vol 1, pp. 97–114. Cambridge, England: Cambridge University Press, 1985b.

Taylor C: Theories of Meaning. In *Human Agency and Language. Philosophical Papers,* vol 1, pp. 248–292. Cambridge, England: Cambridge University Press, 1985c.

White RW: Ego and reality in psychoanalytic theory. Psychol Issues 3(3): monograph 11, 1963.

Wrubel J: Personal meanings and coping processes. Unpublished doctoral dissertation, University of California at San Francisco, 1985.

Zajonc RB: Feeling and thinking: Preferences need no inferences. Am Psychol 35:151, 1980.

Zajonc RB: On the primacy of affect. Am Psychol 39:117, 1984.

A Phenomenological View of Stress and Coping

During the long weeks of trying to induce a remission, when Lara was still doing relatively well, I used a variety of approaches in working with her based on what kind of day she was having. Sometimes we would just joke around and listen to music; other times we would talk about more serious issues—not just her illness, but her personal life, as well as my own. I think Lara was able to open up to me because I shared a piece of myself. . . . There were days when I walked in the room and could tell by Lara and her mother's faces and greetings that it was not a good day. I would sit down and listen, giving Lara unspoken permission to be angry or depressed: to question me about the chemotherapy, about why her white blood count was still so low, or about the possibilities of remission or a bone marrow transplant. I was always open with her, accepted her feelings, and never made light of them.   *Robin Fireman Kramer, Clinical Nurse Specialist*

The phenomenological view of stress and coping presented here grew out of a desire to develop a language that more adequately captured the possibilities lived out by actual people coping with events as divergent as birth, childhood illnesses, aging, and death. After reviewing prior studies of expert nursing practice, we concluded that a phenomenological perspective also more adequately captures the knowledge and notion of good embedded in expert nursing practice. The language of positivistic social science and the natural sciences is too impoverished to give an adequate account of what actually occurs in everyday life. Thus, this work stems from dissatisfaction with atomistic, mechanistic, and strictly utilitarian views of the person. Atomism does not allow for an understanding of the person in the situation and ignores the ways people are constituted by their relationships. Mechanistic accounts do not allow for meanings. In the utilitarian view, the person is an economic agent who bases action on a cost-benefit analysis, or enlightened self-interest at most. Utilitarianism is consequently an impoverished account of human possibility. Although people *can* become economic in their way of being in the world, reducing their involvement with others to exchanges of goods and services is not the *only* possible way of relating to others. Nor is such an economic self-understanding conducive to caring for others and participating in a common humanity.

Sister M. Simone Roach (1984), a Canadian nurse theorist, cites anthropologist Loren Eisley's observations of a Neanderthal man who had lost an arm but still lived because he was cared for. Eisley noted that even in that hard, violent, primitive, and stony world, caring existed, as evidenced by the survival of that injured man. This early evidence has caused anthropologists to suggest that the real beginning of civilization should not be gauged by tool use but by the evidence of healed bones. Healed fractures indicate that the person was cared for, given food, and protected long enough to heal. The goal in constructing an account of stress and coping from a phenomenological perspective is to provide an adequate account of human possibility and the experience of caring and being cared for.

In the previous chapter we argued that the phenomenological view of the person overcomes the limitations of a strictly epistemological (Cartesian) approach and transcends the mind-body, subject-object split by examining the ontological foundations: the existing conditions of possibilities that the person experiences in a situation. If one takes an ontological view of the person's capacities, one considers the taken-for-granted meanings evident in bodily skills, embodied intelligence, and understanding of the situation as well as the concerns of the person. For example, Benner (1984) and Wrubel (1985) found that background meanings and personal concerns actually set up what counts as "stressful" and what coping options are available in terms of understanding, skill, knowledge, values, and access (see also, Benner, Roskies, and Lazarus 1980; Wrubel, Benner, and Lazarus 1981).

This chapter turns to the issues of stress and coping and considers how the phenomenological perspective can inform our understanding of these often used words. First the terms *stress* and *coping* are defined from the phenomenological perspective. Then a number of issues that are often not considered but are central to the concepts of stress and coping are discussed. These include the role of the body; the role of the situation; the role of personal concerns; emotions as lived meanings;

skills; and sources of commonality among and uniqueness of persons and situations.

What Is Stress?

Stress is defined as the disruption of meanings, understanding, and smooth functioning so that harm, loss, or challenge is experienced, and sorrow, interpretation, or new skill acquisition is required. This definition draws on the work of Lazarus and his colleagues (Folkman, Schaefer, and Lazarus 1979; Lazarus 1966, 1968, 1981; Lazarus, Averill, and Opton 1970; Lazarus and Cohen 1977; Lazarus and Folkman 1984; Lazarus, Kanner, and Folkman 1980; Lazarus and Launier 1978). Early work on stress focused on discussions of whether stress lay in the event or in the person's response to the event. Lazarus's theory of stress and coping posits that stress involves both the person and the situation. It results from the person's appraisal of his or her adaptive relationship to the context. This relationship is called a *transaction.*

Lazarus's concept of transaction allows us to take the necessary step away from a representational notion of the person to a phenomenological one. Rather than viewing the stress experience as the accretion of variables reflecting aspects of the environment and the person, the transactional approach views stress as the result of the person's grasp of the meaning of a situation for the self when that meaning conveys challenge, loss, threat, or harm.

Just as in Chapter One we made a distinction between disease and illness, here we must clarify what we mean by stress. As long as one has no symptoms or other disruption of usual functioning, there is no experience of illness, even though disease may be present and the body may be suffering damage at the cellular, tissue, or organ level. Thus, when we speak of stress here, we mean the person's physical, emotional, and/or intellectual grasp that smooth functioning has been disrupted. For example, patients who die before regaining consciousness after a serious accident do not undergo the same changes in the adrenal cortex as those who are conscious after the accident. A part of the stress response is dependent on consciousness (Symington, Currie, Curran, and Davidson 1955). Although the physiological stress response occurs without consciousness, it does not have all the same characteristics that are found when the person is aware of the injury or insult that has occurred. We do not use the term *psychological stress* to make this distinction between the stress response during consciousness and unconsciousness because that term emphasizes the role of mental appraisal, and, by implication, overlooks the role of embodied intelligence (Dreyfus 1979). The role of the body is presented in greater detail in a later section of this chapter.

Stress, in its common use, then, refers to the person's grasp that life is awry, and the term is used in this sense here. But there is another common meaning of stress that is not intended here, and that is the view of stress as the result of not dealing well with a problem. This definition is at the base of most stress-management approaches. The coping prescriptions offered by such approaches probably work well when the issue truly is a problem, e.g., the best way to manage available time to complete required tasks. This view may have limited success when the source of stress is dilemmas, quandaries, and predicaments, but it fails to grasp the essence of such situations as calamities, disasters, and tragedies. Strong feelings experienced over the death of a loved one or the threat of pain, disfigurement, or death can be debilitating, and the person may indeed need to find ways to gain temporary respite. But the feeling must be acknowledged if the person is to work through to a new reality that contains some continuity and connectedness with the past. This relationship between emotions and temporality is addressed further in the discussion of temporality.

Also, stress-management approaches that deal only with altering emotional states by dampening, controlling, or distracting may be helpful in the short term to interrupt a stressful response set, but in the long run, such strategies foster an alienated stance toward emotions. When viewed as "responses" that must be controlled, emotions are foreign, unwanted interruptions to the "business" at hand, namely, staying calm and feeling peaceful while accomplishing one's goals. This is a decidedly instrumental or strategic view of living. Unfortunately, it ignores the content and guidance provided by emotions. In fact, the person who learns to "manage" (ward off, distance) emotions effectively eliminates the guidance and direction provided by those emotions. For example, anger is a signal that something of value is frustrated, thwarted, violated, or threatened. One might learn to control the feeling of anger, but that control is counterproductive if it shuts off awareness of the issue or stake. Emotions alert the person that something important is at stake, even though the person may not have clarity about what is at stake. At advanced levels of skilled performance, emotions allow the person to attend to and recognize "fuzzy resemblances" (Benner and Tanner 1987). Clearly, to be trained not to recognize and attend to feelings is not the best stress-management strategy in the long run. Momentary calm may be gained at the expense of learning from the situation or attending to the issue at hand.

Of course, at times it may be imperative to dampen or alter emotions in order to function. Lazarus and Folkman (1984) call this *emotion-focused coping,* since the goal is to manage one's emotions, often so that one can cope better with the task at hand. The position we are taking is that emotions are not contentless interruptions that must always be managed because they interfere with optimal functioning. We claim that emotions are essential to the highest levels of functioning and provide access to situations that will be blocked if "feelings" are ignored.

We do not view stress as a state that can always be avoided or even one that must always be "cured." Rather, stress is the inevitable result of living in a world in which things matter to one. One might seek to "cure" the tension felt by someone who overschedules time and always has many unfinished tasks, but would one seek to "cure" the anguish felt by the parents of an infant with a life-threatening congenital defect? If we regard these parents' situation as a problem, then the solution is either to cure the infant's defect or convince the parents not to care about what happens to their baby. Although distancing and disengagement are sometimes suggested as coping strategies by stress-management advisers, in the example above, such disengagement is inappropriate. One would not seek to cure the parents' anguish, but rather to ease it.

We posit that stress cannot be "cured," not only because, short of miracles, there is no cure for disasters, calamities, and tragedies but also because, in the phenomenological view of the person, there is no way to step outside of one's own history. The person both constitutes and is constituted by his or her experience. A person with cancer who has a remission beyond the five-year mark may be judged to be cured of the disease, but the experience of having had the disease will inform the rest of that person's life. One might derive strength from the experience and feel that, having survived cancer, one can handle easily the more mundane upsets of daily life. Or, one might feel vulnerable because of the close brush with death and see smaller misadventures as confirmation of the precariousness of existence. In fact, there is a range of diverse ways in which the experience of surviving a life-threatening illness could constitute a person. The only experience that is not a possibility is viewing the world in exactly the same way as before.

One can be rid of the disease but not of the experience of the disease.

It is a premise of this book, however, that nurses can and do make a difference in how a person experiences an illness. Nurses are in the unique position of being able to understand both the disease experience and the meanings that the patient brings to that experience. As a result, nurses can help shape the illness experience for the patient by guiding, interpreting, and coaching. In doing this, nurses do not cure stress, but they help patients survive it. They do this by using many of the stress-management strategies, such as the relaxation response (Benson 1976), visualization, self-hypnosis, desensitization, and progressive relaxation. However, nurses also establish a healing relationship by helping the patient mobilize hope and embrace recovery by appropriating available social, emotional, and spiritual resources. Nurses act as cultural mediators and serve as coaches for patients, making that which is strange and foreign approachable and interpretable (Benner 1984).

What Is Coping?

It should be clear by this point in the discussion that coping is not an antidote to stress. Stress is the experience of the disruption of meanings, understanding, and smooth functioning. Coping is what one does about that disruption.

Lazarus theory of stress and coping (1966, 1981; Lazarus and Folkman 1984) has extended the notion of what it means to "do" something. Lazarus points out that although doing something directly is what is typically thought of as coping, not doing something on purpose is also a way of coping. Other ways of coping are seeking out information relevant to the situation, trying to change the way one thinks about the stressful situation, and attempting to make oneself feel better (or at least different) without changing either the situation or how one thinks about it.

The phenomenological view of stress and coping is a departure from a cognitivist[1] approach, the theoretical position that holds that the mind acts like a computer (see Chapter Two, pp. 35–38). It abandons the cognitivist assumptions that the mind is distinct from and distanced from the external world, that experience is primarily a mental judg-

---

1. "Cognitivist approach" refers to a particular theoretical view of the mind. It does not refer to a use of those intellectual powers that might be termed "cognitive" or conceptual abilities.

ment about the external cause or conditions that gave rise to that "mental judgment." In the phenomenological view of stress and coping, the person is not seen as a rational calculator of external events whose meanings are limited only to the pointing out and designation of objects, facts, and events. Rather, the person is understood both to constitute and be constituted by meanings. This constitutive role of meaning is the ontological basis of perception. That is, the concerns, background meanings, skills, and practices of the person set up what counts as stressful and what the coping possibilities are. In the phenomenological view, coping can never be an unlimited choice from a list of effective and ineffective options. Instead, coping is bounded by the meanings and issues inherent in what counts as stressful. Some choices will always be untenable or unrelated to the person's concerns and most often not easily translated to the person's situation. For this reason, coping cannot be seen as a separate antidote or antibiotic for the "germ" stress.

Once we understand the person as a participant self that both constitutes and is constituted by relationships, we gain a new perspective on the role of the body, the role of the situation, and the role of personal concerns in the processes of stress and coping. The self is not an objective outsider but a participating insider within the situation. The person is enabled to participate by an embodied intelligence, a situation grasped in terms of its meanings for the self and by personal concerns that determine the salience of some of those meanings (Dreyfus 1979). This does not mean that an objective attitude cannot be assumed and that the person cannot achieve a detached, disengaged view of a situation; this "objective attitude" is just one more way of being *in* a situation. However, the detached, objective way of being in the situation yields different possibilities and different options. The way the person is *in* the situation sets up different possibilities. This is an ontological observation. The assumptions of the subject as a particular kind of knower are bypassed.

Thus, to explicate fully the phenomenological view of stress and coping, we also need to discuss the roles of temporality, the body, the situation, and personal concerns.

Temporality

Historicity and temporality are essential for the way human beings understand themselves. Identity and continuity are linked to temporality. The notion of temporality must first be rescued from the notion of a linear succession of moments. For Heidegger, temporality is linked with meaningfulness and having a world:

> We indicated earlier that the phenomenon of the world manifests itself to the Dasein.[2] Given that the Dasein exists, is in a world, everything extant that the Dasein encounters is necessarily intraworldly, held-around (contained) by the world. We shall see that in fact the *phenomenon of time*, taken in the more original sense, is *interconnected with the concept of the world and thus with the structure of Dasein itself* (1982, p. 255).

> . . . When we characterized the concept of the world, [we] saw that in it there is intended a whole of relations having the character of the in-order-to. We designated by the term *significance* this totality of relations of the in-order-to, for-the-sake-of, for-that-purpose, to-that-end. Time as right and wrong time has the *character of significance,* the character that characterizes the world as world in general. It is for this reason that we call the time with which we reckon, which we leave for ourselves, *world-time* (1982, p. 263).

Heidegger clarifies that he is not using a common conception of linear time: "The common conception thinks of the nows as free-floating, relationless, intrinsically patched on to one another and intrinsically successive" (1982, p. 263). The person exists in the present, as influenced by the past, and is projected or "thrown" into the future. In this phenomenological perspective, time has a qualitative dimension and is imbued with intentionality. Time creates a story. This is evident when a new self-understanding or new knowledge causes a person to reinterpret the past. From the new vantage point, different aspects of the situation may now stand out and assume a new importance. A major illness such as cancer or cardiovascular disease can cause an extensive life review and reconsideration of the past so that the past is reinterpreted in light of the disease.

Oliver Sacks (1984) captures this notion of temporality as a form of existence in his description of recovery from a leg injury. He describes the qualitative leaps and transformations in his passage from one stage of recovery to another:

---

2. *Dasein* is a term used by Heidegger (1962, 1982) to depict human being, e.g. that cultural being whose being is in the world, and that being that we ourselves are. Heidegger uses this term instead of *subject* or *self* because Dasein is a different notion of what it means to be a self.

The return of health and strength—convalescence—was intoxicating, and I continually misjudged what I could or should do; and yet it wasn't smooth, it consisted of steps—with no spontaneous advancement from one stage, or one step, to another. When I stole a look at my chart and saw "Uneventful Recovery," I thought: "They're mad. Recovery *is* events, a series of wonderful, unpredictable events: recovery is events, or rather advents—the advent of new and unimaginable powers—events, advents, which are birth or re-births.

Recovery was not to be seen as a smooth slope, but as a series of radical steps, each inconceivable, impossible, from the step below. And, by the same token, one could have not even hope, in the least, for the unimaginable next step (for hope implies some degree of imagining). Thus every step had the quality of miracle—and might never occur without the urging of others.

With each step, each advance, one's horizons expanded, one stepped out of a contracted world—a world one hadn't realized was so contracted (p. 154).

Sacks (1984) captures the quality of losing a perspective and sense of the future as a result of injury and incapacitation. He points up the essential requirement for an expert coach who can help the patient imagine the next step so that the patient can project the self into the future. The expert coach (Benner 1984, 1985) gives the patient the imagination required to try the next step and move into the future. The nurse-coach learns from other patients with similar illnesses and recovery trajectories what to expect including a rough timetable. This sense of forward movement, along with astute descriptions of progress in concrete detail, allows the patient to gain a sense of progress and projection into the future. The patient's world expands to include future capabilities.

When a major life change, such as the death of a loved one occurs, the person may get stuck with old irrelevant concerns that become the background for their current actions, but this resolution of grief is less than satisfactory. For example, a simple task such as going to the grocery store may flood a grieving spouse with memories and "estranged" decisions. Old shopping patterns reflecting the special preferences and diet of the deceased still feel salient but are no longer relevant. New quantities and types of food are now needed, and this fact is usually experienced as one more confrontation that one's life has changed drastically. Shopping has become a myriad of new decisions. All the old, taken-for-granted patterns are no longer relevant. And something as routine as shopping can be experienced as taxing. Merleau-Ponty (1962) describes this as an alteration in temporality:

> Time in its passage does not carry away with it these impossible projects; it does not close up on traumatic experience; the subject remains open to the same impossible future, if not in his explicit thought, at any rate in his actual being. One present among all presents thus acquires an exceptional value; it displaces the others and deprives them of their value as authentic presents. We continue to be the person who once entered on this adolescent affair, or the one who once lived in this parental universe. New perceptions, new emotions even, replace the old ones, but this process of renewal touches only the content of our experience and not its structure. Impersonal time continues its course, but personal time is arrested. Of course this fixation does not merge into memory insofar as the latter spreads out in front of us, like a picture, a former experience, whereas this past which remains our true present does not leave us but remains constantly hidden behind our gaze instead of being displayed before it. The traumatic experience does not survive as a representation in the mode of objective consciousness and as a "dated" moment; it is of its essence to survive only as a manner of being and with a certain degree of generality. I forgo my constant power of providing myself with "worlds" in the interest of one of them, and for that very reason this privileged world loses its substance and eventually becomes no more than a certain *dread* (p. 83).

Dreyfus (1987) has called this view of being caught up with the past "breadth" psychology because the past becomes the atmosphere for the present. One's assumptions, habits, and concerns spread out as a precognitive, taken-for-granted way of being in the world.

Temporality is illustrated in any life experience. For example, a second pregnancy has a different quality of experience than a first pregnancy, in part because the temporality of the event is now understood from beginning to end in a way that was not possible during the first pregnancy. The same is true for the parents' experience of the second child's growth and development. The parents can now understand developmental changes as time-bound phases in a way that was not possible during the first child's development. Similarly, recovery timetables take on different dimensions depending upon the person's past experience with serious illness.

For Heidegger (1982), time is neither spatial nor contentless. Time is relational and directional:

> In contrast to the notion of time modeled after space, Heidegger grounded our understanding of space in the notion of time. As we have

pointed out, the common notion is that time is indifferent with respect to content, because each of its series of points is identical to every other. In Heidegger's view, however, time is *essentially* content: It *exists as* activity, such as concernful dealing and attention, rather than being "filled up" by such activity (Faulconer and Williams 1985, p. 1184).

Temporality is not experienced in the abstract. It is specific and formed by what has gone on before and by what is anticipated. Stress and coping are shaped by one's temporality.

The Role of the Body

In the Cartesian view, notions of the body are restricted to a mental representation of the body, commonly known today as "body image." Notions of "body schema" also fit this representational view of the mind-body relationship. Although it is true that one may have an image of the body, that mind-held image is not the primary way one experiences one's body. The primary experience is one of "ground" or base for action and knowing. All perception stems from the perspective of the body. Our directionality comes from the lived experience of the body. All our prepositional language reflects this locus of the body, e.g., in front of, to the side, and behind, the body. The phenomenological perspective stands in contrast to the cognitivist assumption made by Pennebaker (1982): "The perceptual process required for the encoding of internal sensory information represents the same processes that have traditionally been implicated in the perception of external environmental events" (p. 19).

Pennebaker's perspective is an extreme form of cognitivism that sees the mind as detached and different from the body, reading internal cues just as it reads external ones. This position ignores the way that internal or bodily experience constitutes a perspective. Internal cues can never be experienced as outside-in, they are always experienced as inner. Furthermore, the direction of influence goes in both directions in a constitutive way. A sour stomach may color a sunset, and a particularly beautiful sunset may soothe a sour stomach. The inner environment has a different horizon than the outside environment, which directs our attention outward. In other words, the person does not look out on internal sensations as one looks out on outward events and things. The use of the body to perceive is different for inner and outward attending. For example, fear or anxiety may heighten awareness of the *external* environment under certain conditions, and this focused attention may dampen one's awareness of internal sensations. However, when the internal sensations are the focal point of attention, they may be intensified by attentiveness. In each case, the horizon and attentional focus of perception are different.

In *What Computers Can't Do*, Hubert Dreyfus (1979) outlines the limits of a cognitivist or computational theory of the mind:

> Adherents of the psychological and epistemological assumptions that human behavior must be formalizable in terms of a heuristic program for a digital computer are forced to develop a theory of intelligent behavior which makes no appeal to the fact that a man has a body, since at this stage at least the computer clearly hasn't one. In thinking that the body can be dispensed with, these thinkers again follow the tradition, which from Plato to Descartes has thought of the body as getting in the way of intelligence and reason, rather than being in any way indispensable for it. . . . [However] our ability to be in situations might depend, not just on the flexibility of our nervous system, but rather on our ability to engage in practical activity. After some attempts to program such a machine, it might become apparent that what distinguishes persons from machines, no matter how cleverly constructed, is not a detached, universal, immaterial soul but an involved, self-moving, material body (pp. 235–236).

"Common sense"—situational understanding and embodied intelligence that allow one to respond to global situations and ambiguous circumstances—has been consistently resistant to programming solutions. This is exactly the kind of intelligence that requires embodiment (Benner and Tanner 1987).

The body has an ontological capacity to relate to meaningful situations. For example, Wolf, Cardon, Shepard, and Wolff (1955) found that some blood donors constrict their arterioles *prior* to having their blood drawn in anticipation of the blood loss. Constriction of arterioles in response to loss of one liter of blood is a normal compensatory response that maintains a normal blood pressure. In this case, circulatory adjustments occur in response to a meaningful situation that implies the threat of blood loss. Likewise, Wolf (1981) and his colleagues were able to induce elevated blood pressure and a reduction of renal blood flow in subjects during a discussion of intimate personal conflicts. When subjects were reassured, the blood pressure dropped, although renal flow reduction continued for a time, outlasting the stress. In both cases, the meaning of the situation is embodied and initiates bodily responses.

The body does not require complete understanding or conceptual clarity to respond to a meaningful situation. This capacity to recognize and respond to "fuzzy problems" and "similar situations" has a decided adaptive capacity. It sets up the person to recognize impending threats and danger before the nature of the danger is clear. This capacity can also exact a toll, as in the case of the person's ontological capacity to develop anticipatory nausea upon entering the parking lot before a chemotherapy appointment (see the discussion in Chapter Eight, pp. 279–282).

Schottstaedt, Pinsky, Mackler, and Wolf (1958) demonstrated the embodied capacity to respond to social distress that is especially relevant for nurses. Researchers observed and recorded the social interactions among fifteen to twenty long-term patients on a metabolic unit. At the same time, extensive laboratory studies were also conducted without the knowledge of those recording the social interactions. Schottstaedt and colleagues found that the metabolic deviations correlated with the atmosphere recorded on the unit separately by raters unaware of the laboratory analysis. Wolf (1981) reports the study:

> Even transient disruptions of the equilibrium were found to be associated with substantial measurable metabolic changes in terms of urinary excretion of water, sodium, potassium, calcium, nitrogen, and creatinine. . . . Interpersonal difficulties among those with strong ties were the most common sources of stress to be associated with metabolic deviations, accounting for 28 of the 46 stressful situations associated with such deviations. Interpersonal stresses arising between individuals without strong ties were less often associated with significant repercussions in the metabolic data.
>
> For several days, the whole population of the ward reacted in a similar fashion during a period of severe anxiety among the nurses. The nurses had been asked to submit to a psychological testing procedure and to evaluate the performance of one another in relation to individual patients. They proved to be reluctant and felt personally threatened by the request. Throughout this period of uneasiness among the nurses, all of the patients under study in the ward displayed a metabolic response consisting of a negative balance of all measured metabolites. The atmosphere of the ward was tense and subdued. There was no way to measure or otherwise quantify the psychological stimulus. In fact, the patients were unaware of the circumstances responsible for the nurses' anxiety. This experience illustrates that a bodily response to stress depends not so much on the quantity of the noxious stimulus but, rather, on the quality or configuration of the prevailing circumstances. Thus, looking only

for quantifiable data may cause one to miss the most pertinent evidence (pp. 5–7).

We have thought of mind and body as separate in the Western tradition, and we have thought that the direction of influence was usually from the mind to the body. For this reason, we have missed the ways in which the body responds to meaningful situations without explicit conceptual clarity. The example above also shows the role that concern plays in bodily responses. The bodily responses are stronger when the conflicts are between those having greater involvement and concern (see pp. 78–80). Merleau-Ponty (1962) describes this embodied ability to respond to meaningful situations:

> It has always been observed that speech or gesture transfigure the body. . . . The fact was overlooked that, in order to express it, the body must in the last analysis become the thought or intention that it signifies for us (p. 197).

The body has the capacity to dwell in meanings, as Polanyi (1958) points out. A less objectified view of the body (see Parker 1981) and a fuller appreciation of embodied intelligence has major implications for how we treat our bodies when we and those we care for are sick. For example, from Merleau-Ponty's theory of the body Schilder (1986) has drawn implications for the use of physical restraints on acutely ill patients.

Merleau-Ponty (1962) outlines five dimensions[3] of the ontological capacity of the body: inborn complex; habitual, skilled body; projective body; actual projected body; and phenomenal body. Each of these notions of the body is presented below.

INBORN COMPLEX

This is the precultural body with which the baby is born. This has been studied extensively in recent years (Thomas 1982). Even in utero, the infant has remarkable bodily skills. As Bower (1977) notes, "A newborn thus begins life as an extremely competent learning organism, an extremely competent perceiving organism." The newborn infant recognizes visual patterns and even gives preferential attention to them. The infant prefers complexity, movement, and three-dimensionality over flat static visual stimuli (Frantz and Nevis 1967). The newborn responds to sound and can localize the direction from

---

3. We are indebted to Hubert Dreyfus's commentary on Merleau-Ponty's writing for this interpretation, which was presented in various classes taught by Professor Dreyfus at the University of California, Berkeley, 1977–1985.

which a sound comes (Wertheimer 1961) and has the capacity to grasp a "a spatially relevant, functional relation between audition and vision" (Mendelson and Haith 1976).

Ohnuma (1987) has summarized fetal capacities as follows: As early as fifteen weeks the fetus can grasp, frown, squint, and grimace. The fetus will also suck its thumb and swallow amniotic fluid. The senses of taste and smell are formed by the fifth month, and the sense of touch is developed by the sixth month. Researchers have recorded responses to sound as early as twenty-four weeks. At twenty-five weeks, a light shone on the mother's abdomen will make the fetus turn its head. Almost all fetuses respond to sound by the thirtieth week. During the ninth month, when the walls of the abdomen and uterus are thinner and admit more light, the fetus begins to develop daily activity cycles.

Brazelton's (1973, 1978) Neonatal Behavioral Assessment Scale includes the following behavioral integrative processes of the neonate: a response decrement to repeated stimuli, orienting responses to objects and to the examiner's face and voice, varying quality and duration of alert periods, responses to being cuddled, avoidant reactions to a cloth over the face, consolability, and self-quieting activity. Thus, in addition to an innate capacity to learn, there seem to be complex sets of capacity to respond (a given neurobehavioral organization) already present at birth.

HABITUAL, SKILLED BODY

The habitual, skilled body includes all the culturally and socially learned postures, gestures, and customs, such as distance standing and greetings. These bodily habits are learned early in life through identification and imitation. They are normally not learned through direct didactic instruction. An anthropologist such as Hall (1959) may scientifically chart the typical distance that Americans, Mexicans, or Japanese stand apart, but natives of these countries will not be able to state the correct distances in feet and inches, even though they daily stand the correct distances and become uncomfortable when their personal space is violated. This discrepancy between people's ability to stand the appropriate distance apart from one another according to the situation and their inability to tell someone what that appropriate distance is can be accounted for by the fact that distance standing is not learned by rules. It is learned over time through identification, imitation, and trial and error and becomes incorporated into the habitual body.

These culturally attained habits have been highlighted in anecdotes about spy training. For example, Americans prefer to place the plate so that the pie wedge points directly toward them. The direction of the point may be more American than the traditional apple pie. The "unconscious" repositioning of the apex of the pie wedge could, for a spy, be a dead giveaway of an American habit.

Nancy Doolittle (1985) cites an example of a patient performing an involuntary social gesture to cover a yawn with the hand that has been paralyzed by a stroke. The patient cannot make a willful movement of the hand to the mouth with his paralyzed arm (a case of pure intentionality). However, his habitual body responds in ways not controlled or activated by his voluntary planned actions. Oliver Sacks (1985) points to the useful function of the phantom limb as an aid in successfully using a prosthesis. Although amputees struggle to lose the distressing sensations of the phantom limb, this habitual bodily experience offers a positive benefit for the amputee who wears an artificial limb. As Sacks's patient, "a clear-headed man, with an above-the-knee amputation," explains:

> There's this *thing,* this ghost foot, which sometimes hurts like hell—and the toes curl up, or go into spasm. This is worst at night, or with the prosthesis off, or when I'm not doing anything. It goes away, when I strap the prosthesis on and walk. I still feel the leg then, vividly, but it's a *good* phantom, different—it animates the prosthesis, and allows me to walk (p. 66).

By vigorously rubbing the stump or activating memories of the limb through some meaningful motion, the bodily memory of the limb is evoked so that the person can "take over" or embody the leg.

Both Merleau-Ponty (1962) and Polanyi (1958) cite the example of the blind person's use of the cane. Initially, the blind person feels objective pressure in the palm of the hand. However, with time the person extends his or her bodily awareness to the end of the cane so that there is a bodily takeover of the cane. The skilled blind person no longer feels "objective pressure" in the palm of the hand; instead, he or she feels the curb. All skillful tool use depends on this skilled bodily capacity to take over or extend bodily awareness to the end of a tool, probe, scalpel, IV catheter. In each case, the instrument becomes perceptible, not completely transparent but yet not foreign and alien, as the tool seems to the beginner.

Our cultural assumption of a mind-body separation may have prevented the full exploitation of the habitual body in assisting patients with brain injuries to overcome their limited planned action ability. The habitual body's ability to respond to a situation automatically suggests that we could use the power of former strong situations to assist the patient in old habitual responses and that these responses, when encouraged, could create new bodily memories in the presence of changed bodily capacities. This is a speculative hypothesis supported by Merleau-Ponty's (1962) theory of the body.

Skill acquisition is a good example of the role of the habitual, skilled body. Expert bicycle riders and swimmers rely on embodied intelligence to guide them in the acquisition of these complex skills. We have no adequate formal theoretical account of how swimming and bicycle riding are possible. We daily rely on the habitual, skilled body for opening and closing doors, turning lights on and off, recognizing disparate clinical sights and sounds. Dreyfus and Dreyfus (1986) use the everyday example of driving to illustrate the embodied capacity of skilled know-how:

> Intuition or know-how, as we understand it, is neither wild guessing nor supernatural inspiration, but the sort of ability we all use all the time as we go about our everyday tasks. . . . On the basis of prior experience, the proficient driver, approaching a curve on a rainy day, may intuitively realize that he is driving too fast. He then consciously decides whether to apply the brakes, remove his foot from the accelerator, or merely reduce the pressure (p. 29).

Discussing the expert driver, Dreyfus and Dreyfus (1986) note that if such drivers were given a hypothetical test asking for velocity and decisions made at different points in the above sequence, they, much like the people asked about standing distance, would be puzzled by not being able to specify distances, speed, and decisions.

The habitual, skilled body gives the expert clinician a capacity, a set to act. The habitual, skilled body sets up a particular relationship with the situation, whether it be a complex clinical situation, a situation encountered by an expert pianist beginning a concert, or a situation faced by an expert diabetic responding to the quirks of insulin, glucagon, and glucose metabolism. The habitual, skilled body becomes more visible to us in breakdown due to neurological damage or immobilization. The loss of the habitual, skilled body makes the body feel foreign and objective, like a thing: A stroke victim describes a paralyzed limb as a piece of "dead meat" (Doolittle 1985). Without a habitual, skilled body, people find all activity effortful and deliberate.

The habitual, skilled body is a major coping resource offering flexible fast responses to complex situations. Its loss is a major coping deficit and indeed becomes something to be coped with. We have adequately exploited the potential of the habitual, skilled body neither in rehabilitation nor in acute care settings, where the environment may strip the patient of the possibility of responding in habitual, skilled ways.

We have much to learn from expert patients who have developed habitual, skilled bodies in response to a chronic illness. A respect for the habitual, skilled body of the patient with a chronic illness causes the clinician to respect the patient's knowledge and develop lines of clinical inquiry that go beyond a mere mapping of symptoms onto preexisting explanations. The patient's learning about his or her own illness becomes a source of clinical discovery and inquiry in its own right

PROJECTIVE BODY

The projective body is the virtual body, or the way the body is set to act in normal skilled comportment. For example, most people do not have to think about placing one foot in front of the other for normal walking. People with neurological damage can suffer loss of proprioception, as people with tabes dorsalis do. Instead of having a normal projective body, such a person has to calculate mentally the best placement of the feet. The projective body is one's set to action. It is the bodily know-how that people possess even when they are not activating that know-how. People know how to reach objects with the best approach. Without thinking about it, they know whether to use the right or left hand, to reach over the shoulder, or to execute a full turn. The projective body is limited by the actual experience of skilled performance.

Patients who have a near death experience report a disturbance in their projected body (personal communication from M.J. Sauve 1986, Sauve 1985). Five percent in a sample of 60 talked about having lost an integrated sense of the body, not feeling fully *in* the body. For example, one woman perceived the end of her fingers approximately one inch above where her fingers actually ended.

ACTUAL PROJECTED BODY

The actual projected body is just one's current actual projection. Sitting before a computer, the operator's projections relate to past history and skill comportment related to the keyboard. The nurse caring for a sick toddler in a hospital playroom sets up another whole complex of projected bodily skills that are as flexible and as varied as the situation demands. Because the nurse is experienced in attending to sick toddlers, her or his body is poised to attend to the IV lines while at the same time the nurse encourages the toddler to play and to make transitions before boredom or frustration sets in.

Sudnow (1978) describes the actual projected body in his ethnography of jazz improvisation. After becoming skilled at jazz improvisation, Sudnow experiences his hands and fingers "on the way to" certain regions of the keyboard.

Merleau-Ponty (1962) talks about a bodily sense of maximum grasp. This is when one feels his or her perceptual grasp to be accurate. An athlete performing at maximum grasp of the situation talks about feeling "at one" with the situation or having quick response time. There is no "thinking time," just an immediate and appropriate response.

THE PHENOMENAL BODY

The phenomenal body is the body aware of itself. The person can attend to and describe kinesthetic sensations. All that has been written and studied related to body image fits under this category. It is possible for one to make one's bodily sensations a project of study. It is quite possible for the person to experience and describe his or her sensations quite "objectively." However, this ability does not indicate that *all* one's skillful comportment is conducted in such a theoretical, detached way.

Being a part of one's phenomenal body, one can sense one's body in many of the ways the person is taught to do culturally. For example, one can imagine one's stomach, even the anatomical shape of it, often when one experiences hunger pains. Such a phenomenal body has been culturally available only since dissection ushered in an anatomical understanding of the body. Through biofeedback, one can be taught to recognize which bodily states produce a certain heart rate, blood pressure, or skin temperature. Limited deliberate control of my bodily functions is made possible through creating learning around bodily sensations. This learning is limited to what is available to one's phenomenal and projective body. For example, an elaborate description of intracellular sodium pumps cannot give the person volitional control over the cellular pumping action. Not even visualization will alter the cellular state directly. However, if one's anxiety is decreased, then one's electrolyte balance may indeed be altered directly by one's feeling state. The techniques that have the patient visualize the physiological functioning of the body work not by mechanical instruction to the body but by the pathway of symbolism and resulting feelings (see Chapter Five, p. 163).

The current practice of having cancer patients visualize their killer cells and their immune system may elicit a climate of control and hopefulness that makes the immune system respond (Simonton, Matthews-Simonton, Creighton 1978). This is an intriguing soliciting of the culturally available belief in bodily capacities. The "cure" calls forth a symbolic bodily capacity using the current cultural social body, which is based on anatomy and physiology (see Scheper-Hughes and Lock 1987).

BODILY INTENTIONALITY

In the view handed down from the Enlightenment tradition (Shils 1981)—a view that may be termed a technological understanding of the body—the body is considered raw material to be shaped and controlled, just as the environment is seen as raw material to be harnessed. From the phenomenological perspective, this is an alienated view of the body. In the old view, there is no way to describe the person at home in the body or in the world. In fact, the world is overlooked altogether (Dreyfus in press). By contrast, in the phenomenological view, appetites and emotions are *not* understood as raw material to be shaped and controlled, but as reliable ways of knowing. The phenomenological view makes it possible to explore the wisdom of the body in new terms. Thus, the ability to read vague feeling states and respond to them appropriately need not go unnoticed just because the person cannot readily articulate such knowledge. For example, diabetics may become experts at reading their physical and emotional responses to blood sugar levels without being able to explain this ability.

One of the most pervasive examples of a technological self-understanding is the relatively modern notion of counting calories and designing a diet to meet precise nutritional energy "needs" at the cellular and tissue level. Eating is taken up as a technologically manipulated exercise even for the healthy person, and control becomes the goal, with "willpower" becoming the fulcrum in a delicate balancing act. Scales and calorie counters are used. This is very different from relying on one's own interpretation of appetite and hunger. The technological approach has limited effectiveness. The metabolism slows down to adjust to the limited intake of calories, so the body foils the attempts at control. And because this method relies on constant calculation and manipulation of diet, the dieter is prone to slips. The person may lose awareness of his or her actual physical sensations of hunger and appetite in the process. Even though hunger and appetite are influenced by habits and social conventions, attending to the sensations can provide a basis for altering one's social responses and habitual eating patterns. Several authors (e.g., Wardell 1985) have called attention to this and offer an alternative skill-training approach that encourages persons to regain a sense of actual appetite and hunger, to regain trust in their bodily capacity to regulate their eating patterns. This bodily capacity provides an alternative strategy for people who feel discouraged by the constant calculating and control-oriented approach to eating.

It is common to find a change in posture and embodiment as the person takes up new ways of being in the world as a result of a major life change. Bodily orientation and perceptions actually change with ways of being in the world. Grappling with practical situations, change, and adaptation depends on embodiment and embodied intelligence (Gendlin 1978).

Embodied intelligence and the skillful body are social and historical through and through. The body as a capacity to respond and act responds to meaningful situations and to lived cultural meanings. Barbara Duden (1987) has conducted an extensive study of the notion of the body in seventeenth-century Germany by studying women's understanding of their bodies as reported to a rural German physician. Duden reviewed 2000 cases and concluded that this prescientific understanding of the body created different physical experiences and different physical possibilities. The embodied meanings not only pointed to "facts" but also actually constituted embodied possibilities. She found that pregnancy was experienced much more as a total bodily experience. The metaphors for pregnancy were generativity metaphors not production metaphors, as they came to be during the industrial revolution.

Duden's hypothesis is that these women actually survived physical events that we would find it difficult to imagine surviving without modern medical aid. She attributes the possibility of surviving to embodied social meanings. This historical evidence raises provocative scientific questions, even though the historical data cannot provide definitive answers.

It is now defensible to argue, based upon what we know about the stress response syndrome, that people may have overreacted and through a chain of unfortunate interventions even died from what would now be considered non–life-threatening physical ailments. By the same token, people may have survived life-threatening illnesses because of vigorous immune systems and protection from excessive stress responses through ignorance of the severity of the illness. This is not an argument for a retreat from modern medicine but rather for the recognition that the body is more than a nonreactive machine and therefore can facilitate recovery or cause harm through meaningful responses to socially defined situations.

Fagerhaugh and Strauss (1977) illustrate the strength of social definition on symptom experience by their discovery that health care workers in burn units socialize their patients into the appropriate level of response to pain according to the stage and socially expected amount of pain. The patients soon join the socialization process, and the socially acquired pain expectation, no doubt, alters the pain, just as the degree of healing alters the experience of pain. The person's pain literally becomes shaped (constituted) by social expectations. This is why pain for the cancer patient may be more laden with fear and anxiety if it is thought to be a sign of recurrence (Coyle and Foley 1985). The person with cancer must deal not only with the physical discomfort caused by the pain but also with his or her own understanding of the pain as a probable indication of disease progression or even death. Furthermore, the person is not radically free to "reinterpret" pain in just any fashion.

It is possible through social conditioning to create a "voodoo" death, that is, literally to frighten a person to death. It may be that we have unwittingly created "high tech" voodoo deaths by offering only anatomicophysiological access to one's self-understanding and body (Cannon 1942, Cousins 1983). One such example was given from a nurse in the Midwest. An asymptomatic patient came in for an elective cardiac catheterization performed because of electrocardiogram changes. The cardiologists discovered advanced arteriosclerotic heart disease and scheduled him for a triple coronary artery bypass operation the next morning. The man was duly alarmed and shortly after admission began experiencing excruciating chest pain. The nurse was frustrated in her attempts to relieve the pain because intravenous access was difficult and therefore delayed. He was offered reassurance in an environment of concern and frustration.

It was decided to move him to the coronary care unit. When the patent learned this, his alarm and pain increased. He asked them to call his wife but please to take care "not to scare her to death." He, however, was extremely frightened. Soon after his arrival in the coronary care unit, his pain still uncontrolled, he experienced ventricular fibrillation. In fact, this stood out as a critical incident for the nurse because less-than-effective medical intervention was available and there was excessive conflict during the resuscitation. He was resuscitated in a chaotic poorly functioning team environment and rushed to the operating room, where emergency surgery was done. He did not regain consciousness. There is, of course, a strictly anatomicophysiological explanation for this man's death. The case is cited here only to raise consciousness and pose the question: To what extent did fear and anxiety contribute to this man's death? However, it is not possible in this case to sort out this complex question.

A phenomenological perspective on embodied intelligence has profound implications for the way we set up our healing environments and for our therapies. By placing patients in strange, highly technical environments, or in environments rife with conflict, the net result may be one of terror with disastrous physical-emotional harm. On the other hand, placing patients in reassuring environments may calm fears and promote healing. And finally, by placing people with damaged or debilitated bodies in situations that solicit a whole set or capacity to respond, we may hasten recovery of spontaneous habitual skills. Oliver Sacks (1984) cites the incident of having full range of motion restored to his leg only upon being precipitously pushed into a swimming pool and challenged to swim. His habitual body took over, and he responded with full range of motion. His bodily capacity to respond, or what Merleau-Ponty (1962) calls the set to action, gave him what deliberate willful effort was not able to accomplish (see Chapter Nine, pp. 342–345).

Harriett Lionberger's (1985, 1986) research offers evidence that therapeutic touch functions as a body therapy through restoring a sense of integrity and possibility in the body's capacities and wisdom. Through therapeutic touch, the patient who has come to experience the body as alien and uncooperative may develop a new trust in the body's capacities for restoration and healing.

This notion of embodied intelligence, embodiment as a way of knowing and a means of skillful comportment in the world (Merleau-Ponty 1962) gives new meaning and impetus to the traditional nursing body therapies such as back rubs, bed baths, early ambulation, and moving the patient to more "normal" settings (e.g., trips to the coffee shop, brief walks outside) to encourage and restore forgotten responses and combat the shrinking of perception that occurs with institutionalization.

The Role of the Situation

The term *situation* is used as a subset of the more common nursing term *environment* because the former term connotes a peopled environment. Environment is a broader more neutral term, whereas situation implies a social definition and meaningfulness. To be situated implies that one has a past, present, and future and that all of these aspects of temporality, discussed below, influence the current situation.

Situation implies having a place to stand, a place to be. When a patient wakes up from open heart surgery or any major procedure, the situation is not well defined from the patient's perception. He or she feels quite desituated. Astute recovery room nurses and ICU nurses provide a sense of the situation for the patient, including information about body boundaries, restraints, and tubes as quickly as possible. For the expert ICU nurse, the situation is well defined and familiar. The nurse coaches the patient, helping him or her to understand the rapidly changing postoperative situation. The patients feel "situationless" because the situation is so foreign and ill defined. They remain so until they regain full consciousness and once again have some command of their skilled body. Desituatedness brings about the loss of many central meanings.

Health and illness are always situated in the person's life. When an illness is extreme, it temporarily becomes the whole situation, and the other aspects of the person's life may fade into the background. In contrast, the illness may be defined totally in response to another situation, such as a major performance or other life event. The nursing history usually takes into consideration how the situation is defined for the patient.

The notions of situation and situatedness offer two perspectives: one available from inside the situation and the one available to the outsider looking on. Human scientists have called these two perspectives the "outside-in" and the "inside-out" perspectives. Likewise, the actor may be engaged in the situation or be detached and removed. The coping options available to the person vary depending on how the person is involved in the situation. We can better understand how different ways of being involved in a situation can affect coping options by thinking about situations in the terms Heidegger (1962, 1982,

Dreyfus in press) uses to describe different relationships to tools or equipment.

READY-TO-HAND

When the person is actively involved in the situation, the equipment is ready-to-hand. It is transparent or unnoticed, an extension of the body and the action. A patient may use crutches or a prosthesis in a "ready-to-hand" or taken-for-granted way. Ready-to-hand equipment or bodily extension allow for smooth functioning. The equipment may go unnoticed because it is such an extension of the body, and the focal point of attention is the intended action. When a person is healthy, his or her body is ready-to-hand, unnoticed. Also, the person who has adjusted to a physical disability can experience the body as ready-to-hand after becoming skilled and accustomed to the disability.

UNREADY-TO-HAND

Here the equipment breaks down and therefore is noticed. Smooth functioning breaks down. When one is using a typewriter, a key may become stuck, and the whole keyboard may lose its familiar structure. The unhampered use of a prosthesis may be interrupted by mechanical failure or even by self-consciousness. In the condition of unready-to-hand, the situation is altered, and the person loses the maximum grasp that was available during the ready-to-hand condition. Because the unready-to-hand is more noticeable than the ready-to-hand condition, this state is the one most often studied by scientists. It is a situation that is "problematized" by the breakdown. However, as Heidegger (1975) points out, an account of the unready-to-hand state does not yield an accurate view of the ready-to-hand state.

PRESENT-AT-HAND

The present-at-hand is the most detached objective view of the situation. Here, the person stands outside the situation and looks on. From the Cartesian tradition, this stance is the closest to "truth" because it is more objective and less involved. The referential context of equipment is lost, as well as the action. Relational aspects of the situation cannot be adequately studied from this stance, nor can the actual lived experience because the present-at-hand analysis can only provide static snapshots of the particular states of the situation at particular points in time. Smooth functioning over time, or the ways the elements of the situation are related are not captured in a present-at-hand analysis. Instead of terms describing what it is like to have a cane or a prosthetic limb function as an extension of the body, now the descriptive terms capture the objective properties of the cane and device. Density, size, color, and length of the cane are examples of present-at-hand properties that can be studied from this objective vantage point. Characteristics of the situation can be studied from the present-at-hand vantage point. Important descriptive terms are duration, frequency, intensity, novelty, pervasiveness. But notice that these terms are not descriptive of the lived situation. They are not an inside-out description.

THE PERSON IN THE SITUATION

The way the person is engaged in the situation creates different possibilities. For example, for one who is fully committed to the situation, as a parent might be to a sick child, questions about abandoning the child or leaving the situation simply do not show up as options. The parent does not feel "brave" or courageous for staying in the situation because there is just no other way to be. The parent has a world-defining relationship with the child that does not allow for even imagining a life without the child. However, for the distant relative or stranger whose affectional bonds to a child are weak, staying with a child through a difficult illness or handicap may call forth major efforts to cope with staying in the situation. The way the person is involved in the situation calls forth different coping issues.

Extrapolating a bit, Heidegger's terms *ready-to-hand, unready-to-hand* (breakdown), and *present-at-hand* may be used to describe one's level of involvement and absorption in the situation. A person's descriptions of a situation may offer clues as to how involved the person is in the situation and what the coping issues are for the person. For example, for the person who is having difficulty staying in the situation, the description may sound more "objective" and may be given in a detached way.

Involvement can be understood only in relation to particular situations. There is no situationless involvement. Accounting for the situation (along with the role of the body, personal concerns, and temporality) offers a solution for the human science dilemma of the limits of formalization. The human situation is sufficiently complex with capacities, meanings, and equipmental and social context that it is not possible to completely formalize every aspect that a complex skilled activity entails. However, understanding the situation and constraining attention to "the situation" as understood by the person *in* the situation avoids the problem of considering the situation as an endless list of separate variables and problems. When the person/situation are analyzed into objective lists, meaningful distinctions are lost and it is hard to determine which aspects of the situation are most important. The situation determines what options are available and salient. The situation limits the proliferation of variables and issues to consider. Understanding the situation encourages a relational and contextual account. We are able to move around in the everyday world because our understanding is always situated and our actions are typically only as orderly as the situation demands (Dreyfus 1979).

Different phases in an illness are literally different situations. For example, the prediagnostic situation is rife with ambiguity. It is a time of limbo. The options and outcomes can proliferate endlessly. Although it may seem feasible to cope with any one outcome, the consideration of multiple outcomes and multiple contingencies is extremely distressing to the vigilant person who copes by seeking information and trying to master the situation. The less vigilant person may cope extremely well with a prediagnostic situation because the person simply does not consider the alternative outcomes that may be pending. Similarly, patients with recurring cancer may experience their periods of remission as a kind of limbo because symptoms are vague and it is unclear what bodily sensations might be ominous signs (see Chapter Eight, pp. 284–285).

One of the major limitations of the cognitive and behavioral theories of stress and coping is that the way that the person is in the situation cannot be seriously considered. In both views, the private subject stands in opposition to the situation. The person's way of taking up his or her particular concerns and the way the person is involved in the situation are central in the Heideggerian phenomenological perspective presented here. From the phenomenological perspective, the person is not a private subject standing over against (in opposition to) an "objective" situation. Although it is true that a situation is always interpreted, the interpretations available to the person are neither completely private nor under the complete control of the individual. One might choose to "put the best face" on a bad situation, but there is a limit to this form of willful optimism. The person cannot just choose to be cheerful in the face of the loss of a major self-defining relationship and maintain a sense of personal identity and integrity. One can choose to stop acting in "caring ways," but if one cares, deliberately choosing not to care does not immediately or automatically erase the concern for the one cared for.

Another problem with the extreme views of radical freedom and extreme subjectivism ("thinking makes it so"), other than being poor accounts of reality, is that the person who actually takes up this self-understanding is prone to vacillate between feelings of omnicompetence (complete autonomy and freedom) and the opposite extreme complete incompetence or powerlessness. Glass (1977) noted this vacillation in the type A personality, which is a caricature of extreme individualism and radical freedom (see Chapter Seven). It is as if any evidence of the limits of control and individual freedom undermines any sense of control.

Personal interpretation of the situation is bounded by the nature of the situation and the way the individual is *in* it. Someone who is in a committed relationship with a spouse experiences divorce differently from someone whose world is not defined by the relationship with the spouse. However, when the situation is totalizing, as was the extreme case of the Nazi concentration camps, the range of personal coping diminishes greatly and no one escapes unharmed (Benner, Roskies, and Lazarus 1980). There is no set of omnicompetent coping strategies for all the circumstances of life. Even though every holocaust survivor must be credited with extraordinary strength, courage, and perseverance, no survivor escaped unharmed. Epidemiological studies have shown that survivors have subsequently suffered higher morbidity and mortality rates than those who are living under similar circumstances but are not holocaust survivors (Benner, Roskies, and Lazarus 1980).

A rational view of good coping like Haan's (1977) or Weisman's (1979) holds that coping is only healthy when the person can be said to have an objectively accurate assessment of reality. These models of mental health break down when they are used to understand coping in extreme situations. Mastery, control, rationality, and autonomy without regard to situation and relationships tend to be the cultural ideals underlying most versions of "ideal" coping or ideal mental health. Mastery, autonomy, and rationality were not real options in the concentration camps (Benner, Roskies, and Lazarus 1980). When a committed couple must weather an extreme illness of a partner or parents must face a devastating illness of their child, autonomy, mastery, control, and rationality are not the salient issues. In the extreme situation, the person *in* the situation must be studied, and a normative view of ideal mental health accompanied by a list of deficiencies may even make help giving and help receiving impossible.

Lazarus (1985) has written about this unfortunate tendency to apply normal mental health standards to situations of extreme deprivation or suffering. He calls it the trivialization of distress. Lazarus's article also points out the cultural problem of prescribing a meaningful solution for a particular person under particular circumstances (a particular patient with a particular world). Another person cannot just adopt that person's experience or world. Such an approach is an instrumental takeover of issues of significance. Such an instrumental takeover is also evident in the unwarranted conclusion that people should develop friendships "for their health's sake." Making friends to improve one's health is not the same as having friends. Friends for friendship's sake set up a world and are a way of knowing oneself (Sandel 1982). Friendships of this nature are constitutive. "Possessing friends" or establishing contacts for one's health does not ensure that friendships will develop, nor does such a strategic approach necessarily combat loneliness or provide emotional and social support.

Kestenbaum (1979) points out that the paradoxical quest for "healthy dying"—a consumer demand for a death experience that exceeds ordinary life—may at first appear to glamorize death. However, the end result may be trivialization or a sense of defeat and failure. Such a quest is not new. As Kestenbaum points out, Jeremy Taylor's *The Rules and Exercises of Holy Dying,* originally written in 1665, has recently been reprinted (1977). However, the modern revival of the significance of dying may focus on the psychological experience without a social and cultural context for attending to the meaning issues. "Why" questions are no longer considered productive or accessible and are replaced with "how" questions. "Consumers" may be left with vague expectations to have a "self-actualizing" experience in their dying that exceeds their prior experience in ordinary living. This instrumental takeover, making a goal of further self-development out of dying, can be excessively demanding for the patient. It may deprive the dying person of what comfort he or she can find in the mystery, finiteness, and kinship of the human experience of death. It is unclear what the expert might reasonably prescribe for a "healthy" death and under what circumstances such prescriptions would provide comfort and help for the dying (see Chapter Eight).

A purely structural or process view of extreme events such as the holocaust overlooks the *content* of the event. However, the person living through such an event makes alterations and has changed perspectives that are not eradicated by time. For example, Nelly Sachs (1967) captures the extent of the devastation and deprivation experienced in the concentration camps in her poem "Chorus of the Rescued:"

> We, the rescued,
> The worms of fear still feed on us.
> Our constellation is buried in dust.
> We, the rescued,
> Beg you:
> Show us your sun, but gradually.

Yet even in the Nazi holocaust, the role of varying situations is evident. Different experiences yielded different sequelae. For example, those who suffered severe work torture had greater difficulties with work adjustment than those who suffered the privations of confinement and other forms of abuse. Those who spent years running and hiding suffered yet different long-term effects; they tended to be more anxious (Benner, Roskies, and Lazarus 1980).

The Role of Personal Concerns

CONCERN AS MOTIVATION

Traditional psychological accounts of motivation, intentionality, and agency have overlooked the role of concern, that is, the ability to have people, events, and things matter to the person in a constitutive and motivating way. These traditional accounts of motivation are based on a Cartesian subject-object notion of the relationship between the person and his or her world. As Sandel (1982) describes this view, one's personal characteristics and significant others are viewed as possessions and attributes rather than as constitutive of the self. It is, in Taylor's (1985) terms, a strategic view of the person, rather than a significance view.

In the phenomenological view, the person is not motivated in a subject-to-object way toward or away from some thing, person, or goal, nor is the person in the world merely in a spatial sense. The person is in the world in an existential way so that the person is involved in his or her world (see discussion in Chapter 2, pp. 48–49). Being-in is a way of summing up an essential aspect of human existence. He calls this peculiarly human way of being involved "concern" (Heidegger 1962).

Thus, concern is a way of being involved in one's own world. It describes a phenomenological relationship wherein the world is apprehended directly in terms of its meaning for the self. Since the person is in the world in an involved sense, and since the person also apprehends meaning for the self directly, there is no subject-object division. The subject-object division creates the problem of understanding motivation. Without a direct relationship between person and context, motivation must be seen as arising either from people's own internal drives, needs, or structural traits or else from external prods or rewards in the environment.

Because of the involvement that concern creates, the world, that is one's own world, engages one. Concern attunes one to cues and signs that relate to or affect that concern. A commonplace example is a mother's awareness that her baby is crying. It is an everyday occurrence for someone, other than the mother, to comment, "Is the baby crying? I didn't hear anything." What people are really unaware of is that everyone has the equivalent of many crying babies in his or her life. Where there is a concern, anything that touches on that concern has salience for the person. We are all like the legendary Indian trackers moving through the forest, noting that a racoon passed through here last night, and three deer came the same way this morning. Signs that are insignificant to others are filled with significance for us. And like the actions of the woman who jumps up and runs out of the room, our actions may be puzzling to others until they learn that "the baby was crying." Then, what we do makes perfect sense to someone else, perfect human sense.

THE HEALTH CARE PROVIDER AS INTERPRETER

Concern is a meaning term that defines an involvement. Since it is not linear or quantitative, it cannot be measured. As a meaning term, it is qualitative, and so individual concerns can be interpreted and described. Because concern defines an involvement, in trying to understand an individual concern, one wants to ask "in what way is the person involved" rather than the quantitative question "how much."

There are many different arenas of concern. Spouse, family, work, and our physical, mental, and spiritual self are some of the commonly investigated ones. Within each arena of concern are many different ways of caring. Ways of caring are not limitless because our cultural possibilities are finite. But, even within these limits, there is a wide range of possible ways to be involved in one's world. When illness strikes, the illness and the possible ways to cope with it are understood in the light of personal background meanings, the situation, and the ongoing concerns in the patient's life.

Because personal concerns determine what is at stake for the person in any situation, the challenge for the health care provider is to interpret those concerns that influence the person's understanding of his or her own illness. Just as with background meaning, because we share a culture we have shared meanings. Even when those meanings are not personally held by the interpreter, they are understandable as possible ways of being in the world because of shared culture. Caring for a patient enables the expert nurse to be a participant in the sub-culture of being a patient. In this way, the expert nurse can have access to a patient's meanings and concerns without directly having the illness experience.

The ability to interpret concerns enables the health care provider to help patients deal with their illnesses. The nurse may also act as a guide at a time of transition, when a concern is changing for a patient. This is particularly crucial when the central concern at the time of the illness prevents the patient from accepting medical care. Benner (1984) describes the case of an executive who had to be coached to give up temporarily his need to be in control and allow himself to be cared for. Acting as a guide in changing concerns may not take long discussions. In fact, long discussions may be precluded, as patients are often unable to talk because of fatigue, medication, or intubation. Nurse Mary Cucci in the example below shows that, by being aware of the patient's transitional state and conveying to the patient that she understands how the person feels, the nurse can, with a few words and actions, help the patient take up a new meaning.

> I am able to tune in to where patients are at. For example, a woman came in yesterday with respiratory distress, a history of emphysema, and heart failure. Her PCO_2's were 80 when she arrived. Her O_2 was just on two liters. (She had responded to therapy well and was looking perkier.) This health problem may have been exacerbated by the news that her daughter, who had been hospitalized for a heart attack, had just died. Her daughter was fifty-one years old. So we talked a little bit about it. She immediately said to me when I walked into the room, "My daughter died," and she was still wheezy and rumbly. It seemed that she just had to tell somebody. She told me all about her daughter. I just listened commenting: "She sounds very special."

Interviewer: How did you form such an alliance with this patient so quickly?

I told her I was taking charge. I let her know that she didn't have to worry and that I was going to take care of her, so she could let go a little bit and trust me. She did well until her family came in early in the evening and she got upset, maybe because she could see their grief. It was just as I was leaving. She was intubated about midnight. This morning when I went in she was in discomfort. She was scared, but she looked as though she was willing to go through it. In other words, she was pointing (not just looking, but pointing) to things that were wrong. They were specific little things. It wasn't as though the whole thing was overwhelming. So I could deal with the little things, but she was frustrated; she was physically restrained.

Interviewer: You made a clinical judgment: "She looked as though she were willing to go through it." I'm not sure what you mean by that.

She had some strength in her. She had some strength and energy and was willing to participate in her illness, I guess. It seemed that she was going to cooperate with what was going on. I was looking for clues: Had this lady really lost it in her grief? Had she sunk? That was one of the things I was wondering about as I entered the room this morning. Was she so emotional that she was not going to be able to be coached along through this illness? Or was she going to be so uptight that we were never going to get her comfortable or maybe achieve some things in terms of rest and relaxation, and giving her breathing treatments and suctioning today? Was she going to be available? And she was going to be available.

Interviewer: You could tell that she was available to you, that she was with you somewhat.

Yes, you could see it in her eyes. They were focused, and she was restful looking in the bed. She looked at me when I said, "Good morning. It looks as if you've had a rough night." [The interview continues. Mary Cucci gives detailed information about the explanations that were given to the patient, and the decisions to take the restraints off and to give the patient pen and paper for writing.] (Benner and Tanner 1987, pp. 25–26)

Another important role of the nurse is to interpret the patient's concern to the physician or to the family. Physicians and families have their own concerns in relation to patients, and these may be at odds with what the patient wants. Or a patient's concerns may shift, and neither the physician nor the family may be aware of it or be able to hear it. The following exemplar reveals how crucial this role can be:

PARADIGM
A Quiet and Peaceful End
Judith DeChristopher, BS, RN

The "critical incident" took place on a "quiet" night on the unit. There were four RN's on duty, each of us with a module of patients (nine to ten people) to care for. We tended to work autonomously, unless we needed assistance with a "heavy" or "acute" patient. On this night I had in my charge nine patients, one of whom was J.V., a fifty-year-old black woman whose belly was swollen from ascites. The swelling of her abdomen and lower extremities greatly inhibited her mobility; she required nursing assistance in turning from side to side and in transferring from bed to chair. She was most comfortable sitting up in a recliner, where the weight of her belly impinged less on her breathing. She experienced little pain from her condition, but she did suffer from extreme fatigue and bouts of nausea and vomiting that were only minimally responsive to antiemetics. She had recently completed a third essentially unsuccessful round of chemotherapy and RT and was midway through a fourth course of both.

J. was aware of the terminal nature of her disease and spoke freely with me (her primary nurse) of her acceptance of her impending death. Her goal was to die peacefully and as comfortably as possible, with no medical heroics to postpone the inevitable. As J. tended to sleep little during the night (she napped a lot during the day), I would stop in her room and talk when my work with other patients ebbed. She spoke much of the strength of her religious convictions and of the love and support she received from extended family members and church friends. She also talked at length about her second husband, a man who was not yet willing to accept the terminal nature of her disease and who was insistent to her and to all caregivers that she live "at all costs." They had no children.

I was comfortable talking with J. about her disease and impending death and felt strongly that her grasp of the situation was congruent with the limitations of medical therapy. I came, through caring for this woman for several weeks, to both admire and respect her quiet strength and dignity and to love her as a person. I wanted for her what she wanted for herself—a quiet and peaceful end with those she loved in attendance. I had spoken briefly with her attending physician on several occasions about her desire to end the medical therapies (which even he agreed were not working) so as to spare her the side effects that made her days so uncomfortable. We had also spoken about "DNR" status, but he was unwilling to write such an order without her husband's acquiescence.

On the night in question, J. and I had talked extensively about what would happen as her condition deteriorated and death seemed inevitable. She was horrified at the prospect of spending her last hours or days connected to a respirator in an ICU setting. She stressed to me that it was *her* life, not her husband's, that hung in the balance and that she should be allowed to control how she lived or died. I agreed.

I stayed late the next morning and paged her attending oncologist. I insisted that he see her that morning; that he listen to her desires, not her husband's; that *she* was his patient, not her husband. I recounted our conversation of the previous night and insisted that to deny her wishes was tantamount to treating her as less than a person. I had never before spoken so insistently to an attending physician. I was quite used to being assertive with the interns and residents who abounded in our medical center, but in my interactions with private physicians I tended to be more aloof, less substantive, more deferent to traditional roles. Interns and residents, however, could not terminate therapy initiated by attending physicians nor could they write DNR orders.

This was the first time I had gone out on a limb to serve as a patient's advocate with an attending physician. I felt angry at a system in which the individual patient is left to the mercy of caregivers who are often more interested in legality than ethics. I felt powerless to do more than argue my patient's case. At the same time I felt proud that I had risked incurring an attending physician's wrath to protect what I saw as my patient's right to die with dignity.

Surprisingly, he came up within the hour, spoke with her privately, then wrote orders to discontinue the chemo and RT and made her an official DNR. She died peacefully, with her cousin present, a few evenings later.

This incident taught me several things about nursing. It taught me first, and foremost, that we must include a patient's desires in the goals of medical/nursing therapeutics. We treat not just a diseased body, but a whole person. To formulate a plan of care that does not incorporate input from the patient is to create a gulf between us and those we would serve. It also taught me that simple human interaction (talking, touching, sharing a cup of tea) is as valid a nursing function as participating in the resuscitation of a patient with cardiac arrest. (Though one certainly takes precedence over the other, both are necessary and valid.) I also learned that much of what I (we) perceive as nursing's powerlessness is rooted in our own beliefs about our role, rather than the role itself. The power to persuade and influence can be as important as the authority to write orders.

THE CONCERNS OF HEALTH CARE GIVERS

As individuals, nurses' lives are ordered by their own networks of concerns. As nurses, they have nursing concerns, and the nature and role of these concerns are crucial to the effectiveness of their nursing practice. The concerns of nurses, that is, what matters to nurses, clearly differ from nurse to nurse and from situation to situation. What matters for one is providing a certain kind of nursing care. For another, it is seeing that a patient has the best quality of life possible. For a third, it is the individual patient himself or herself.

Whatever form the concern takes, it is crucial that there be concern. Without it, different patients and aspects of their situations would not have salience for the nurse. Concern is essential for the nurse to be situated, that is, to be placed in a way that makes sense to the nurse and of which the nurse can make sense. Without some form of concern, there can be no knowledge of the situational features that make a difference, no attunement to the cues that signal a change in status.

A nurse's concern arises out of her or his own personal history, professional history, and the situation. Empathy, that is, the vicarious experiencing of pain, distress, and so on, is not a form of concern. However, empathy may be a path nurses can take to develop a concern. Concern allows the nurse to tune into the otherness, the singularity of the patient. In interviews, expert nurses describe what is both unique and yet recognizably human about their patients. Recognizing the individual expression of human qualities is not the same thing as looking for types. When one looks for types, one engages in a reductive activity that allows distancing and dismissal. (One "knows the type," or "has someone's number," or "has someone pegged.") Nurses describe discovering qualities in their patients, qualities such as motivation, courage, independence, willingness to go on. Although nurses certainly know about and are familiar with such qualities, they have completely unique expressions in their particular patients. Because nurses see them in this light, recognizably human and yet unique, individual features and behaviors can stand out as signaling progress or illness. Only from this stance of concern can the patient be interpretable and knowable to the nurse.

The knowledge that concern makes available is both generalizable and specific. Nurses need both generalizable and specific knowledge to help most patients. Generalizable knowledge comes from experience across many situations so that a specific situation is readily interpretable. For example, different patients tolerate different cardiac outputs. Specific knowledge has to do with the individual patient. It can be based on either long-term or short-term experience with the patient.

I'm taking care of one girl who was here several months ago. I *know* her and she knows me; she's one of my primary patients. And I can walk in and tell that things aren't right with her because we have a long-term relationship.

I think one big thing (in knowing a patient) is just how the patient *looks,* especially if you have seen that patient before, even the day before.

A nurse has some form of concern to begin with. But each new situation can elicit its own particular concern. In some cases it may have less to do with the patient as a known individual, than with his or her medical situation.

PARADIGM

A Classic Case

Gail L. Marculescu, RN[4]
El Camino Hospital, Mountain View, California

Jim was transferred to our unit after experiencing an esophagogastrectomy for removal of an esophageal lesion. Jim had been transferred to our unit from ICU the evening prior, after his recovery necessitated a prolonged stay in the ICU because he had difficulty being weaned from the respirator. I noticed Jim sitting upright in bed, oxygen cannula and IV tubing moving vigorously, gesturing with his right hand for me to move toward his bed. I was immediately aware that Jim was short of breath and struggling to talk. I could hear the bubbling Argyle chest tube apparatus and observed the dry, intact dressing on his right chest wall with brown tubes protruding from the site and connected to water seal drainage. Jim explained, "I've been in terrible pain all night, and no one's come in to see me. In ICU they checked me all the time. Can't you do something?"

I began to talk to Jim in the most soothing, quiet voice I could muster, reassuring him that I would try to help him feel better with some pain medication just as soon as I assessed him further by taking his vital signs and "checking him over." My assessment indicated a fever of 100.00, pulse 100, respirations 24–26, with rales in lung bases bilaterally. Just as I was telling Jim I would return with pain medication, his physician came in and heard the same story repeated. I decided to give IV morphine in small, frequent doses every 10–15 minutes until Jim had received a total of 8 mg of morphine in 1 hour and 15 minutes. Finally he expressed feeling as though he could "breathe easier, without hurting."

---

4. An abridged version of this paradigm case was published in Am J Nurs 87: 1556–1558. December, 1987.

Jim's wife and daughter came in to visit and expressed pleasure at seeing him "resting so comfortably." I was not so satisfied with Jim's condition and continued pain. I administered 2 mg of morphine just prior to assisting Jim to ambulate for the first time. After instructing him in techniques for getting out of bed and obtaining the portable oxygen tank to make ambulation easier for him, Jim and I (and another nurse) began our journey of just ten steps. Jim shortly became dusky in color and extremely short of breath. I hurriedly moved him toward the bed to allow him to rest. I was concerned about what I observed, and my brain silently told me "pulmonary emboli."

Jim's facial color returned to almost normal when he finally was resting in bed, but my assessment of his vital signs alarmed me. Jim's pulse rate was 124 and his respirations were 40 and labored at rest. I immediately attempted to telephone his physician, who was not on call that weekend. The physician on call was in the O.R. I requested a stat order for electrolyte panel and blood gases, which was accomplished. Jim's blood pressure was dropping slowly, his pulse was now 140, and his respirations continued at 40 and labored. I knew Jim was in deep trouble. I delegated my other patients to my colleagues on the unit. I called back to the O.R. with the results of my new assessment, plus the added information of abnormal blood gases; I thought them to be incompatible with life!

I informed the surgeon that I was going to notify the original physician at home and transfer the patient immediately to critical care. I called respiratory therapy to assist with respirations during transfer. I informed his family of my concern for Jim's respiratory status and the need for transfer to ICU, requesting their assistance to gather his personal belongings and to take his flowers home. Jim's original physician met me in the hallway during the transfer and I related my findings. I volunteered: "It feels like a classic case of pulmonary embolus right out of my nursing textbook."

I followed Jim's progress in ICU by requesting information regarding his status from the physician every time I saw him. It was determined that Jim had (previously unknown) underlying lung disease that was exacerbated by the morphine administered for pain. However, a lung scan or arteriogram had not been done, and I continued to wonder if Jim didn't have more to teach us.

Jim returned to our unit. I watched his lack of progress for three days and wondered why Jim continued to need oxygen, was anorexic, lethargic, and short of breath with activity. One day prior to his scheduled discharge date I had the opportunity to care for Jim once again. I did not feel comfortable preparing Jim for discharge knowing in "my gut" that he was not ready to manage at home. When Jim's physician came on the unit, I spoke to him about my concerns. He responded with: "All right Gail, I'll get in a pulmonary specialist—that's what you've wanted all the time, isn't it?" I did not intend for him to feel challenged, but I just knew I could not in good conscience send Jim home in the condition he was in.

Jim was seen by a pulmonary specialist that afternoon and had a pulmonary arteriogram the next morning. The results of the arteriogram indicated multiple pulmonary emboli. The surgeon came back to the unit during the afternoon to tell the patient and me. I was surprised when the physician sought me out to say: "You were right all along, Gail. This has been one of those experiences that reminds me that I can sometimes be too relaxed. Thanks for your help." Jim's discharge was delayed by ten days of heparin therapy, but when he returned home he was ready to be discharged and to return to his previous lifestyle (Marculescu 1987).

Gail Marculescu's concern situated her so that certain aspects of her patient's condition stood out as relevant. This patient's health problem strikes her as a "classic case of pulmonary emboli," but it is only possible to recognize a classic case from a situated stance that grasps certain aspects as salient. Her concern embeds her in the situation so that she perserveres and persists in questioning the physician's treatment and assessment.

In other cases, the patient as a person becomes part of the nurses concern:

Some patients complain a lot. He didn't. He was just very hopeful that something would be found, that he would feel better. So he was really searching, I think. And it just made my heart go out to him.

I don't know what engaged me, but I got very engaged. I think that I got engaged by his struggle to be independent. His determination not to be dependent even in the face of these terrible surgeries, and constantly having to be tube fed.

Concern has a way of breaking through routines and preset plans. Against the background of concern, certain things stand out as significant. The press of that sense of significance, that knowledge, leads nurses to make themselves available, regardless of the inconvenience or upset it may cause.

He wanted some one there. He kept pulling me back. So I decided to stay. I had another patient, and we had someone else take over that assignment.

A nurse's concern is what brings her or him into the profession in the first place. It changes and multiplies with new situations. It forms the basis for both medical knowledge and human knowledge, because it directs attention and it determines the salience of aspects of the patient's situation. And concern, whatever form it takes, enables the nurse to attend to the patient's concerns.

> It was like she had to tell somebody. She told me all about her daughter. I was just listening.

> He made a point to share a lot of personal aspects of his life. And not everybody does that.

> The thing they say about me is that I'm able to talk with my patients about anything. What I try to do is not feel self-conscious, because I figure these are things that are important to them.

In sum, concern is a way of caring about patients that enables taking care of patients. Concern situates the nurse so that what is salient about the patient and about the patient's situation is apparent. Concern determines salience and is the basis for gaining knowledge that is both generalizable and yet specific. A nurse's concern can make both the patient and the patient's medical situation interpretable. A nurse's concern can make medical interventions possible for and understandable to a patient. And a nurse's concern can lead her or him to understand a patient's concern and champion that patient when further interventions are known to be painful and useless. Concern is caring, and without caring there can be neither cure nor comfort.

Conclusion

In concluding this chapter, we turn to two issues that must be considered when discussing any theory of stress and coping but that could not have been addressed here before the full approach had been discussed and illustrated. First we turn to the issue of the role of emotions, and then to the matter of seeing commonalities among people. We end with a summary.

THE RELATIONSHIP BETWEEN LIVED MEANINGS AND EMOTIONS

In the phenomenological view, emotions have qualitative content. They are the language of embodied intelligence. They link the person with the lived situation. Emotions gain a new respectability because they no longer are considered a source of interruption, loss of rationality, or a barrier to "objectivity." Emotions allow the person to be engaged or involved in the situation. Emotions create the possibility of attunement that does not require precise elemental bits of information. Emotions give access to global recognition of whole situations as similar and dissimilar to past whole situations. Emotions in this view are essential to effective coping. They are no longer always considered entities to be *coped with,* although one's responses to feelings may create the need for coping with the emotion so that one can attend effectively to the situation. The emotion can be attended to for the clues and guidance it offers. Even when an emotion is unwanted or disruptive, and the person engages in coping actions to dampen the particular emotion, the very capacity for emotion sets up the possibility for coping with (e.g., dampening, distancing, denying) the disruptive, unwanted emotion.

Attending to the emotion offers the possibility of bringing a past interpretation of the situation into the present, where past history can be reinterpreted and reconstituted. This has a distinct transformative advantage over *always* avoiding the content of the emotion because reinterpretation in light of present circumstances and knowledge offers the possibility for growth or new understanding, or new coping options.

As was illustrated in Chapter Two, our view of the person is not strictly strategic and instrumental. In the phenomenological view, the person is seen as attuned to and concerned with a world of significance. This fact does not imply a libertarian, expressive, "let-it-all-hang-out" view of emotion. Rather, it generates a respect for the knowledge and wisdom to be gained from allowing emotions to direct attention and thoughts. Emotions are no longer viewed as "interruptions"; they have significance and content in their own right. The cognitivist question of which is first, the emotion or the thought, becomes a nonissue, since the two are seen to be mutually constitutive of one another.

The alienated, detached view of emotions as unruly bodily responses that must be controlled actually cuts the person off from being involved in the situation in a complete way. Rigid, consistent dampening of emotions may preclude attaining higher levels of expertise. Expertise depends on intuitive grasp, and intuitive grasp requires reading of whole situations (see Benner 1984, Benner and Tanner 1987, Dreyfus and Dreyfus 1986).

SOURCES OF COMMONALITY AND UNIQUENESS BETWEEN PERSONS AND SITUATIONS

The transition away from Cartesianism is made difficult because even the best thinkers are culturally drawn to translate what is not "objective" to a "subjective" view. This whole chapter will be misunderstood if the reader considers the phenomenological account a subjectivist account. The intent of the phenomenological project is to dissolve the false dichotomy of objective versus subjective.

A major objection to phenomenological research has been the question of whether or not commonalities can reliably be discovered if the rational bases of commonality, i.e., laws and mechanisms, are abandoned. This is a valid objection only if meanings are thought to be private and subjective. Indeed, the more commonly followed school of phenomenology in the United States, which is based on the work of Edmund Husserl, proposes a systematic approach to the study of "mental content." Heidegger, who was a student of Husserl, saw the limitations of a private individualistic view and proposed the notion of common meanings (see Dreyfus and Hall 1982). The Heideggarian, phenomenological perspective on the role of temporality, the body, the situation, and the role of personal concerns offers a relational view of the person that is not wholly private and idiosyncratic.

The scientific study of stress and coping from a phenomenological perspective can uncover both commonalities and uniqueness. The sources of commonality will, however, not be uncovered through positing general laws, mechanisms, or universal and atemporal "processes." The expectation that sources of commonality exist is based on the premise that human beings inhabit a common world and participate in common meanings. Therefore common themes, common meanings, and even common personal concerns are expected in a study of human beings who have common cultural backgrounds and are in common situations. Further, commonalities can be anticipated because of common capacities and the common experience of being embodied and having a temporal structure to existence.

"Subjectivity" and "objectivity" are no longer the central terms of concern, and a "new kind of objectivity" is achieved through discovering what can be consensually validated in the study of human beings who are temporal, relational, and contextual, through strategies that seek timely, atemporal, and noncontextual truths.

SUMMARY

The first three chapters have set up a new vantage point for understanding stress and coping. In philosophical terms, this vantage point includes an ontological perspective and is not restricted to common epistemological assumptions about the person. These two philosophical distinctions are of more than mere academic interest. When stress and coping are studied from an epistemological perspective, the only questions addressed have to do with knowing. Furthermore, there are built-in assumptions about the knower and about what can be known. The knower is a subject who generates hypotheses and makes more or less accurate observations about the world. From a traditional epistemological position, what is known is limited to more or less accurate *representations* in the mind. The body is external to the mind and is also known by the mind in a similar way as other "external" objects.

This epistemological stance, which assumes a mind-body split, is intimately linked with our Western notions of knowledge, freedom, and the conditions for verifying knowledge. For example, in this view, doubt is prevalent. One cannot directly assume that a representation of the outside world is accurate. Thus, "objective" data are preferred to "subjective" data. Objective data are created by setting up a special "data language" that decontextualizes and removes any "interpretive" element from the data.

Charles Taylor (1985) has called this notion of an objective data language "brute data." However, Taylor (1985) and other philosophers of science (Heidegger 1982, Kuhn 1970, Polanyi 1958) have called this assumption of an interpretation-free data language into question. They reason that what can be perceived is *always* determined by preconceived notions, cultural meanings, skills, language, and instruments.

The human background practices—culture, language, skills—of even the scientific tradition set up the very conditions of possibility for anything at all "showing up" for the human being. The background meanings, practices, and expectations handed down in the culture of seventeenth-century science have been termed the "received view" in nursing literature (Suppe and Jacox 1985; Webster, Jacox, and Baldwin 1981). These authors have called into question logical positivism, the name given to the traditional epistemological assumptions that are very much tied to the mind-body split and subject-object thinking (Collins 1985). The implications of the phenomenological view of the person and the roles temporality, embodiment, the situation, and personal concerns guide all the discussions of stress and coping in health and illness in the subsequent chapters.

REFERENCES

Benner P: *From Novice to Expert: Excellence and Power in Clinical Nursing Practice.* Menlo Park, Calif.: Addison-Wesley, 1984.

Benner P: Quality of life: A phenomenological perspective on explanation, prediction, and understanding in nursing science. Adv Nurs Sci 8:1, 1985.

Benner P, Roskies E, Lazarus RS: Stress and coping under extreme conditions. In Dimsdale JE (ed): *Survivors, Victims, and Perpetrators: Essays on the Nazi Holocaust.* Washington, D.C.: Hemisphere, 1980.

Benner P, Tanner C: Clinical judgment: How expert nurses use intuition. Am J Nurs 87:23, 31, 1987.

Benson H: *The Relaxation Response.* New York: Avon, 1976.

Bower T: *A Primer of Infant Development.* San Francisco: W.H. Freeman, 1977.

Brazelton T: Introduction. In Sameroff A (ed): *Organization and Stability of Newborn Behavior.* Monograph Society for Research in Child Development. 43:1, 1978.

Brazelton T: Neonatal behavioral assessment scale. Clin Devel Med 50:1, 1973.

Cannon WB: Voodoo death. Am Anthropol 44:169, 1942.

Collins CE: The last dogma of empiricism. Unpublished dissertation, University of California at Berkeley, 1985.

Cousins N: *The Healing Heart.* New York: W.W. Norton, 1983.

Coyle N, Foley K: Pain in patients with cancer: Profile of patients and common pain syndromes. Semin Oncol Nurs 1(2):93, 1985.

Doolittle N: A phenomenological study of stroke victims. Unpublished doctoral paper, University of California at San Francisco, School of Nursing, 1985.

Dreyfus HL: *Being-in-the-World: A Commentary on Heidegger's Being and Time, Division I.* Cambridge, Mass.: MIT Press, in press.

Dreyfus HL: *What Computers Can't Do: The Limits of Artificial Intelligence.* Rev ed. New York: Harper & Row, 1979.

Dreyfus, HL: From depth psychology to breadth psychology: A phenomenological approach to psychopathology. In Messer, SB, Sass LA, Woolfolk RL (eds): *Hermeneutics and Psychological Theory.* New Brunswick, New Jersey: Rutgers University Press. 1987.

Dreyfus HL, Dreyfus SE, with Athanasiou T: *Mind Over Machine: The Power of Human Intuition and Expertise in the Era of the Computer.* New York: The Free Press, 1986.

Dreyfus HL, Hall H: *Husserl, Intentionality and Cognitive Science.* Cambridge, Mass.: MIT Press, 1982.

Duden B: *Geschicchhte unterder Haut.* Stuttgart: Germany, 1987.

Fagerhaugh S and Strauss A: *The Politics of Pain Management.* Menlo Park, Calif: Addison-Wesley pp. 101–112, 1977.

Faulconer JE, Williams RN: Temporality in human action: An alternative to positivism and historicism. Am Psychol 40(11):1179, 1985.

Folkman S, Schaefer C, Lazarus, RS: Cognitive processes as mediators of stress and coping. In Hamilton V, Warburton DM (eds): *Human Stress and Cognition: An Information-Processing Approach.* London: Wiley, 1979.

Frantz R, Nevis S: Pattern preferences and perceptual-cognitive development in early infancy. Merrill-Palmer Q 13:77, 1967.

Gendlin ET: *Focusing.* New York: Bantam Books, 1978.

Glass, DC: *Behavior Patterns, Stress and Coronary Disease.* Hillsdale, NJ: Erlbaum 1977.

Haan N: *Coping and Defending: Processes of Self-Environment Organization.* New York: Academic Press, 1977.

Hall ET: *The Silent Language.* Greenwich, Conn.: Fawcett Publications, 1959.

Heidegger M: *The Basic Problems of Phenomenology,* Rev ed. Hofstadter A (trans). Bloomington: Indiana University Press, 1982.

Heidegger M: *Being and Time.* Macquarrie J, Robinson E (trans). New York: Harper & Row, 1962.

Kestenbaum R: "Healthy Dying": A paradoxical quest continues. J Soc Iss 35:185–206, 1979.

Kuhn T: *The Structure of Scientific Revolutions,* 2d ed. Chicago: University of Chicago Press, 1970.

Lazarus RS: Emotions and adaptation: Conceptual and empirical relations. In Arnold WJ (ed): *Nebraska Symposium on Motivation.* Lincoln: University of Nebraska Press, 1968.

Lazarus RS: *Psychological Stress and the Coping Process.* New York: McGraw-Hill, 1966.

Lazarus RS: The stress and coping paradigm. In Eisdorfer C, Cohen D, Kleinman A, Maxim P (eds): *Models for Clinical Psychopathology,* pp. 177–214. New York: Spectrum (Medical and Scientific Books), 1981.

Lazarus RS: The trivialization of distress. In Rosen JC, Solomon LJ (eds): *Preventing Health Risk Behaviors and Promotiong Coping with Illness,* Vol 8. *Vermont Conference on the Primary Prevention of Psychopathology.* Hanover, N.H.: University Press of New England, 1985.

Lazarus RS, Averill JR, Opton EM Jr: Toward a cognitive theory of emotions. In Arnold M (ed): *Feelings and Emotions.* New York: Academic Press, 1970.

Lazarus RS, Cohen JB: Environmental stress. In Altman I, Wohlwill JF (eds): *Human Behavior and the Environment: Current Theory and Research.* New York: Plenum, 1977.

Lazarus RS, Folkman S: *Stress, Appraisal, and Coping.* New York: Springer, 1984.

Lazarus RS, Kanner AD, Folkman S: Emotions: A cognitive phenomenological analysis. In Plutchik R, Kellerman H (eds): *Theories of Emotion,* vol 1. *Emotion: Theory, Research and Experience.* New York: Academic Press, 1980.

Lazarus RS, Launier R: Stress-related transactions between person and environment. In Pervin LA, Lewis M (eds): *Perspective in Interactional Psychology.* New York: Plenum, 1978.

Lionberger HJ: An interpretive study of nurses practice of therapeutic touch. Unpublished doctoral dissertation, University of California, San Francisco, 1985.

Lionberger HJ: Therapeutic Touch: A healing modality or a caring strategy? In *Nursing Research Methodology Issues and Implementation.* Rockville, Maryland: Aspen, 1986.

Marculescu GL: Early warning: A dialogue with excellence. Amer J Nurs 87:1556, 1987.

Mendelson M, Haith M: The relation between audition and vision in the human newborn. Monographs Social Res Child Dev 41:1, 1976.

Merleau-Ponty M: *Phenomenology of Perception.* London, England: Routledge & Kegan Paul, 1962.

Ohnuma K: Making senses. *Hippocrates* 1(2):73, 1987.

Parker J: Cancer passage: Continuity and discontinuity in terminal illness. Unpublished doctoral dissertation, Monash University, Australia, 1981.

Pennebaker JW: *The Psychology of Physical Symptoms.* New York: Springer-Verlag, 1982.

Polanyi M: *Personal Knowledge.* London: Routledge & Kegan Paul, 1958.

Roach MS: *Caring: The Human Mode of Being: Implications for Nursing. Perspectives in Caring.* Monograph 1. Toronto: University of Toronto, School of Nursing Faculty, 1984.

Sachs N: *O The Chimneys.* New York: Farrar, Straus & Giroux, 1967.

Sacks O: *A Leg to Stand On.* New York: Simon & Schuster, 1984.

Sacks, O: *The Man Who Mistook His Wife for a Hat and Other Clinical Tales.* New York: Simon & Schuster, 1985.

Sandel M: *Liberalism and the Limits of Justice.* London: Cambridge University Press, 1982.

Sauve MJ: Survivors of sudden cardiac death: The medical and psychosocial factors related to self-report of physical health, mental health and perceived health status. Unpublished doctoral dissertation. University of California, San Francisco, 1985.

Scheper-Hughes N, Lock MM: The mindful body: A prolegomenon to future work in medical anthropology. Med Anthropol Q 1:6, 1987.

Schilder E: The use of physical restraints in acute care settings. Unpublished doctoral dissertation, University of California at San Francisco, School of Nursing, 1986.

Schottstaedt WW, Pinsky RH, Mackler D, Wolf S: Sociologic, psychologic and metabolic observations on patients in the community of a metabolic ward. Am J Med 25:248, 1958.

Shils E: *Tradition.* Chicago: University of Chicago Press, 1981.

Simonton OC, Matthews-Simonton S, Creighton J: *Getting Well Again.* Los Angeles: J.P. Tarcher, 1978. Distributed by St. Martin's Press, New York.

Sudnow D: *Ways of the Hand: The Organization of Improvised Conduct.* Cambridge, Mass.: Harvard University Press, 1978.

Suppe F, Jacox AK: Philosophy of science and the development of nursing theory. In Werley HH, Fitzpatrick JJ (eds). *Annual Review of Nursing Research.* New York: Springer 3:241, 1985.

Symington T, Currie AR, Curran RC, Davidson JN: The reaction of the adrenal cortex in conditions of stress. Wolstenholme GE, Cameron MP (eds): *CIBA Foundation Colloquia on Endocrinology,* vol 8. *The Human Adrenal Cortex.* Boston: Little, Brown, 1955.

Taylor C. *Hegel and Modern Society.* Cambridge, England: Cambridge University Press, 1979.

Taylor C: *Philosophical Papers,* vols 1 and 2. Cambridge, England: Cambridge University Press, 1985.

Taylor J: *The Rules and Exercises of Holy Dying.* New York: Arno Press, 1977. First published 1665.

Thomas A: Current trends in developmental theory. Annual Prog Child Psychiatry Dev 82:7, 1982.

Wardell J: Austin B: *Thin Within: How to Eat and Live in a Thin Person.* New York: Simon & Schuster, 1985.

Webster G, Jacox A, Baldwin B: Nursing theory and the ghost of the received view. In Grace M, McCloskey N (eds): *Current Issues in Nursing.* Scranton, Pa.: Blackwell Scientific Press, 1981.

Weisman AD: *Coping with Cancer.* New York: McGraw-Hill, 1979.

Wertheimer M: Psycho-motor coordination of auditory-visual space at birth. Science 134:1692, 1961.

Wolf S: The role of the brain in bodily disease. In Weiner H, Hofer MA, Stunkard AJ (eds): *Brain, Behavior, and Disease,* pp. 1–9. New York: Raven Press, 1981.

Wolf S, Cardon P, Shepard EM, Wolf HG: *Life Stress and Essential Hypertension.* Baltimore: Williams & Wilikins, 1955.

Wrubel J: Personal meanings and coping processes. Unpublished doctoral dissertation, University of California at San Francisco, 1985.

Wrubel J, Benner P, Lazarus R: Social competence from the perspective of stress and coping. In Wine JD, Smye MD (eds). *Social Competence* 61–99. New York: Guilford Press, 1981.

CHAPTER FOUR

Coping with Illness Across the Adult Lifespan

I was comfortable talking with J. about her disease and impending death and felt strongly that her grasp of the situation was congruent with the limitations of medical therapy. I came, through caring for this woman for several weeks, to both admire and respect her quiet strength and dignity, and to love her as a person. I wanted for her what she wanted for herself—a quiet and peaceful end with those she loved in attendance. *Judith DeChristopher, RN, BS*

As individual as our lives are as adults, we nevertheless share a number of experiences that change our understanding of ourselves and our world and serve as markers in our journey through life. Where an individual is in relation to these markers and what effect they have had on his or her personal meanings are what we mean by experience in this chapter.

Thus, when we talk of life experience, we mean the way in which a life history affects understanding across time. Experience does not mean simply a passage through time, it means the way in which one is changed, for bettter or for worse, by what happens to one. Life experience changes meanings, understanding, and skills. Much of life experience is individual and is experienced personally. But what happens and what is taken in, and the way in which what happens is understood, are greatly affected by the possibilities available in a culture. For example, suttee, the self-immolation of a widow on the funeral pyre of her husband, is not a cultural possibility for us, but dying of a broken heart is (Averill and Wisocki 1981, Clayton 1979, Schulz 1978).

The common experiences of adult life—first job; career path; marriage; children; illness and loss of parents, spouse, and friends; one's own aging—all lead us into certain realms of demand and possibility.

Illness at any point in this course through life will have different meanings, depending on where one is and what the experience has meant.

It should be noted that this approach to lifespan development differs from the Freudian view. In that view, one is determined to experience all adult life experience from the perspective of meanings derived from unresolved childhood experiences that exist in the unconscious. In our view, adult life experience is as important as childhood experience in shaping understanding and personal meanings. The range of possibility that situations offer as one enters them as an adult is not limited by one's childhood traumas.

This chapter is devoted to an overview of notions of adult development and a demonstration of how an understanding of adult development can widen our understanding of the meaning of illness for people and the nature of coping with illness across the adult lifespan. We first discuss some theories of life course development to pave the way for understanding how this field has become more phenomenological in its approach. Then we discuss a phenomenological approach to lifespan development, paying particular attention to the issues of context and temporality. Finally, we discuss how an understanding of lifespan issues can help health care professionals in their dealings with patients.

Theories of Lifespan Development

Up until the 1960s, adulthood was, for the most part, viewed as a relatively static time developmentally. Researchers focused on the early years of life up to adulthood. In infancy, childhood, and adolescence, all development (social, emotional, and cognitive) is rooted in biological development. Adulthood, from one perspective, can be seen as the endpoint of that developmental thrust. Before 1960, if adult development was considered at all, it was thought of in the light of the later years of life. Old age was the next time in the lifespan that biological changes appeared related to other, especially cognitive, areas of human functioning. Theories of decremental change were propounded to describe this time of life.

Originally, social science research in adult development reflected an outgrowth of these ideas of the decrements that accompany aging. Now, researchers view the adult years as a time of continuing development and the entire lifespan as a time of continuing growth and change. In recent years, researchers in the field of human development have begun to focus on the very issues that are central to a phenomenological theory of stress and coping: the issues of the role of context as constitutive and the nature of temporality as not being mere passage of time but as having the content of experience.

Jung (1933) was one of the first theorists of lifespan development. His view differs from Freud's, who posited that one is determined to experience all adult life experience from the perspective of meanings derived from unresolved childhood conflicts. These conflicts, according to Freud, continue to direct adult behavior from the person's unconscious. Jung proposed that the human life course is marked by a shift in middle age from an outwardly directed to an inner focus of concern. He saw human development as having two distinct phases, from puberty to mid-adult years, then from those years to death. The first phase is expansive and focused on tasks, goals, and achievements. The second phase is an unconscious and undramatic time of turning inward and self-reflection, a balancing of feminine and masculine forces within the self, with the ultimate attainment being self-actualization.

Erik Erikson (1963) is probably one of the best-known theorists of lifespan development. He saw the human lifespan as divided into eight "epigenetic" stages: basic trust versus basic mistrust, autonomy versus shame and doubt, initiative versus guilt, industry versus inferiority, identity versus role confusion, intimacy versus isolation, generativity versus stagnation, and ego integrity versus despair. The first four stages are faced in childhood; the fifth, in adolescence; and the last three, in adulthood. Each stage is a psychosocial crisis. The resolution of the crisis offers possibilities for further growth and development, and the failure to resolve leads to maladjustment. The name of each stage reflects the polarity of success and failure.

Both Jung's and Erikson's approaches to the human life course have a certain appeal. There is a general sentiment that we have either experienced ourselves or witnessed in others some or all of the phases outlined. But both approaches are essentially theoretical, that is, they do not arise from large normative studies but rather from the individual author's own thinking on the subject and encounters with individuals in clinical settings. And they are psychological theories, that is, they describe a process of development that all individuals can be expected to undergo regardless of their life circumstances. Life circumstances may enhance or limit the individual's chances of Jungian self-actualization or Eriksonian crisis resolution, but the drive to self-actualize or the unfolding of the stages will occur despite life context.

Erikson's (1963) epigenetic theory of life course development is less purely intrapsychic than the Jungian formulation, which, in its researched aspects (see Havighurst, Neugarten, and Tobin 1968) is independent of actual life course events. Erikson's stages reflect struggles appropriate to particular ages but are not themselves tied to specific life cycle occurrences. From the perspective of these theorists, appraisal would shift across the life course both according to what stage predominated and to how successfully one had resolved the struggle of the earlier age. Thus, supposedly one needs to resolve the issue of intimacy versus isolation before one can deal with the crisis of generativity versus stagnation.

Although Jung did not conduct normative studies using his theory, studies have been conducted that seem to reflect a Jungian intrapsychic shift. For example, Havighurst, Neugarten, and Tobin (1968), reporting on their Kansas City study, found an increased inward directedness with aging reflected in Thematic Apperception Test protocols. (The Thematic Apperception Test or TAT is a projective measure somewhat like the Rorschach that uses realistic but ambiguous drawings rather than inkblots as the projective stimulus.) This inner-directed focus of concern preceded disengagement (where disengagement occurred) and was not correlated with level of activity or morale at any age.

Buhler (1968) presents a theory of passage through the life course, which she sees as a fusion of the biological and the biographical. In some ways, this is a more transactional view than the other psychological approaches. The individual life is seen as the interplay of internal determinants and external occurrences. With Coleman (Buhler and Coleman 1964), Buhler developed a research instrument to assess both normative and pathological adaptation at different ages. She sees each age as characterized by a different pattern of goals and concerns. However, even though Buhler credits external events with playing a role in individual change over time, she, like Jung and Erikson, posits that this shift in concerns over the life course has some internal basis.

That there is such a change in people over time is almost a truism. Individuals, in varying ways, do appraise life experiences differently at different points in life. But whether they do so because of an intrapsychic shift or for some other reason has been at issue as long as social scientists have concerned themselves with lifespan development.

Sociologists offer another way of understanding how people change across the life course through their concepts of socialization, social roles, and social norms. Neugarten (1973) notes that "from the sociological perspective, personality is generally seen as an emergent of the interaction between the biological organism and the social context, and the task of the sociologist has been to explore this interaction from the standpoint of social organization" (p. 54). The taking on of social roles, then, can be seen as a way to account for the intraindividual changes across the life course. As one takes on a social role, it becomes salient to one, and the basis of appraisal shifts.

The social role approach to lifespan development has held, for the most part, that the latter part of adult life is marked by loss and crisis. This view depends mainly on the notion that we take on social roles much more easily than we shuck them off. Research findings, as we shall see in a later section, contradict this notion. Furthermore, there are different ways and degrees of being "in" a social role, so that the mere tenure of a role is not an indication of the kind of concern it generates.

Havighurst (1952) offers a variant of the social role approach. He does not characterize the life course as a passage through roles but rather as a continuing encounter with different tasks. The tasks grow out of both individual and societal needs. Although the tasks Havighurst outlines as being appropriate for different ages appear at this distance of time to represent a heavy bias for middle-class values, the idea of tasks (which was influenced by Erikson's approach) is more flexible than the notion of social roles. The former offers a greater sense of individualization while still emphasizing the importance of social meanings.

Socialization is the term sociologists use to describe the interaction between person and society that leads to the assumption of social roles or the perception of developmental tasks. Socialization provides one with the norms and values that facilitate appropriate social behavior. The following discussion of research concerning age-grading and social supports in old age provides an example of how socialization is seen to work developmentally and of what impact it can have on health and mortality.

Neugarten, Moore, and Lowe (1968) found that there is a consensus as to what constitutes age-appropriate behavior. Moreover, as age increases, there is greater correspondence between what the individual believes other people think is age-appropriate and what the individual believes is appropriate. This consensus is called age-grading, and it operates as a norm that changes across the life course.

Rosow (1967) conducted a study of population density of the elderly in different residential situations. He concluded that age-grading profoundly influenced the access to social supports among the elderly, particularly among the working class. He found that people do not generally make friends across generations. Thus, elderly people who do not venture far from their neighborhoods, as tends to be the case with the working-class elderly, need a certain proportion of other elderly in the neighborhood to develop an adequate social network.

It is important to distinguish between social networks and social supports (Cobb 1976) and also to realize that neither networks nor supports are uniformly important for everybody (Lowenthal 1964, Townsend 1963). Nonetheless, research has shown that just a social network measure, without a weighting for degree of support, proved to be a powerful predictor of mortality (Berkman and Syme 1979). Thus, because of age-grading, elderly people who live in areas where the elderly are of low density tend to have limited social networks. As a result, they could be at greater risk of mortality.

Even here, though, we must attend to the creative and various adaptive modes of which humans are capable. Berkman and Syme (1979) found that people who lacked one part of a social network (a spouse, for instance) could balance that lack by extensions of another part, for example, many close friends. Shanas, Townsend, et al. (1968) found the same compensatory network system among the elderly. For instance, people who never married maintained close ties to siblings. In these cases, the "substitute" social tie was as protective as the conventional one.

The above discussion of psychological and sociological approaches to lifespan development is not meant to be exhaustive. The point is to illustrate the kinds of theories that have been proposed. The aim of these theories is to describe and explain the processes of development.

Psychological theories of development like Jung's and Erikson's are structural, that is, they are based on the idea of the priority of mental structures to experience. The term *structure* in this sense refers to a mental framework that determines how the world is to be understood as well as what behavioral response is to be given. In the structural approach, the task for the researcher is to identify structures that all people have in common or that are shared by groups of people. Structure cannot be thought of in terms of the specific content of personal meanings because content is too situation specific. The point of a structure is that it is appplicable to different contents. For example, according to a structural approach, all of the activities of a person in the throes of the Eriksonian intimacy versus isolation developmental crisis will reflect that level of development. Erikson's historical case study, *Young Man Luther* (1962), is an example of this view.

Thus, a mental structure is like a set of rules for how to act. An understanding of the structure can be gained by observing it in actual situations, but the structure itself is understood as applying across situations. Because cognitive structures are ideas, forms, or organizers, they cannot themselves be conceived of or understood in terms of contextually relevant particulars. And since they apply across individuals and are used as a way of grouping individuals, they cannot be thought of in terms of individual life experience.

The structural approach is appealing because it offers an alternative to the mechanistic social-learning way of accounting for how people change across the life course while still seeming to account for individual consistency. But the structural approach still has the problem of not connecting the person to the situation. Although the person is seen as active (in a mental sense) rather than as the passive recipient of stimuli from the environment, the Cartesian dualism remains intact. There is no direct connection between the person and the situation. Not many developmentalists address this particular issue, of course, because Cartesian dualism is so deeply embedded a notion that it is taken as a given. But Piaget, a seminal structural theorist and researcher of childhood development, makes clear in his writing that thinking is representational. And as long as all thinking is conceived of as representational, there cannot be a direct connection between the person and the situation.

Phenomenological Approach to Lifespan Development

In the 1970s, interest turned away from theories of developmental processes to metatheoretical considerations of the bases for the theories themselves. Developmental theories were described as being either "mechanistic" or "organismic" (i.e., structural) in orientation. The differing assumptions behind each approach were seen to lead to differing ideas of the processes of development, of the methods of studying development, and of the criteria for what constitutes development. These two contrasting approaches were seen to be mutually exclusive (Overton and Reese 1973, Reese and Overton 1970).

These philosophical considerations of the developmental theories opened up the field to other approaches. As developmentalists reflected on the available theories, which conceptualized the person as either developing because of internal/psychic leaps or because of mechanistic responses to external/environmental stimuli, they began to produce formulations in which both the person and the context were seen as having active roles in lifespan changes (Lerner and Busch-Rossnagel 1981). Theoretical interest focused on the connection between person and context, and this connection was viewed varyingly as relational (Looft 1973), transactional (Sameroff 1975), or dialectical (Riegel 1975, 1976).

What the structuralists were trying to describe was the way in which people change in dramatic shifts over time. Piaget became the model for this approach because he documented these kinds of changes in the cognitive leaps that children make as they develop. (See Chapter Two, p. 39, for an example of such a stage.) Once children make the leap, they never again see things in the same way as before. There is no "regression."

A similar shift in how things look happens to people across the lifespan. Becoming a parent, falling gravely ill, and losing a dearly loved person are examples of life experiences that have the same impact on people as moving from one cognitive stage to another has on children. Things never look the same again. But simply because the result is similar, that is, a radically reorganized way of thinking or experiencing, it does not necessarily follow that the cause is the same. A child's understanding of constancy of number may be the result of a mental structural change or of a neurological structural change, but other developmental changes across the life course can have other causes.

In Chapter Two we described aspects of humanness that make it possible for a person to grasp a situation in terms of its meaning for the self—embodied intelligence, background meaning, concern, and the situation itself. Here, we discuss how these aspects fit into new notions of temporality and context so as to contribute to a phenomenological perspective of adult development.

TEMPORALITY

The issue of temporality is necessarily at the heart of any notion of life course development. And yet there is little understanding by social scientists of the meaning of temporality in human life. The influence of positivism in social science is in large part to blame for this. In an empiricism based on the model used in natural science, history, or the passage of time, is viewed as a variable that must be controlled. If you want to test two groups of people to see if an intervention makes a difference, you test them, do the intervention to one group, don't do it to the other, then re-test them and measure the statistical difference between time one and time two. History, that is, anything else that happens to those people besides the intervention between the first test and the second test, can contaminate the purity of the results.

Within the field of human development, researchers have often stressed the importance of attending to *cohort effects,* that is, the effect of a shared history on a group of people that makes them incommensurable with another group. Living through the Great Depression in one's teenage years is an example of such a shared history.

These caveats about the effects of the passage of time on people make sense within the confines of a positivistic approach for two reasons. First, if human behavior is to be analyzed into its law-like elements, then these lawful properties have to operate independent of time. Second, if people have a Cartesian mind-body duality, the study of people has to be "objective." In order to study people objectively, they must be objectified, that is, seen as frozen images apart from the flux of time.

We have already presented the case against Cartesianism and positivism in Chapters Two and Three. In brief, a Heideggerian phenomenological approach proposes that the person is not a mind-body duality, but a self-interpreting being, that is, a being who is an embodied intelligence brought up in a world of meaning, who has concerns, all of which provide embeddedness (connection) in a situation grasped in terms of its meanings for the self. Such a being cannot be studied objectively, because such an objective, de-situated, ahistorical study will always miss the essential aspect—the self-interpretation, the lived meaning.

For such a being, temporality is fundamental because, as discussed in Chapter Three, pp. 63–67, temporality does not refer to mere passage of time or to a series of events arranged historically. Temporality means being anchored in a present made meaningful by past experience and one's anticipated future. The present moment is connected to all the past moments of a person's life, because the present moment is infused with the personal understanding of past lived experience. And this meaningful connectedness of past and present enables the emergence of the possibilities of the future.

This view of temporality does not reduce the social scientist simply to the study of flux. To the contrary, this approach, unlike the positivist one, enables us to grasp the person as a person, and not as an object. It provides a vantage point, not the natural scientist's objective view, but a human scientist's meaning-filled understanding. Faulconer and Williams (1985) describe this phenomenological view of temporality as transcendental:

> In spite of the problems associated with the traditional insistence on transcendence as necessary to knowledge, there is a very real sense in which that insistence is correct. Something transcendental, something going beyond the mere moment, some continuity is necessary for there to be understanding—but not metaphysical transcendence. That has a long history of failure, from Parmenides in 600 B.C. to positivism in the present. However, given a Heideggerian/Gadamerian view of temporality—a view in which time is not modeled on geometric space—transcendence of the moment is not a problem because time is not a series of dimensionless and, therefore, contentless points. The moment is, thus, itself transcendental; it has at once giveness and openness. Temporality does not need to be transcended by atemporal principles, because it is transcendental: As what it is, it has content and direction (p. 1187).

It must be noted that although, at a casual glance, this may resemble a deterministic view, it is at base very different. The Cartesian model of the person in which the mind is seen as separate from the external world with access only through representations, has produced two approaches to human futurity. One is a deterministic view in which the person is seen as almost a pawn in the hand of past experience. The future is determined by the past. The other is the radical freedom view (Sartre 1948, 1957; Follesdal 1981) in which the person is seen as capable of choosing meanings without regard for past experience or present understanding. In the phenomenological view, the person is neither determined nor free. The person both constitutes and is constituted by meaning. Past experience infuses understanding and limits the range of what is possible in the present without determining which of the available possibilities will be chosen. Furthermore, present experience can open up new possibilities for the person in the future.

CONTEXT

Context describes all the ways the person is connected in the world. Temporality is one of those connections. The person in the present moment is connected to all past moments. And this connectedness enables futurity. Temporality is part of context, because temporal-

113

ity describes a life course passage that is informed by meaning. The term *context,* then, implies temporality, because the person brings to each present moment all the relevant understandings of his or her past.

Background meaning is also part of context. Background meaning is the Heideggerian phenomenological term for how a person understands the world. It is temporal in nature because it is the result of a person being reared in a particular culture, subculture, and family at a particular time. Background meaning is a part of context in that it permits perception of the factual world. Background meaning is not itself a thing. It is not propositional knowledge. It is, as Merleau-Ponty (1968) has analogized, like a light. One does not see the light but what it illuminates. Without the light, one can see nothing because there is no basic, "objective" world, only the interpreted one. Thus, background meaning enables one to live in a context.

Concern is another way one is connected to context. *Concern* is the Heideggerian term used to describe the involvement people have when things matter to them. Concern also clearly has a temporal aspect, since concern changes across time and situation. For example, parental concern changes as the child grows and matures. A parent may always love the child with a deep caring—but the shape of that caring, the kind of involvement—will shift across their shared life course.

Concern in particular allows us to see how the connectedness to one's world connoted by the term *context* is not a link simply from the person to her or his world. It is a two-way connection. As a concern is born within the person, formerly unnoticed things take on a new relevance. For example, it is common for women experiencing infertility to see pregnant women everywhere they go. They may wonder if they are witnessing a population explosion since they do not recall noticing so many examples of fertility before their own became a concern. This heightened awareness increases the emotional burden of the experience of infertility:

> Pregnancy was so much on my mind that I became acutely perceptive in identifying the possible signs in myself and others. Even before pregnancies were announced and no one else had an inkling of the situation, I often was aware of others being pregnant. Little signs, invisible to most, stood out like beacons to me. For example, when my sister was only two weeks pregnant and hadn't even had a pregnancy test yet (although she suspected she was with child), I "knew" about it. I noticed during that visit that she chose to drink soda, not wine, and that one morning she went back to bed "not feeling well." Other minor cues leapt out at me and

I grew increasingly depressed without one word about pregnancy ever being mentioned. For the rest of the visit, I acted like a zombie and no one even knew why (Salzer 1986, p. 41).

Thus, concern is not just an understanding that allows the person to define the situation in a certain way. The situation itself defines the person because of the way concern involves the person in it. For example, it is commonly understood that romantic love provides one with a seemingly whole new vision. To the person in love, the whole world may seem rosier, lovelier, or more full of possibility. To the person outside the situation, the person in love may seem unusually unperceptive of the faults and limitations of the loved person.

Temporality and Context over the Lifespan

THE LIFE CYCLE EVENT APPROACH TO LIFE COURSE RESEARCH

Life cycle events, that is, the culturally expectable events that can occur across the lifespan, provide a point from which to examine the issues discussed above. They also provide access to the possible cultural meanings that may inform a life interrupted by illness. Life cycle events cut across the concerns of psychology, biology, and sociology because these events can be explored both as individual experiences or biological developments and as social phenomena. They allow us to approach the person normatively and also force us to face the major issue of individual variation.

As noted earlier, theories of adult development have often been built on the premise of decrement. Aging brings decrement in physical capacities, psychomotor speed, social role involvement, and so on. Approaches to life cycle events are not different. Theory and research in adaptation to these events propose that they will be perceived as involving loss and generating crisis. Parkes (1971), for example, argues that life cycle change involves radical revision of one's world view, and such revision is perceived as involving loss. In this way, even gains can engender a sense of loss in the individual. Parkes proposes that this equation of change with loss holds true for the entire life cycle.

More usually, theories that life cycle events involve loss focus on the events associated with the middle and later years (e.g., Berblinger 1966, Cath 1963). Whereas Parkes's notion is based on the premise of an internal mechanism whereby the revision of one's world view is always perceived as a loss, these other approaches assume that the "decremental" events of middle and late life are always perceived as loss. Thus, attainment of middle age means loss of unlimited futurity; menopause, loss of ability to bear children; empty nest, loss of children; retirement, loss of job; widowhood, loss of spouse. All of these taken together represent loss of status in the social system.

Research has not proved the loss hypothesis. These theories have suffered the fate of so many others. As Sameroff (1977) sums up:

> Whenever retrospective research has indicated a variable thought to be causal to some adverse behavioral outcome, prospective research has shown that individuals with exactly the same characteristics or experience have not had the adverse outcome (p. 61).

The decremental approach to aging and the loss hypothesis concerning life cycle events propose that all people will understand these events as demands requiring coping. But current research indicates that these events are not equally stressful for all people. This finding makes sense in the light of the phenomenological theory of the person proposed earlier. One's understanding of situations as threatening or benign is constantly changing as events change and as one acts or refrains from acting to change events. Understanding also changes as people reinterpret their past in the light of the present. But it is important to reiterate that in the phenomenological approach, the situation has its own impact. No amount of reinterpretation will erase the content of the situation itself.

Pearlin and Lieberman (1977) illuminate this issue of the situation's contribution to demand level by discriminating among those aspects of life cycle events that contribute to emotional distress. They conclude that it is not the life cycle transition itself that leads to symptoms of distress, but the life circumstances in which people find themselves once they have made the transition. If the posttransition life context presents a high level of demand, symptoms of distress are quite likely to appear. However, if the new conditions are benign, the people are as likely to enjoy good mental health as those who have not undergone a transition.

In sum, then, the adaptive demand of a life cycle event depends, to speak transactionally, on both the person and the situation. The basis for making appraisals changes over the life course. In this way, a particular event will have a different meaning and a different relevance for well-being at different times in life. When the passage through a transition is completed, the new life context can be threatening or benign. This distinction between the meaning of the passage and the nature of the destination allows us to see more clearly how people cope with life cycle events. The event may not be perceived as threatening, and the new life circumstances may also not present threat. This may be what happens in smooth transitions. Attending to the changing bases for perception and to the impact of situational features on level of demand is part of the phenomenological approach that includes meaning and context as central to human understanding.

A study of relocation of the elderly provides a good example of the crucial roles played by both meaning and context. Tobin and Lieberman (1976) studied three groups of elderly people: those on a waiting list for admission to a home for the aged, a matched group of community-based elderly with no plans for relocation, and a group of institutionalized elderly. They found that those who had decided to enter a home for the aged closely resembled the institutionalized group in mood and cognitive constriction. Features that have generally been attributed to the effects of institutionalization were prevalent in the group facing institutional life but still living in the community. The waiting list group, however, suffered no more physical illnesses or personal losses than the community group did. The meaning of the impending institutionalization, especially in terms of limited futurity and hope, accounted for the change in cognitive and affective function.

However, once the people were relocated, the individual meaning of the event did not predict whether they would experience crisis. Rather, the amount of change involved predicted the negative outcome. Prior to relocation the meaning of the event was the source of distress. Once the relocation had taken place, the situational demand, measured simply by degree of change, was the important determinant (Lieberman 1975).

LIFE CYCLE SITUATIONS AS AN ALTERNATIVE TO EVENTS

At this point, we are in a position to see that the language used to describe what happens across the life course shapes how we might think about it. The very phrase *life cycle events* is a reflection of decontextualized, spatial sense of temporality. In this sense of temporality, continuity is seen as a series of snapshots, a succession of unconnected moments. Viewing temporality in this way, rather than seeing the present as an integration of the past that offers possiblity for the future, means that research interest will more naturally turn to how well people survive these events rather than to how living through these situations shapes understanding.

In its crudest sense, the event view of the life course is like the classic steamroller scene in a Tom and Jerry cartoon. In one scene Tom is flattened by a steamroller, but in the next scene he is his former shape and again chasing Jerry. This notion of how to get through life has cultural roots for us. We admire the person who "springs back" after living through a devastating situation.

Another view of the life course also has a cultural basis for us. This view is that what happens to a person makes a difference in his or her life and shapes future understandings. With age, many people find out that they can, somewhat like Tom, be "flattened" by a devastating experience yet live through it. Often, as with, for example, bereavement, friends and others look for signs that the person has returned to his or her "old self." The person does eventually recover from the immediate and overwhelming aspects of the loss, but the person is really never the same again. Nor would he or she want to be. For just as people are constituted by their concern, by their love for another, so they are also constituted by the loss of that loved person. This is not a pathological state. To return to some former condition, some earlier constitution of the self before the other had entered one's life, with no new condition for future possibility, that is real pathology.

Researchers have also been interested in the phenomenon of resiliency. In their studies, they are often caught up in naming healthy and unhealthy responses rather than describing the different ways different people go through life. This view has led to various predictions about the effects of life cycle events. Subsequent research has not shown these predictions to hold true.

For example, a ten-year study of divorced families (Wallerstein and Kelly 1980) has shown that younger children are less vulnerable to the stresses of major changes in family structure than older children. In recent years, counselors have advised against staying unhappily married "for the sake of the children." This research shows that it could be even more damaging to the child than previously thought.

Another example is found in a study of working women (Pearlin 1975). It was thought that working women would show greater depression than nonworking women because of the greater demands on their lives. It was found, however, that depression was linked to the number and age of children, independently of whether the women worked or not. The larger the number of young children at home, the more likely the woman was to be depressed. This finding reinforces the notion of how one is constituted by one's situation.

The view of the person as a personality structure that understands experience and acts on the basis of structural traits misses the phenomenological point of how one reciprocally constitutes and is constituted by both one's meanings and one's situation. This reciprocal constitutiveness is clearly seen in the passage through the life course. In the example above, depression is seen to be an emotional condition one experiences when one is involved in the world created by a certain family stage. As the children mature, the family moves into another stage in which there is less need for constant caretaking. The parents experience less fatigue, and the possiblity appears of sharing household responsibilities with the children. Gaining a picture of how people's perspectives are organized by their particular life stage and family stage means gaining a grasp of the role of the situation.

COPING WITH LIFE COURSE SITUATIONS

Although it now seems clear that the decremental view of life cycle events is inaccurate, it seems equally true that a smooth, unstressful passage through the life course is a near impossibility. Just by existing in time, one is subject to losses. But we do more than just exist. Things matter to us, and because of this we are involved in a world whose meanings for us are shaped by our concern. However, there are ways of being in a situation, ways that our culture makes available to us, that can affect the smoothness of a passage through a life stage. The following sections are concerned with different stances that can affect the ease or difficulty of living through life course situations. These stances have been identified by research.

EXPECTATION, ANTICIPATION, AND REHEARSAL. Living in a culture informs one of a certain number of expectable situations. Leaving home, working, getting married, having children, having one's parents die, having one's children leave home, retiring from work, and having one's spouse die are all culturally expectable situations. Not all people experience all situations, nor do the situations arise in the same order. And in some cases new subclasses of situations have arisen that are becoming possibilities in current-day culture, for example, adult children returning home, single parenting, sharing custody of children, and following multiple-sequential careers.

119

Whatever the path of one's own individual life, the participation in the general culture prepares one to expect to encounter certain situations. And part of one's ability to be comfortably situated in one's own life can be attributed to the general expectation that some events are part of the natural order of life. Because of this expectation, one anticipates the situation as a preparation for its occurrence. Lowenthal, Thurner, and Chiriboga (1975), for example, debunked the myth of the empty nest in their study of four major life transitions. The empty-nest women happily anticipated their release from parental responsibilities. Neugarten, Wood, Kraines, and Loomis (1963) saw anticipation of menopause as an important factor in their respondents' ability to deal with its difficulties.

Anticipation of an expected life situation has also been observed in preretirement people. Wrubel (1985), for example, found that preretirement men and women anticipated retirement through rehearsal. Some women had begun to set up routines that they felt would protect their free time from their husbands' demands. Others regarded vacations as a foretaste of what retired life would be like. Some men did a mental rehearsal of retirement, imagining what a typical day might be like for them after retirement.

It is easy to see how anticipation could foster smooth adaptation to a life situation such as menopause or retirement, but evidently anticipation also performs a protective function for a major loss like bereavement. Rees and Lutkins (1967) report finding a significantly greater death rate among bereaved relatives when the death occurred in the street or some similar place than when the death occurred at home or in a hospital. Parkes (1975) found a similar association using mental disturbance one year postbereavement as an outcome variable.

There are limits to the effectiveness of anticipation, however, particularly when the posttransition life context presents a high level of demand. Cowan, Cowan, Coie, and Coie (1978) illustrate this in their study of the transition to parenthood. A measure of attitudes toward child-rearing provided the basis for discussions among the couples, particularly in those cases in which the husband and wife disagreed sharply. The prenatal discussions, however, did not forestall conflict over appropriate child-rearing techniques once the child was born.

ON TIME/OFF TIME. Expectation that one will encounter predictable situations, then, is one stance that makes major life changes, even changes that involve loss, easier. Experiencing the expectable life changes makes one a member of one's own cultural community. One can draw on the experiences of others as support or guidance in one's own life. Just simply knowing that others have experienced the same life changes can be felt as supportive.

Expectation and anticipation are not uniformly useful in easing the experience of life cycle stress, however. A life cycle situation that does not take place when expected can itself be the source of stress. Neugarten (1968) calls this experience being "on time or off time:"

> Men and women are not only aware of the social clocks that operate in various areas of their lives, but they are also aware of their own timing and readily describe themselves as "early," "late," or "on time" with regard to family and occupational events (p. 143).

> The middle-aged and the old seem to have learned that age is a reasonable criterion by which to evaluate behavior; that to be "off-time" with regard to life events or to show other age-deviant behavior brings with it social and psychological sequelae that cannot be disregarded (p. 146).

Sometimes the expected does not come early or late; it does not come at all. We are aware of some of these "nonevents" and the pain that their nonoccurrence causes because they have been taken up recently in the popular press. Particular emphasis has been focused on marriage and child-bearing for women. Other expectations that are sometimes not realized include becoming grandparents, being promoted, or living out a retirement dream.

REAPPRAISAL AND REINTERPRETATION. Anticipation is not always useful at smoothing the path of the life course. Anticipation that leads to rehearsal or anticipation that leads one to see how others handle a situation can help. But there are definite limits to what can be anticipated. The situation itself has its own power to constitute one, to present possibilities, and this cannot be experienced in the abstract or outside of the experience itself. For example, Cowan et al. (1978) found that anticipating the birth of a child through discussions of attitudes toward parenting proved useful. No amount of anticipation, however, can prepare parents for the overwhelming love and tenderness they will feel for their baby or the extreme fatigue they will experience.

Although sometimes the situation presents demands no amount of anticipation can prepare for, at other times the anticipation is much worse than the reality. Once involved in a situation, people often can live with it, even though ahead of time they could not imagine being able to do so. This experience, sometimes called reappraisal, has been documented in life cycle research. Researchers (Streib and Schneider 1971, Streib 1975) conducting a longitudinal study of 2000 retirees reported that the majority found retirement not to be as bad as they had anticipated. In some respects, the retired men had overestimated how bad retirement would be, and the actual experience of it came as a pleasant surprise. But in other respects, this reappraisal occurred in spite of negative situational change. For example, income dropped drastically (56%) after retirement, but the men reported being satisfied with their financial level.

Britton and Britton (1972) also report a similar finding in their nine-year study of personality changes in a group of community-based elderly. The researchers were struck by their respondents' ability to adapt to circumstances they had formerly considered unthinkable and to find those circumstances "not so bad."

Bray, Campbell, and Grant (1974) give us further insight into the reappraisal process in their longitudinal study of management recruits. By examining a life cycle nonoccurrence, these authors offer insight into the constitutive power of the situation. In this case, the occurrence or nonoccurrence was promotion into upper management positions. The awareness that they were not going to move any farther up the corporate ladder could be a bitter experience for these men, since they were recruited and trained with the expectation that they would achieve at least middle-management positions. The researchers found that nonpromotion was not generally felt to be so terrible, and outcome measures independent of this personal assessment bore out this conclusion. Bray et al. found that the values of the nonpromoted men shifted more to wife, family, religion, and humanistic pursuits. The values of the promoted men shifted more toward work and community involvement.

This finding is supported by the work of Pearlin and Schooler (1978), who describe the shift in values as a useful coping strategy for occupational role demands.

> With relatively impersonal strains, such as those stemming from economic or occupational experiences, the most effective forms of coping involve the manipulation of goals and values in a way which psychologically increases the distance of the individual from the problem (p. 18).

From the phenomenological perspective, the change in goals and values that results in this psychological distance cannot be chosen in a "purely intentional" way. Values are not simply like garments to be put on and taken off at will. The possibility for change develops out of the transaction between the person and the situation.

What Pearlin and Schooler call "psychological distance," we would term a shift in concern, a change in how something matters to one. People who can cope with this kind of problem in this way undoubtedly experience less stress. But this points out the impossibility of thinking of coping as a context-free, concern-free list of options that people should choose from to reduce the stress in their lives. A different way of understanding one's experience arises from a shift in concerns. The shift in concerns grows out of experiencing different situations across the life course and out of being made open to possibility by one's concerns and one's experience in actual situations. The shift in concerns creates a new understanding or a reinterpretation of one's experience.

Here it is possible to illuminate the distinction between coping and the effectiveness of coping. How one copes is determined by the person's concerns and the situational possibilities. Whether the choices made work to alleviate distress or change the situation is another issue. Being situated so that one's concern changes and leads to a reinterpretation of a situation appears to have adaptive value. For example, Clark (1967) points out the maladaptive nature of failure to shift concerns and hence be unable to reappraise. She researched first admissions of elderly people to a psychiatric hospital and a control group of elderly community residents. The mentally ill elderly clung to values of competition and aggression that the researchers viewed as appropriate for a younger age level, whereas the healthy community residents had adopted values of cooperation and harmony.

FUTURITY AND FINITUDE. Because we live temporal lives, we have futurity. That is, our present lives contain the content of past experience in such a way as to open to us certain possibilities in the future. One future possiblity is death. Our awareness of death is our sense of finitude, and it necessarily changes as we pass through the life course.

Change and progress are importantly meaningful in our culture. In the United States these meanings have had tremendous impact on many levels of our social structure, from the continual incorporation of immigrant ethnic groups into the cultural mainstream to the rapid shifts in and proliferation of technology. On an individual basis, the background meaning of change and progress has been taken up in terms of self-improvement.

Just as in the larger society these background meanings lead people to improve their station in life and their economic position, so on a personal level they lead people to make themselves better wives, husbands, lovers, parents, employers, workers, or just better people. A negative result of emphasizing progress on a personal level is that the experience of being can be sacrificed to the goal of becoming. But since there is a terminus to each life, there must also be a terminus to becoming. One's sense of futurity and finitude will be greatly shaped by how these meanings are taken up in one's life.

As people enter middle age, they take on a perspective of time left to live as opposed to the perspective of years one has lived (Neugarten 1968). But having a sense of finitude, that is, having a sense of being anchored in a finite life cycle with a beginning, middle, and end, does not preclude a sense of futurity. Finitude puts an end to futurity only if one holds the notion of radical freedom as a personal background meaning, that is, the idea that anything is possible. Because a sense of finitude gives one a sense of limited possibility, the lived meaning of radical freedom could well lead to despair.

However, we propose in this book that people live with a sense of situated possibility. They do not define their lives negatively, that is, in terms of everything that is not available to them, but in terms of what is possible within the situation. Thus, even terminally ill people have possibility.

Without a sense of finitude, one may think that one has unlimited possibility yet act on the basis of situated possibility. It could be that as people age and experience finitude, they also experience this sense of situated possibility. This could account for a shift in concerns and greater self-acceptance with aging. Butler (1968) exemplifies this notion in his discussion of the "life review," a process that he sees as normative in the elderly and that can enable an elderly person to see his or her life as meaningful and fulfilled.

In conclusion, by looking at coping with life cycle situations in the large scale, through the processes of expectation, anticipation, rehearsal, being on time or off time, reappraisal, reinterpretation, futurity, and finitude, we have noted a way that people change and are changed by their life experience. All of these developmental processes involve shifts in the way people grasp meaning, understand the world, and interpret events. The coping process, then, is part of the process of development. Coping involves not just how one struggles with situational demands or how one's life is affected by one's changing situation. It also involves personal change through the incorporation of new meanings.

Illness Across the Lifespan

Throughout this book we have emphasized the importance of both the person's own understanding and the context in which the person lives in determining how a situation will be interpreted. In viewing illness across the lifespan, it is possible to see how these two aspects, that is, personal meanings and the person's context, affect the meaning a serious illness will have for the individual. In this section, as in the earlier ones, the issues of context and temporality are addressed. First, we describe the life cycle, paying particular attention to both the family life cycle and the work cycle of adulthood. Then we examine the time frame of illnesses, noting particularly the differing demands of each phase. Finally, we consider the issue of the meaning and meaningfulness of illness.

THE LIFE CYCLE: WHAT AN ILLNESS INTERRUPTS

Illness is always an interruption, and one of the major things it interrupts is an ongoing life course. What is going to be interrupted depends on where the person is in his or her own personal life journey. Traditionally, we think of life as moving through infancy, childhood, adolescence, young adulthood, middle age, and old age. And more recently, old age has been divided into young-old and old-old, since in recent decades an increasing proportion of the aged population have lived beyond age eighty. Indeed, an increasing proportion has been in the older age bracket. In 1940, 42% of the elderly were 65–69 years old, and 13% were 80 or older. In 1979, 35% were 65–69 and 21% were 80 years or older (Fingerhut 1982).

We have tended to think of these life stages as occurring within the parameters of fairly specific chronological ages. Certainly, the earliest stages are very age-defined. However, in the world now, judging life stage by chronological age, except for infancy and childhood, is becoming increasingly difficult. As Neugarten and Neugarten (1987) observed:

> Adults of all ages are experiencing changes in the traditional rhythm and timing of events of the life cycle. More men and women marry, divorce,

remarry and divorce again up through their 70's. More stay single. More women have their first child before they are 15, and more do so after 35. The result is that people are becoming grandparents for the first time at ages ranging from 35 to 75. More women, but also increasing numbers of men, raise children in two-parent, then one-parent, then two-parent households. More women, but also increasing numbers of men, exit and reenter school, enter and reenter the work force and undertake second and third careers up through their 70's. It therefore becomes difficult to distinguish the young, the middle-aged and the young-old—either in terms of major life events or the ages at which those events occur (p. 30).

And it is not just in adulthood that the predictability of life events is becoming obscured. The timing of the move from adolescence into adulthood is also shifting. The traditional indicators of adult status—leaving home, work, marriage, and parenthood—no long occur at predictable ages or in a predictable order. Many more teenagers are becoming parents and in various ways are taking on the roles of mother and father. At the same time, more young adults are reestablishing dependency on family, moving back into the family home when they cannot be economically independent or else attain desired material goals on their own. Others find their entry into a profession delayed because of the years of education required.

The shifting timing of life cycle passages does not render the study of such passages meaningless. It does mean, though, that one must be very careful in generalizing about groups on the basis of either chronological age or life passage. For the health care giver, the lack of a clear correspondence between chronological age and life stage means that great attention must be paid to the person as an individual. The nurse must discover the particular shape that person's life course has assumed and understand the possible role of that person's life stage in the meaning of the illness for the person.

One approach that can provide some access to such personal meanings is to think of the lifespan more in terms of specific life cycle situations than in terms of generalized age groupings. In the breakdown given above, we spoke of young adulthood, middle age, young old age, and old old age. Social scientists find it useful to think of the adult life course in terms of more specific categories of family stage and work stage.

FAMILY STAGE. Various authors have provided divisions of the family life cycle for the health care worker. Among them are Duvall (1967), Glick (1955), Hennen (1980a), and Medalie (1979). Although they differ on the number of stages the family goes through, the essential divisions boil down to premarriage, marriage, childbearing, child rearing, child launching, empty nest, and widowhood. Each stage in the family life cycle brings with it its own demands and concerns.

As with all "normative" phases of life, it is important to recognize that these family phases are not prescriptive. Increasingly in our culture we are seeing mixing, reordering, and reentering of family life phases. More young women bear and rear children before marriage; more older men with grown children father new families; more divorces and remarriages create new family organizations with stepchildren. In fact, divorce, remarriage, and stepparenthood could possibly be added to the list of "normative" family life phases. Furthermore, not only does everyone not experience all these phases in a prescribed order, but also not everyone is in the situation in the same way. Marriage and family concerns can be such that they could be central or peripheral to a person's life, or they could be in balance or even in competition with other concerns, such as concerns about work or the self.

The premarriage time involves issues of relationship and commitment. The marriage stage, which involves just the husband-wife dyad, can have its own stages, depending on when or if children arrive on the scene. And shifting bases for satisfaction in marriage across the marriage life cycle appear to be different for women than for men. For example, in a 1960 study of 800 couples, Rollins and Feldman (1981) found that patterns of marital satisfaction for wives reflected stages of family life, with the childbearing and child-rearing phases engendering greater dissatisfaction and negative feelings about the marriage. Patterns of marital satisfaction for husbands corresponded more closely to their career trajectory, with the low point occurring just prior to retirement.

The arrival of the first child changes the relationship not only because now there are three instead of two members of the family, but also because an entirely new situation with its own demand level is encountered. The childbearing phase of family life is particularly demanding because the current children are often still quite young and requiring attending at a time when new and totally dependent family members are being added. For working parents, and especially those working outside the home, this can be an extremely demanding time.

The child-rearing phase of family life presents a less demanding context. The children are older and more independent. It is during the child-rearing phase that those mothers who took time off from work or career to bear children tend to reenter the work world.

The child-launching phase has undergone a number of shifts in recent decades. Marriage was often the occasion for both male and female children to leave home. Now education, work, or career are often the reasons for leaving the parental home. Also, some children are returning home after having been launched because they have difficulties in establishing economic independence. During the child-launching phase, the dynamics of the family shift somewhat because of the absence of one or more of the members. Second and third children get an opportunity to be the eldest or the only child.

The empty-nest phase of family life, during which the couple is again a dyad, is a fairly recent phenomenon. It was not until the mid-nineteenth century that life expectancy rose enough to allow even one parent to survive until the last child was married. One gerontologist (Cain 1968) estimates that even in the 1880s either the husband or wife would die less than a year after the marriage of the last child. Increased life expectancy has thus dramatically changed family life. As discussed in an earlier section, the empty-nest phase was once thought to be a traumatic and depressing time of life for women. Now researchers have found that couples with stable marriages often experience it as a "honeymoon." It is a time of relief from the demands of parenting and a time to renew the companionship experienced earlier in the marriage or premarriage time, before children arrived on the scene (see Lowenthal, Thurner, and Chiriboga 1975).

Death of a spouse creates another phase of family life. Losing a husband or wife creates a context of demand that goes far beyond the issues of grieving, although grieving itself is a central process. Depending on the ages of children, the surviving spouse may have to take on a greater parental responsibility. Many aspects of mutual life that were divided up or shared must now be shouldered alone. Even small, everyday requirements, such as balancing a checkbook, doing the laundry, or having the car serviced, can be experienced as major demands, not only because one is unaccustomed to doing them but also because the need to do them is a poignant reminder of the loss.

The value of understanding family life stages for the health care worker lies not in the handy labels such knowledge gives, but rather in the possible access to personal meanings, demands, and resources the individual patient lives with. The world created for a person by his or her family and marital concerns can be a powerful force in recovery from illness. Most certainly, it will influence recuperative needs. The family demands contribute to the illness experience and the recovery trajectory. That is why discharge planning that only considers disease and not illness, such as the diagnostic related groups (DRGs) form of reimbursement, creates problems. For example, a man who has delicate ear surgery may find early discharge desirable but treacherous if he needs quiet and there are very young children at home.

WORK STAGE. Understanding work stage also gives access to personal meanings, demands, and resources. One of the first questions we ask new acquaintances is "What do you do?" In our culture, work and career stage are central parts of adult identity (Erikson 1963, Friedman and Havighurst 1954, Holland 1973, Super 1957, Super and Bohn 1970, Tausky and Piedmont 1967–68). A serious illness at any point in a person's career has major implications for what demands and constraints are placed on the person and what resources are available. For example, finances are always a central consideration in a serious illness, not only because of the cost of the hospitalization and treatment but also because the ill person is not capable of producing income. The long-term impact of the illness on the person's ability to work is another example of a central concern during an adult's illness. However, other meanings arise out of the individual's particular work situation, and one aspect of that particular situation is work stage.

Career entrants face different adjustment demands than people at later stages do. Regardless of chronological age, people in the first stage of their careers typically feel the need to prove themselves. Career entrants test themselves, seek feedback on how they are doing, and are generally concerned about what kind of workers they are and want to be (Benner 1974, Benner and Benner 1979, Schein 1964). At this stage, one's work identity is not yet formed. An interruption of work life, such as by a serious illness, can derail the process of creating a work identity.

The issues of mid-career workers center around the concerns over their actual accomplishments versus what they had hoped to accomplish. Various researchers have described this stage as one of crisis involving rethinking goals (Brim and Wheeler 1966, Levinson et al. 1974, Levinson, Darrow et al. 1978), but it is not yet clear whether this crisis actually affects career workers on a large scale. The longitudinal study of management recruits by Bray, Campbell, and Grant (1974) seems to indicate ways that the situation can exert its own pull in constituting workers' lives. All of the men in the study started out with the possibility of promotion to upper management positions, but only some actually were promoted. The researchers found that those who were not promoted beyond middle management became involved in family and community life, while those who were promoted became more involved with work.

Even though it is not inevitable that the mid-career stage involve crisis, it is quite possible that a serious illness at this point in a person's career trajectory could precipitate, if not a crisis, at least a major rethinking of goals and ambitions. It is not at all unusual for a major illness to have an effect on one's sense of purpose. Even people who do not change their main goals and ambitions often, as the result of a serious illness, change something about the way they live their lives. For instance, they take time out for the things that matter to them, such as family or spiritual development.

Treatment of an illness such as coronary heart disease requires that the person make changes in lifestyle. Finding new meanings is an important step in such recovery, because "lifestyle" is really based on personal background meanings, and people cannot flourish when deprived of meaning. The health care giver who can guide the taking on of new meanings in such circumstances performs a life-saving function. (See Mary Cucci's story in Chapter Seven, pp. 247–250.)

The preretirement stage is a time of gradual shifting of concerns away from work. Over a period of years, the person begins to think about, then mentally rehearse, and then finally make plans for activities during retirement. Many factors—how dissatisfied the person is with attainments versus expectations, what kinds of shifts in meaning have occurred over the years, what expectations the person's social and work milieu set up for the person—influence how this stage goes for the person. However, a serious illness in this stage very often precipitates retirement, even when the person has the physical capacity to continue working (Mages and Mendelsohn 1979). But sudden retirement without the preparation and shift in meanings away from work goals can leave the person without the base for engaging in meaningful activity. In this situation, the illness itself can become self-defining, and the person's life becomes circumscribed and ordered primarily by the requirements of the illness rather than by his or her pre-illness concerns and involvements.

Work life, like family life, is a constitutive situation. As work changes over time, as the person becomes better at his or her work, as the person is promoted or passed over, as the person adjusts to the realities of work life or rebels against them, so the transactional relationship to the work situation shifts. The meaning of work shifts likewise. An awareness of work meanings and the relationship between work stage and work meanings can give the health care giver useful insight into what the patient has to cope with.

THE TIME FRAME OF ILLNESS

Here, as elsewhere in this book, we emphasize that illness has particular meanings to the person. In fact, illness is the disease understood in terms of its meaning for the self. This understanding is a bodily as well as a mental grasp. Also, each particular illness has its own temporal nature. In the earlier discussion of the life course, we attended to the importance of understanding temporality as being the content of a life. The person's present experience is understood in terms of all past meanings as well as in terms of present situatedness. This connection of past and present sets up the way the person understands and is oriented toward the future.

One access to the meanings of an illness for a person is to understand the temporal nature of the illness itself. In chapters devoted to different kinds of illness, we indicate what kind of temporality that disease has. The following section discusses some of the general aspects of the illness experience based on an overall temporal scheme.

DIAGNOSIS. The diagnostic stage of an illness has its own situational features that differ from other stages of an illness. The revelation of the presence of disease always has its own story. In the extreme, it can be long and arduous, or it can be brief and shocking. An example of the former is the forgetful spouse who, after several years of various diagnoses and increasing decline in functioning, is finally diagnosed as having Alzheimer's disease because the assessing neurologist has ruled out everything else. An example of the latter is the seemingly healthy father who is felled by a heart attack while out hiking with his family. These are extreme examples, but they clearly illustrate that the temporality of the diagnostic stage sets up the conditions for coping.

Hennen (1980b), following McWhinney (1972), Mechanic (1968), and Zola (1973), outlines ten stages in the career of a patient. Six of these stages *precede* consulting the physician. They are as follows:

1. Some *discontinuity* is perceived in usual function.
2. The discontinuity is perceived as *illness*.
3. Some form of *self-care* is attempted.
4. *Family* serves as the first-line *external resource*.

5. Other *external nonprofessional resources* are tried.
6. *Professional, nonmedical resources* are consulted.
7. *Physician* is consulted.
8. *Diagnostic assessment.*
9. *Management plan.*
10. *Cure* or *chronic illness* or *death* (p. 34).

It is apparent that the diagnostic phase of an illness does not begin when the patient enters the doctor's office. From the first understanding of discontinuity as illness, the patient is engaged in a diagnostic process. By the time the patient sees the physician, he or she already has at least one possible diagnosis in mind and may also have already ruled out others. Thus, one aspect of the diagnostic phase is the development of the person's own interpretation of his or her illness, an interpretation that may have been informed by the opinions of family, friends, or informal medical contacts. Sometimes, family or friends take on the diagnostic role and seek medical help on behalf of the patient. This can occur when personal meanings prevent the seeking of medical help or when the disease process inhibits or destroys normal mental functioning.

Another feature of the diagnostic stage is the movement of a bodily awareness into the foreground of awareness, in which the discontinuity or anomolous symptom is noticed and thought about. Part of the experience of stress associated with the diagnostic stage derives from this breakdown of smooth functioning. The normally taken-for-granted bodily functioning is noticed, checked on, and reflected on many times a day in an exhausting process of assessing the seriousness of the symptom. Regular activities may be curtailed or abandoned altogether, or else, normal life goes on in addition to, even in competition with, the new life of self-diagnosis.

The concern over the meaning of the symptom is usually experienced emotionally as fear, worry, and anxiety. The person may become involved in yet another wearing task, that of trying to reduce both the experience of these emotions and their impact on the rest of his or her life.

Another emotional feature of the diagnostic stage is the experience of uncertainty. The sense that something is seriously wrong, without knowing quite what, is stressful for the patient and family alike. This experience of uncertainty can sometimes keep both the patient and the family vacillating between hope and despair. And this see-saw of emotions can go on both before and after medical help is sought.

One damper on hope, however, even during the diagnostic stage, is the fact of being taken seriously by the physician and other medical personnel involved. Once the person consults a physician, and the physician shows concern by ordering diagnostic tests or even hospitalization, the possibility of clinging to the hope that the symptom is not serious is greatly diminished. Each situation, however, offers its own possibilities. Among the possibilities for hope at this point in the diagnostic stage are that the patient does not have the worst possible disease but another, less painful or less deadly one, that the disease is at an early, treatable stage, that the disease is curable, or that the current disability is temporary and return to full functioning is possible.

The medical diagnostic experience presents a new situation to be coped with. The patient with a difficult-to-diagnose illness who is in pain can be offered only palliative measures. Sometimes even palliation is contraindicated when the pain is an important clue in diagnosis. This latter experience can be central in shaping the meaning of an illness for a person, since people expect that, once they are in the hands of medical experts, relief will be forthcoming. Expert nurses recognize this distress and offer any nonpharmacological comfort measures possible, such as relaxation techniques. The expert nurse is always careful to elicit the patient's and family's understanding of the pain. The nurse offers interpretations of symptoms and tests and explains the plans and intentions to relieve the pain. Just acknowledging the pain is a form of comfort.

Sometimes diagnostic tests are themselves painful and/or intrusive and require that the patient remain conscious throughout the test. Medical technology has succeeded in providing astounding access to patients' bodies so that symptoms can be linked to disease processes. Expert nurses provide the coaching and support necessary for patients to survive and understand the assaults of that technology. Excessive fear and anxiety can potentiate pain and increase the risk of physiological responses as diverse as hemorrhage and cardiac arrhythmias.

Uncertainty is experienced throughout the trajectory of an illness. Until the illness is identified, the patient is in limbo; his or her life is put on hold. Once the diagnosis is determined, there still remains uncertainty about the nature, degree, and projected outcome of the illness. A frank, open discussion with one's physician, even a thorough search of the relevant medical literature, can usually only define the parameters of effectiveness of treatment, length of illness, or degree of disability.

Medical researchers have concerned themselves with the issue of whether a person "accepts" or "denies" a diagnosis. Weisman (1972), for example, describes acceptance and denial as complementary processes that patients use to regulate the flow of information.

> This process is in the service of preventing the paralyzing sense of loss and depression that would be disorganizing to the individual if information were not regulated. However, slowly the individual and family must integrate the diagnosis, its meaning, its course, and its outcome (Mailick 1984, p. 87).

This view of the nature of acceptance reflects all the problems inherent in the cognitive-mechanistic model of the person described in Chapter Two. That model assumes that clarity about the implications of the illness is available in advance. It assumes, from the medical perspective, that there is a concrete, unequivocal "thing," a diagnosis of a disease that can be accepted or denied in totality at any one point in time. However, all diseases and treatments actually have multiple courses, and all illnesses present multiple realities that unfold over time in a social context.

A diagnosis of a chronic, seriously acute, or disabling illness affects the patient's entire world. All the ways in which that person is connected to his or her world are likewise affected. Concerns may shift or be given up altogether. The patient has to find new ways of living out concerns but cannot do so in advance because the situation itself reveals its own possibilities to the person involved in it.

For example, the person with serious but asymptomatic or mildly symptomatic cancer can really have no grasp of how debilitated and sick he or she will be once treatment has begun. A "mental acceptance" of the fact that treatment will seriously interfere with that person's ability to continue usual life involvements is not even a close approximation of what it is actually like not to be able to move from one's bed, or what distinctions that person will make between a "good" day and a "bad" one. In fact, one of the difficulties experienced by health care workers is how and what to communicate of their understanding of possible effects and possible futures of the disease. This understanding of possible and probable courses of the disease can be a burden to the health care giver who assists the patient and family with understanding the implications of the illness for their future. Here there is no one truth to tell, but a host of possibilities. Most often, the present and the near future are all the patient and family can cope with.

Accepting a diagnosis means that the person (as well as all the people closely connected to that person) becomes constituted in a new way by his or her illness. In the best of worlds, this new constitution permits the patient to redefine meaning for the self in the situation, and the situation allows the possibility of new ways of expressing old concerns. In the constricted world of the severely ill, even small connections can help sustain a sense of continued meaning.

For example, a sixty-six-year-old woman who held an office at the state level in a philanthropic organization was rather suddenly crippled by a bone tumor in her cervical spine. At the time of her hospitalization, all records and relevant materials for ongoing activities had to be turned over to her replacement in the organization. Her sister-in-law performed this task, but she held one thing back, a small ongoing fund-raising project. The patient had organized this project herself, and it took only a short time at home each month to manage. The sister-in-law took care of this small task until the woman was home from the hospital and strong enough herself to do it.

There is a tendency to speak of what the sister-in-law provided as "symbolic," that is, not the real thing itself but just some sign of the thing that bears the same meaning as the real thing. Rather than offering a symbolic relationship to the patient's former life, the sister-in-law offered the patient her world in terms of present possibilities. Thus, acceptance of diagnosis cannot really mean simply a mental grasp of information. It has to mean somehow finding connectedness to one's world in terms of what is possible in the present situation.

ILLNESS. The diagnostic stage eventually ends. But the line between the diagnostic phase and the illness phase is often blurred. Certainly the person is ill all along. What makes illness a separate phase is that, after diagnosis, the meaning of the illness for the person takes on a new shape. Uncertainties remain, of course, but they are much more specific and delineated; they have to do with the success of a drug or other medical treatment, for example, or with the length or degree of recovery. The illness now has a name, the degree of illness has been ascertained, and the prognosis for recovery has been estimated. This new understanding of the illness domesticates or tames it. Certain specific possibilities are opened up, while others are closed off.

The shape that the meaning of the illness will take depends in part on the nature of the situation. The task in this section is not to name all the possible illness situations that a person might encounter but to indicate in broad strokes the nature of the interruption of an ongoing life. Roughly speaking, there are five types of interruption. An illness can be acute, but brief, with the person returning to normal life and former level of functioning. An illness can be long-term, but at some point the person recovers fully. An illness can be chronic, that is, either continually needing to be treated and managed or only intermittently requiring treatment. An illness can result in disability, although otherwise health is restored. And an illness can result in death. Each one of these forms of illness places the person in a different situation, each with its own possibilities and constraints.

A person with an acute, but relatively brief illness, can put his or her life on hold. This situation is essentially a crisis, and crisis modes of coping can be used. Family and close others can temporarily take on new roles or overextend themselves. The crisis mode works much less well with extended illness, even when the person eventually recovers full functioning, because extended illness calls for regrouping and reorganization. A person with a long-term illness does not simply take a temporary leave-of-absence from life. One is forced to let go of the life as it was lived. The person is left with the need to find an ongoing way of maintaining meaning during a long recovery. The illness becomes both one's occupation and preoccupation.

There is a similar shift in chronic illness, but with the difference that the person knows that he or she will never be able to return to life as it was before. The life is not so much interrupted as reshaped. The illness, no matter how well managed, becomes woven into the fabric of that person's world and into that person's meanings. For example, Kerson (1985) notes that all of the diabetics she interviewed, when asked to describe themselves, would first answer, "I am a diabetic." This held true for even the most active and well-adjusted people in the sample.

The knowledge that the illness is terminal creates yet another situation. We all know that our days are numbered, but without knowing exactly what that number is, we live with a sense of either unlimited or indefinite futurity. Knowing that one has a terminal illness, even though one has the hope of beating the odds and surviving, lends the present a weight that it does not have for other people.

THE TERMINATION OF AN ILLNESS. An illness may end because of cure, because of remission, or because of death. However, as with the shift from the diagnostic phase to the illness phase, the cessation of an illness or of an episode of illness is rarely clear cut. Even in the case of a definite pronouncement of cure with no possibility of recurrence or of permanent disability, the person still faces the convalescent period of regaining strength and stamina, of taking up again family and work responsibilities, and of reintegrating meanings.

Just as upon entering the diagnostic phase the person begins a process of understanding the illness in terms of its meaning for the self, so as the illness ends, the person has to understand wellness in terms of its meaning for the self. One aspect of this understanding involves the habitual body and bodily ways of being in the world. The habitual body can be affected by illness and by long periods of inactivity, and a person can be constantly frustrated by the disparity between what he or she precognitively expects the body to do and what is actually physically possible. A long time may pass between the day the doctor pronounces a person cured and the day that person realizes that he or she "feels like my self again." In some cases, people develop a habitual sick body and need to relearn a well body that is now possible.

Another aspect of understanding illness and wellness in terms of its meaning for the self involves the integration of the illness episode into the personal meanings of the individual. Viewing illness across the life course in temporal terms makes clear the reciprocally constitutive nature of person and situation. Different life issues are at stake for a person at different points in the life course, and illness jeopardizes these life issues. For example, a serious illness in the young adult just setting out from the family nest jeopardizes his or her aspirations for an independent life. Thus, the young adult's life situation can set up, in part, what about the illness counts as stressful. For a young adult, a serious illness could be interpreted in terms of the meaning of the loss of independence at a crucial juncture. But the situation itself of living through a serious illness can create new meanings for the person, new meanings that can in turn create new possibilities. As the illness episode ends, the meanings of that illness continue to be lived out in terms of the possibilities it opened or closed for the individual. One important coaching role of expert nurses is recognizing what could be possible within that person's meanings and pointing it out or otherwise facilitating it.

Not every patient is so fortunate as to have a clear-cut statement that he or she is cured. Very often, when an episode of illness ends, there is concern that there might be a recurrence. In the case of heart attack and stroke, one might be put on a drug regimen and make changes in lifestyle to forestall the possibility of recurrence. With cancer, one is said to be in remission until the passage of a certain time beyond which recurrence is statistically unlikely. It is in these cases that the issue of our temporality comes to the fore. As Mailick (1984) aptly puts it:

> In essence, "remission" is a retrospective word. It is only at the end of a remission that there is certainty that it was a temporary cessation of illness rather than a permanent "cure." A major task for the individual and the family is dealing with this uncertainty and the regulation of hopefulness. To gain no relief from even a temporary respite from illness and to focus only on the likelihood of its recurrence despoils a period which would otherwise allow for a replenishment of emotional and physical resources. Yet to completely deny the possibility of another episode of disease may lead to renewed crisis and despair when it occurs. Thus, balancing requires that the family as well as the patient hold both possibilities in mind, assigning more importance to present improvement and capacities to return to normal functioning, and yet accepting the inevitability of further possible episodes of illness (pp. 91-92).

The situation of uncertain cure is made even more difficult by the fact that it is not simply a situation of mental uncertainty in a stable situation. While on the one hand the person takes up normal life as much as possible, on the other hand drug treatments, required lifestyle changes, and regular monitoring of status are part of the situation to be coped with, and all constantly remind the person of the possibility of recurrence. Living with an uncertain cure can greatly affect the person's passage through normative life situations when those situations involve personal choice. For example, marriage and child-bearing may be deferred, or retirement may be taken early.

LIFE STAGE, SOCIAL CONTEXT, AND ILLNESS

Up to this point the discussion has focused on illness across the life course of separate individuals. In fact, however, illness is rarely simply an individual experience. The life stages and life situations discussed throughout this chapter describe a person in terms not only of the other people present or absent from the life context, but of the way in which they are present or absent. A person is said to be unmarried, married, widowed, or divorced. Or a person is childless, has children, has grown children not living at home, and so on. In short, the context of a person's life is peopled, and the concerns that connect the individual to others shift with time. The family concerns of a seriously ill mother of preschool children differ greatly from those of a seriously ill grandmother.

What meanings the illness has for the person, what resources are available for dealing with the illness, and hence what it is that the person has to cope with are shaped in large part by the social context. This context usually includes both a family and a work context in which that person lives. Although this chapter treats the issues connected to adult development and illness, the rich research literature on childhood illness is revealing on the issue of the importance of family context and coping with illness. Studies of the influence of family context on the mental health of chronically ill children (Pless, Roghmann, and Haggerty 1972), the association between kinds of family problem solving and level of adjustment in the child (Kucia, Drotar, Doershuk, Stern, Boat, and Matthews 1979), and the relationship between family cohesion and psychosocial adjustment (Moos and Moos 1976) all illustrate the value of understanding the coping of a patient in the context of his or her social world.

In addition to the social world the person inhabits prior to becoming ill, once ill the person automatically takes up membership in a new community—that of cancer patient, or heart patient, stroke victim, and so on. Wherever that person or that person's family goes, whomever they encounter, they will always find people with the same or similar illness, or they will find people who know or are related to others with that illness. Even very rare diseases have become part of common parlance because of well-known people who have had them. For example, many people are familiar with myasthenia gravis because of Aristotle Onassis and ankylosing spondylitis because of Norman Cousins. Membership in this community of shared diagnosis brings with it both advantages and disadvantages.

On the one hand, one can feel less stigmatized by illness when one knows that others share the same fate. In recent years the rapid growth of self-help groups based on shared illness (e.g., breast cancer, colostomy) has shown that people often feel that only others who have experienced the same illness can understand and that understanding is therapeutic. On the other hand, one experiences a deprivation of community when one's sole identification is in terms of one's disease. This new identity can be taken on by the person, or it can simply be how he or she is perceived by others, usually because of reduced activity in certain life arenas such as the workplace.

CONCLUSION: ILLNESS, MEANING, AND MEANINGFULNESS

A premise of this book is that the meaning of an illness arises out of the transaction of the individual's personal/cultural meanings and the illness situation. In this chapter we have focused on the personal meanings related to passage through the life course, meanings that even if not shared are at least interpretable by us because of our participation in a common culture. Particular attention has been paid to the role of temporality not as a simple passage of time, but as an integrative force that fuses personal meanings and life experience to allow at once for self-transformation and unity of life over time.

Attention has also been paid to the issue of illness as an interruption of an ongoing life course, as a disruption of meanings and smooth functioning that requires coping. In proposing a phenomenological approach to the person and to stress and coping, we have taken pains to point out the dangers inherent in the view that stress equals disease and coping equals antidote. A corollary of this view, which we also wish to counter, is that while too much of the wrong kind of stress accompanied by the wrong kind of coping is bad, some stress with the right kind of coping is good. This view of the benefits of stress is proposed to explain the observed fact that people often endure hardships, live through extreme deprivation, survive tragedies and emerge not only intact but also sometimes and in some ways better. An example of research in this area is provided by studies of chronically ill children. It has been shown that a marked number of families of seriously chronically ill children (e.g., hemophiliacs and leukemics) were strengthened in family unity and adaptation by their experiences (Markova, MacDonald, and Forbes 1979; Obetz, Swerson, McCarthy, Gilchrist, and Burgat 1980; Pless and Satterwhite 1975).

An extension of the view that stress is beneficial is the notion that all families would be better off if they had a chronically ill child. This, of course, is an absurd extension that no one would seriously support, but it makes the point that in this view stress and coping are externally imposed and unrelated to the meanings and world of the individual or family. However, when stress and coping are viewed as an integral part of what matters to us, as the expression of our deepest concerns and connections, then we can see that out of loss and suffering can come the possibility for new expressions of concern and connection.

REFERENCES

Averill JR., Wisocki PA: Some observations on behavioral approaches to the treatment of grief among elderly. In Sobel H. (ed): *Behavior Therapy in Terminal Care: A Humanistic Approach*. Cambridge, Mass.: Ballinger, 1981.

Benner P: Reality testing a reality shock program. In Kramer M: *Reality Shock: Why Nurses Leave Nursing*. St. Louis: C. V. Mosby, 1974.

Benner P, Benner RV: *The New Nurse's Work Entry: A Troubled Sponsorship*. New York: Tiresias Press, 1979.

Berblinger KW: Problems of the middle years. In *Mental Health in a Changing Community*. pp. 111–117. New York: Grune & Stratton, 1966.

Berkman L, Syme SL: Social networks, host resistance and mortality: A nine-year follow-up study of Alameda County residents. Am J Epidemiol 94:105, 1979.

Bray DW, Campbell RJ, Grant DL: *Formative Years in Business: A Long-Term A.T.& T. Study of Managerial Lives*. New York: John Wiley & Sons, 1974.

Brim OG, Wheeler S: *Socialization after Childhood*. New York: John Wiley & Sons, 1966.

Britton JH, Britton JO: *Personality Changes in Aging: A Longitudinal Study of Community Residents*. New York: Springer, 1972.

Buhler C: The general structure of the human life cycle. In Buhler C, Massarik F (eds): *The Course of Human Life: A Study of Goals in the Humanistic Perspective*. New York: Springer, 1968.

Buhler C, Coleman W: Life goals inventory. Manual and scoring devices, private mimeograph print.

Butler RN: The life review: An interpretation of reminiscence in the aged. In Neugarten BL (ed): *Middle Age and Aging*, pp. 486–496. Chicago: University of Chicago Press, 1968.

Cain LD: Aging and the character of our times. Gerontologist 8:250, 1968.

Cath SH: Some dynamics of middle and later years. Smith Coll Stud Social Work 33: 97, 1963.

Clark MM: The anthropology of aging, a new area for studies of culture and personality. Gerontologist 7:55, 1967.

Clayton PJ: The sequelae and nonsequelae of conjugal bereavement. Am J Psychiatry 136:1530, 1979.

Cobb S: Social support as a moderator of life stress. Psychosom Med 38:300, 1976.

Cowan CP, Cowan PA, Coie L, Coie JD: Becoming a family: The impact of a first child's birth on the couple's relationship. In Miller AB, Newman LF (eds): *The First Child and Family Formation,* pp. 296–324. Chapel Hill: Carolina Population Center, The University of North Carolina at Chapel Hill, 1978.

Duvall EM: *Family Development*, ed 4, Philadelphia: Lippincott, 1967.

Erikson EM: *Childhood and Society*, ed 2, New York: Norton & Simon, 1963.

Erikson EM: *Young Man Luther*. New York: Norton, 1962.

Faulconer JE, Williams RN: Temporality in human action, an alternative to positivism and historicism. Am Psychol 40(11):1179, 1985.

Fingerhut LA: *Changes in mortality among the elderly.* Hyattsville, Md.: US Dept of Health and Human Services, Office of Health Research, Statistics and Technology, 1982.

Follesdal D: Sartre on freedom. In Schilpp PS (ed): *The Philosophy of Jean-Paul Sartre,* pp. 392–407. LaSalle, Ill.: Open Court, 1981.

Friedman EA, Havighurst RJ: *The Meaning of Work and Retirement.* Chicago: The University of Chicago Press, 1954.

Glick P: The life cycle of the family. Marriage and Family Living 17:3, 1955.

Havighurst RJ: *Developmental Tasks and Education.* New York: Longmans, Green, 1952.

Havighurst RJ, Neugarten BL, Tobin SS: Disengagement and patterns of aging. In Neugarten BL (ed), *Middle Age and Aging.* pp. 161–172. Chicago: University of Chicago Press, 1968.

Hennen BK: The family life cycle and anticipatory guidance. In Shires DB, Hennen BK (eds), *Family Medicine: A Guidebook for Practitioners of the Art.* pp. 26–32. New York: McGraw-Hill, 1980a.

Hennen BK: Illness behavior. In Shires DB, Hennen BK (eds): *Family Medicine: A Guidebook for Practitioners of the Art,* pp. 33–37. New York: McGraw-Hill, 1980b.

Holland JL: *Making Vocational Choices: A Theory of Careers.* Englewood Cliffs, N.J.: Prentice-Hall, 1973.

Jung CG: *Modern Man in Search of a Soul.* New York: Harcourt, Brace & World, 1933.

Kerson TS, with Kerson LA: *Understanding Chronic Illness: The Medical and Psychosocial Dimensions of Nine Diseases.* New York: The Free Press, 1985.

Kucia C, Drotar D, Doershuk C, Stern RC, Boat TF, Matthews L: Home observations of family interaction and childhood adjustment to cystic fibrosis. J Pediatr Psychol 4:479, 1979.

Lerner RM, Busch-Rossnagel NA: Individuals as producers of their development: Conceptual and empirical bases. In Lerner RM, Busch-Rossnagel NA (eds): *Individuals as Producers of Their Development: A Life-Span Perspective,* pp.1–36. New York: Academic Press, 1981.

Levinson DJ with Darrow CN et al: *The Seasons of a Man's Life.* New York: Knopf, 1978.

Levinson DJ, Darrow JC, Klein E, Levinson M, McKee B. The psychological development of men in early adulthood and the mid-life transition. In Hicks DF, Thomas A, Roff M (eds): *Life History Research in Psychopathology,* vol. 3. Minneapolis: University of Minnesota Press, 1974.

Lieberman MA: Adaptive processes in late life. In Datan N, Ginsberg LH (eds): *Life-Span Developmental Psychology: Normative Life Crises,* pp. 135–159. New York: Academic Press, 1975.

Looft WR: Socialization and personality throughout the life-span: An examination of contemporary psychological approaches. In Baltes PB, Schaie KW (eds): *Life-Span Developmental Psychology: Personality and Socialization.* New York: Academic Press, 1973.

Lowenthal MF: Social isolation and mental illness in old age. Sociol Rev 29:56, 1964.

Lowenthal MF, Thurner M, Chiriboga D: *Four Stages of Life.* San Francisco: Jossey-Bass, 1975.

Mages NL, Mendelsohn GA: Effects of cancer on patients' lives: A personological approach. In Stone GC, Cohen F, Adler NE (eds): *Health Psychology: A Handbook,* pp. 255–284. San Francisco: Jossey-Bass, 1979.

Mailick M: The impact of severe illness on the individual and family: An overview. In Aronowitz E, Bromberg EM (eds), *Mental Health and Long-Term Physical Illness*. pp. 83–94. Canton, Mass.: PRODIST, 1984.

Markova I, MacDonald K, Forbes C: Impact of hemophilia on childrearing practices and parental cooperation. J Child Psychol/Psychiatry, 21:153, 1979.

McWhinney IR: Beyond diagnosis: An approach to the integration of behavioral science and clinical medicine. New Eng J Med 287:284, 1972.

Mechanic D: *Medical Sociology: A Selective View*. New York: The Free Press, 1968.

Medalie JH: The family life cycle and its implications for family practice. J Fam Practice 9(1):9, 1979.

Merleau-Ponty M: *The Visible and the Invisible*. Lingis A (trans). Evanston, Ill: Northwestern University Press, 1968.

Moos R, Moos B: A typology of family social environments. Family Process, 15:357, 1976.

Neugarten BL, Adult personality: Toward a psychology of the life cycle. In Neugarten BL (ed): *Middle Age and Aging*, pp. 137–147. Chicago: University of Chicago Press, 1968.

Neugarten BL: Sociological perspectives on the life cycle. In Baltes PB, Schaie KW (eds): *Life-Span Developmental Psychology*. New York: Academic Press, 1973.

Neugarten BL, Moore JW, Lowe JC: Age norms, age constraints and adult socialization. In Neugarten BL (ed): *Middle Age and Aging*, pp. 22–28. Chicago: University of Chicago Press, 1968.

Neugarten BL, Neugarten DA: The changing meanings of age. Psychology Today 21(5):29, 1987.

Neugarten BL, Wood V, Kraines RJ, Loomis B: Women's attitudes toward the menopause. Vita Humana 6:140, 1963.

Obetz WS, Swerson WM, McCarthy CA, Gilchrist GS, Burgat EO: Children who survive malignant disease: Emotional adaptation of the children and families. In Schulman JL, Kupst MJ (eds): *The Child with Cancer*. Springfield, Ill.: Charles C. Thomas, 1980.

Overton WF, Reese HW: Models of development: Methodological implications. In Nesselroade JR, Reese HW (eds): *Life Span Developmental Psychology: Methodological Issues*. New York: Academic Press, 1973.

Parkes CM: Determinants of outcome following bereavement. Omega 6:303, 1975.

Parkes CM: Psycho-social transitions: A field for study. Social Sci Med 5:101, 1971.

Pearlin LI: Sex roles and depression. In Datan N, Ginsberg L (eds): *Life-Span Developmental Psychology: Normative Life Crises*. New York: Academic Press, 1975.

Pearlin LI, Lieberman, MA: Social sources of emotional distress. In Simmons R (ed): *Research in Community and Mental Health*. Greenwich, Conn: JAI Press, 1977.

Pearlin LI, Schooler C: The structure of coping. J Health Social Behav 19:2, 1978.

Pless IB, Roghmann K, Haggerty RF: Chronic illness, family functioning, and psychological adjustment: A model for the allocation of preventive mental health services. Int J Epidemiol 1:271, 1972.

Pless IB, Satterwhite BB: Chronic illness. In Haggerty R, Pless I (eds): *Child Health and Community*. New York: Wiley, 1975.

Rees WD, Lutkins SG: Mortality of bereavement. Br Med J 4:13, 1967.

Reese HW, Overton WF: Models of development and theories of development. In Goulet LR, Baltes PB (eds): *Life-Span Developmental Psychology: Research and Theory*. New York: Academic Press, 1970.

Riegel KF: The dialectics of human development. Am Psychol 31:689, 1976.

Riegel KF: Toward a dialectical theory of development. Human Devel 18:50, 1975.

Rollins BC, Feldman H: Marital satisfaction over the family life cycle. In Steinberg LD (ed): *The Life Cycle: Readings in Human Development,* pp. 301–310. New York: Columbia University Press, 1981.

Rosow I: *Social Integration of the Aged.* New York: The Free Press, 1967.

Salzer LP: *Infertility: How Couples Can Cope.* Boston: G.K. Hall, 1986.

Sameroff A: Concepts of humanity in primary prevention. In Albee GW, Joffe JM (eds): *Primary Prevention of Psychopathology,* vol 1. The Issues. pp. 42–63. Hanover, N.H.: University Press of New England.

Sameroff A: Transactional models in early social relations. Human Devel 18:65, 1975.

Sartre J-P: *Existentialism and Humanism.* Mairet P (trans). London: Methuen, 1948. Originally published 1946.

Sartre J-P: *The Trandscendence of the Ego* Williams F, Kirkpatrick R, (trans). New York: Noonday Press, 1957. Originally published 1936.

Schein EH: How to break in the college graduate. Harvard Business Review 42:68, 1964.

Schulz R: *The Psychology of Death, Dying and Bereavement.* Reading, Mass.: Addison-Wesley, 1978.

Shanas E, Townsend P, et al: *Old People in Three Industrial Societies.* New York: Atherton, 1968.

Streib GF: Changing perspectives on retirement: Role crises or role continuities. In Wirt RD, Winokur G, Roff M (eds): *Life History in Psychopathology,* vol 4, pp. 301–325. Minneapolis: University of Minnesota Press, 1975.

Streib GF, Schneider CJ: *Retirement in American Society.* Ithaca: Cornell University Press, 1971.

Super DE, Bohn MJ: *Occupational Psychology.* Belmont, Calif.: Wadsworth, 1970.

Super DE: *The Psychology of Careers.* New York: Harper & Row, 1957.

Tausky C, Piedmont EG: The meaning of work and unemployment: Implications for mental health. Int J Social Psychiatry 14:44, 1967–68.

Tobin S, Lieberman MA: *Last Home for the Aged.* San Francisco: Jossey-Bass, 1976.

Townsend P: *The Family Life of Old People,* abridged ed. London: Penguin Books, 1963.

Wallerstein JS, Kelly JB: *Surviving the Breakup: How Children and Parents Cope with Divorce.* New York: Basic Books, 1980.

Weisman A: *On Dying and Denying.* New York: Behavioral Publications, 1972.

Wrubel J: Personal Meanings and Coping Processes. Unpublished doctoral dissertation, University of California, San Francisco, 1985.

Zola IK: Pathways to the doctor—From person to patient. Social Sci Med 7:677, 1973.

CHAPTER FIVE

Health Promotion

Volumes are now written and spoken upon the effect of the mind upon the body. Much of it is true. But I wish a little more was thought of the effect of the body on the mind. You who believe yourselves overwhelmed with anxieties, but are able every day to walk up Regent Street, or out in the country, to take your meals with others in other rooms, &c, &c, you little know how much your anxieties are thereby lightened. . . .

. . . the symptoms or the sufferings generally considered to be inevitable and incident to disease are very often not symptoms of the disease at all, but of something quite different—of the want of fresh air, or of light, or of warmth, or of quiet, or of cleanliness, or of punctuality and care in the administration of diet, of each or of all of these. . . .

The reparative process which Nature has instituted and which we call disease, has been hindered by some want of knowledge or attention, in one or in all of these things, and pain, suffering, or interruption of the whole process sets in   *Nightingale, [1859]1980, pp. 60 and 8.*

Until about two hundred years ago, health was understood as soundness of mind, body, and spirit (Foucault 1973; Seedhouse 1986). Then, as the science of medicine began to discover the bases of contagion and infection, means of preventing the spread of disease were developed through antisepsis and inoculation. Then drugs were created to combat bacterial infections. In the current ambiance of medical high technology, we have in some ways lost sight of these amazing achievements. No one is immunized against smallpox anymore. Because of the success of worldwide efforts, the deadly microorganism has been eradicated. But this advance in combating infectious diseases gave us another legacy, the medicalization of health. Health came to be understood as the absence of disease.

This view persists. For example, an editorial in the *Journal of Public Health Policy* (1986) has observed that the health promotion

145

chapter in the Surgeon General's 1979 *Report on Health Promotion and Disease Prevention* treats issues primarily related to disease prevention when speaking of smoking, nutrition, physical fitness, and stress control. However, in recent years there has been a movement to view health in a new way, to see a distinction between health promotion and disease prevention. Health promotion becomes a broader, more comprehensive area because it includes not just individuals' health but also family, community, and environmental contributions to health. The editorial argues for the broader view of health promotion in the following way:

> Health promotion refers primarily to the development of healthful living standards. . . . The achievement of physical, mental and social well-being and ability to function, i.e. positive health, requires public health workers to go beyond their concern with preventive and treatment services. . . . The logic of our discipline makes it necessary to support a healthful standard of living through full employment and adequate family income; improved working conditions; decent housing, including the elimination of urban and rural slums and the grim spectacle of thousands of homeless Americans; effective protection from environmental discomforts such as excessive heat and cold, smog, noise and noxious odors; good nutrition that will foster optimal physical and mental development; increased financial support to public education and elimination of financial barriers to higher education; improved opportunities for rest, recreation, and cultural development; greater participation in community activities and decision-making; an end to discrimination against minority groups based on race, gender, age, social class, religious belief, national background or sexual preference; and freedom from the pervasive fear of violence, war, and nuclear annihilation (pp. 150–151).

A value of the broader view of health promotion is that it corrects the mistaken idea that it has been the medical advances that have saved the most lives. McKeown (1979) points out that since the second half of the nineteenth century, most of the decline in mortality has been primarily due to improvements in hygiene and to rising standards of living, especially better nutrition.

Also, medical preventions and cures have not been able to undo the inequities in who is at risk for death and disease. Public health research has repeatedly demonstrated that people in the lowest socioeconomic groups have the highest morbidity and mortality rates. For example, Antonovsky (1967) reviewed thirty studies and found low socioeconomic status to be consistently related to higher morbidity and mortality rates since the twelfth century. However, it is not understood what aspects of lower socioeconomic status create the morbidity and mortality rates (Syme 1986).

Another limitation of the medical approach to health promotion is that it is by nature disease specific, whereas the prevention of disease needs to be multilevel in order to work. Thus, prescribing specific prevention measures for individuals has not had long-lasting and effective health-promotion results because of the difficulty of getting people to maintain behavior changes over time, because of the hidden social and environmental sources of disease, and because of the prevalence of diseases that these intervention programs address (Syme 1986). For example, Syme (1986) reasons that a smoking-cessation program aimed at individuals ignores the environmental factors that influence smoking:

> These factors include cultural themes associated with smoking, such as relaxation, adulthood, sexual attractiveness, and emancipation; the socioeconomic structure of tobacco production, processing, distribution, and legislation; explicit and continual advertising by the smoking industry depicting values that favor smoking; subtle advertising by recording, TV, and movie stars; and the influence of siblings, peers, and other significant persons. In addition, cigarettes are almost always easily accessible and available to everyone (p. 495).

We present the following case study[1] before discussing the different theoretical approaches to health promotion to give the discussion of theory a reference point in the real world. This case study clarifies for us the limitations of many current ideas of health and health promotion. We present it before we discuss various theories of health promotion so that the reader may have an opportunity to decide how each theory might account for Mark's story.

Mark's Story. Mark, a forty-two-year-old man with cerebral palsy, first came to the support group for the disabled somewhat unwillingly. He had been admitted to the hospital with pneumonia secondary to a viral infection. He was severely spastic, and his speech was readily understood only by close family members. He was ADL-dependent and lived with his widowed father in a new condominium. He could toilet himself but could not walk to the toilet unaided. In emergencies, he could crawl. He could feed himself if his food were cut for him. He could partly dress himself if his clothes were laid out in a

---

1. This case study is based on Judith Wrubel's conversations with Mark, his family, and a physical therapist who worked with him.

certain way. Buttons were beyond him, but he could manage some zippers. He had moved into the area two years previously but had not visited a doctor. The physician who took on his care in the hospital called in the physical therapist for an assessment of Mark's condition so that he would know what follow-up care would be appropriate.

The physical therapist was upset by Mark's general condition. She saw that he was in many ways born too soon, because current approaches to physical "habilitation" would have allowed less severe contractures, greater strength, and greater range of movement and control. She was certain that the pneumonia was an inevitable result of general lack of physical movement and shallow breathing. She was amazed that he hadn't been sick sooner. After her assessment, she remarked to him:

"You know, we have a support group for disabled people that meets here at the hospital. You might be interested in joining after your discharge."

Mark's reply (which she could not understand until his father interpreted) was: "But I'm not disabled." She came to understand how he could have this self-understanding after she learned his story.

Mark was born into a midwestern family of Scandinavian extraction. His father and mother still could speak their parents' native tongue. His father was a blue-collar worker. His mother was a housewife. He had one younger sister. The family moved to the Southeast to get special schooling and medical care for him when he was a child. In his teenage years, they moved back to their midwestern hometown. Cerebral palsy was associated with great stigma at that time. Because his speech was comprehensible only to his mother and his sister, strangers assumed he was mentally retarded. So as to appear "normal," he never used a wheelchair around the house. He usually sat in the living room and read. His favorite topic was cars, especially racing cars.

His mother was his support, mainstay, and advocate. She recognized his need and desire to have some independence and had her husband adapt a three-wheel motorcycle for his use. He drove it around the country roads near their home. One evening the motorcycle slipped into a ditch and overturned. Mark was unhurt, but could not right the cycle. He crawled a mile to a farmhouse and finally convinced the family there he was not crazy and had them call his parents. His father wanted to declare the motorcycle off-limits as too dangerous. But his mother said, "No, he has to have it."

His sister was his closest friend. But she went to college, married, and moved abroad for awhile. When he was thirty-eight, his mother died. His father was devastated by the loss. In addition, he and his wife had had a traditional division of roles in the family, and he was entirely undomestic. He had to take on the full-time care of Mark, and he couldn't even understand what Mark was saying. After two very unhappy years for both of them, they moved to the West Coast, where Mark's sister and her young family had settled.

In the new surroundings, life improved for both Mark and his father. Their condo was new and comfortable. They visited Mark's sister once a week for a day plus dinner. And most special for Mark, they lived one block away from a racing car garage. His father took him by at first to look at the cars. The mechanics, owners, and drivers soon found out that this very disabled man, who because of his garbled speech and twitchiness appeared retarded, knew almost as much about cars as they. He could discuss knowledgeably all the internal workings of the various racing car engines. He knew the speeds they could be expected to attain in certain brief spans of time. He could predict what would most likely go wrong with the car first. He became a sort of mascot of the garage. He drove there often on his three-wheeler. And he and his father would travel to some of the big races. The rest of the time, he sat in the living room reading as he always had.

Mark did not think of himself as disabled because being disabled meant being mentally retarded. His mother had tried to protect him from stigma. She helped him develop his undoubted intelligence, and she enabled him to achieve a small measure of freedom and independence at great cost to her own peace of mind.

He did finally start to attend the disabled support group, and there, at last, he found what he had never had: friends. He was dear to his family. His father, sister, brother-in-law, and nephews all loved him, but they were not the same as friends. The men at the garage regarded him with fond tolerance. The liked him and admired his amazing knowledge of cars, but they would never invite him out for a beer after work.

With this group of people, Mark went to movies, day trips, and even week-long vacations to Hawaii and Mexico. They called each other on the phone. And as a group they shared the pain and frustrations of their lives with others who understood.

One day they decided they would each tell the others their impossible dreams, the one thing they always longed to do but knew they would never be able to do. This was painful and yet somehow warming because of the complete understanding that flowed through the group. Then came Mark's turn. "Drive a car," he said. "But that's not impossible," one member of the group protested, "You're supposed to tell us the really impossible thing you want to be able to do." I won't detail the ensuing argument or even the later difficulties, hassles, and red tape. One year later, Mark had his license and a new car specially adapted for his use.

Mark enrolled in special classes for disabled people at a nearby junior college designed to improve strength, flexibility, breathing, and motor control. He began to prepare to take a series of computer classes that would qualify him for employment producing specifications for machinery parts manufacture. Four months before the classes were slated to begin, Mark died of ventricular fibrillation brought on by coughing. The funeral was well attended. All his friends were there.

Theories of Health Promotion

We agree that health promotion should be seen in a wider context than the medical model permits. Quite a few theorists hold the same position. We will not describe each theory individually but will describe five main types of health-promotion theories. First we will summarize them briefly. Then we will discuss and critique them in more detail.

The first type of theory holds that health is an ideal state. This is the Socratic view of perfect well-being in every respect. In the ideal view, health is an end in itself and is only present if disease, illness, handicap, and social problems are absent. The second kind of theory proposes that health is the ability to fulfill social roles. This is a sociological theory in which health is viewed as "the state of optimum *capacity* of an individual for the effective role and tasks for which he has been socialized" (Parsons 1981, p. 69). The third group of theories view health as a commodity that can be bought or given. This is a goods-and-services view of health and is based on a technological self-understanding. In this view, health cannot exist in the presence of disease, illness, pain, or any malady. Health is to be restored piecemeal based upon science and technology. It is, in sum, a biomedical view of health. The fourth group of theories views health as a human potential, that is, a personal strength or resource that may be either physical, metaphysical, or intellectual. In this group of theories, the strengths and abilities called health cannot be bought or given. They are personal tasks that can be lost, facilitated, or encouraged. Health is not an ideal state. To this list of four groups of theories, we will add a fifth based on Antonovsky's (1979, 1987) notion of health as coherence. Antonovsky takes the view that having one's life fit into coherent meaning and social systems is salutogenic, that is, promotes health. He opposes salutogenesis to "disease prevention," noting that the prevention of disease does not necessarily promote health. Antonovsky (1987) is careful to separate the notion of coherence (a significance stance) from a mere measure of control. He differs from our position in that he still views stress as something that can and should be "managed"—as the sub-title of his latest work, *How people manage stress and stay well*, indicates.

HEALTH AS AN IDEAL STATE

This is a utopian, perfectionistic view of health. It is the dream of extreme well-being. It is captured by the famous definition of health offered by the World Health Organization in its constitution in 1946:

> Health is a state of complete physical, mental and social well-being and not merely the absence of disease and infirmity.

The major problem with the definition is the static view of completely achieved physical, mental, and social well-being. The ideal of health sets up a decontextualized standard that ignores personal and social resources, constraints, and possibility. Most people cannot measure up to "complete" physical, mental, and social well-being and are left with a deficit view of their health. The ideal, of course, cannot spell out what is meant by "complete physical, mental and social well-being" in different cultural contexts. Health becomes all-encompassing and essentially the definition for the notion of the "good life." The notion that health can be fully explicated as a complete statement of an ideal state ignores temporality and the limits of formalism. The ideal condemns the person to view life in deficit terms (how far or near am I to the ideal) without providing a way to understand health in the context of the person's meanings, concerns, and community.

HEALTH AS THE ABILITY TO FULFILL SOCIAL ROLES

Parsons (1981) posits that health is: "the state of optimum capacity of an individual for the effective role and tasks for which he has been socialized" (p. 69). This, too, is a normative view of health, but the norms are the established societal roles. It is an ideal view since the goal is one of "optimum capacity" for effective role performance. This theory assumes that the society is "healthy" and that the roles one performs will not cause disease. Degrees of health are not considered (Seedhouse 1986). This, of course, is a serious flaw, since many jobs are hazardous, as are many ways of working, such as the type A behavior pattern (see Chapter Seven). This view of health focuses on doing rather than being and ignores the person's sense of fulfillment and well-being.

HEALTH AS A COMMODITY

This is an advanced position of a technological self-understanding. It is a medicalized view of health. The self and body are understood as

151

raw material to be shaped and controlled in accordance with principles of science and technology (Dreyfus in press). The transition from health as soundness of mind and body to a correction of deficits is traced by Foucault (1973):

> Generally speaking, it might be said that up to the end of the eighteenth century medicine related much more to health than to normality; it did not begin by analysing a "regular" functioning of the organism and go on to seek where it had deviated, what it was disturbed by, and how it could be brought back into normal working order; it referred, rather, to qualities of vigour, suppleness and fluidity, which were lost in illness and which it was the task of medicine to restore. To this extent medical practice could accord an important place to regimen and diet, in short, to a whole rule of life and nutrition that the subject imposed upon himself. This privileged relation between medicine and health involved the possibility of being one's own physician. Nineteenth century medicine, on the other hand, was regulated more in accordance with normality than with health; it formed its concepts and prescribed its interventions in relation to the standard functioning and organic structure, and physiological knowledge—once marginal and purely theoretical knowledge for the doctor—was to become established . . . at the very centre of all medical reflexion (p. 35).

In this transition the positive project of restoring the healthy qualities of "vigour, suppleness and fluidity" was replaced by correcting the identified deficits, those aspects of functioning that did not measure up to the norm. Health becomes a lost commodity that can be replaced by medical intervention.

> According to this way of looking at life (health as a commodity) health can be given or purchased without personal involvement in the process. For example, "medical health" can be purchased by buying surgery or drugs to cure a person's heart disease. The use of a drug gives health. . . . Health is seen as somehow substantial. . . . Health appears to be a thing which exists apart from people, which may be captured if right procedure is followed. This sort of health can be lost if a person has a diseased organ, but with appropriate treatment it can be restored piecemeal (Seedhouse 1986, p. 34).

Making a commodity of health is at its center a technological self-understanding. Borgmann (1984) notes that a technological self-understanding is based on the premise that disburdenment is preferable to engagement and that means can be separated from ends, indeed the means can become subordinate, invisible, and devalued. Borgmann states that a technological self-understanding

. . . first comes into relief when past and present are seen as times of toil, poverty, and suffering and when at the same moment a new natural science emerges from which great transformative power can be derived. On the basis of this power, a promise of liberation, enrichment, and of conquering the scourges of humanity is issued. The promise leads to the irony of technology when liberation by way of disburdenment yields to disengagement, enrichment by way of diversion is overtaken by distraction, and conquest makes way first to domination and then to loneliness. . . . Things in their depth yield to shallow commodities, and our once profound and manifold engagement with the world is reduced to narrow points of contact in labor and consumption (pp. 76–77).

Health as a commodity promises "instant" cures without personal effort. This view of health is false on two levels. First the "commodities" promised are not positive strengths, e.g., suppleness, strength, and fluidity. Rather, they are replacements for identified deficits. Shoring up deficits is necesary to health but not sufficient to create wholeness or positive well-being. Second, the means of health (healthful living) are detached and devalued, so that the person is given the illusion of being "disemburdened" with the "mere means" of rest, exercise, good nutrition, membership and belonging through relations with others, and living out of one's concerns. The deficits of one's means (e.g., smoking, alcohol consumption, and overwork) can supposedly be overcome by replacement of damaged bodily parts or medications.

Borgmann (1984) suggests that we do violence to things when we separate means and ends. Certainly this is the case for health and health promotion. For example, the instrumental takeover of leisure as a means of achieving health is fraught with problems because leisure loses its inherent meanings when it is subordinated to the pursuit of health. Lewis Thomas (1975) describes the problem in the following way:

Tennis has become more than the national sport; it is a rigorous discipline, a form of collective physiotherapy. Jogging is done by swarms of people, out onto the streets each day in underpants, moving in a stolid sort of rapid trudge, hoping by all this means to stay alive. Bicycles are cures. Meditation may be good for the soul, but it is even better for blood pressure. As a people we have become obsessed with health. There is something fundamentally, radically unhealthy about all this. We do not seem to be seeking more exuberance in living as much as staving off failure, putting off dying. We are losing confidence in the human form. The new consensus is that we are badly designed, intrinsically fallible, vulnerable to a host of hostile influences inside and around us, and only precariously alive. We live in danger of falling apart at any moment, and are therefore always in need of surveillance and propping up (pp. 1245–1246).

Thomas captures the loss of faith in our bodies and in our lifestyles in his description of an unhealthy quest for health. His description points up why health promotion cannot be addressed without addressing our understanding of health. In the view above, health is technically created by prescribing precise levels of exercise and calculated diets. This is the technical view of health created by rational control. Meditation to reduce blood pressure is less satisfying than meditation for its own sake, whether sacred or secular. This fact is increasingly recognized by those "prescribing" meditation (Borysenko 1987).

The instrumental stance of "controlling blood pressure" through meditation is a disengaged stance and actually interferes with achieving a meditative state and enjoying the qualities of meditation on its own terms. The problem of instrumental takeover is also evident in the recommendations that people develop friends because "friends are good for your health."[2] But developing friends for your health (an instrumental takeover) is not the same thing as having a friend. Thus what may appear to be holism, addressing the whole person, can in fact be one more instance of striving to make up for a deficient self, an incoherent society, and a body that is not trustworthy. This background stance is inherently incoherent and unhealthy.

In its most advanced form, the consumer-commodity view of health makes the instruments ends in themselves.

> Abstract general ends—health, safety, comfort, nutrition, shelter, mobility, happiness, and so forth—become highly instrument-specific. The desire to move about becomes the desire to possess an automobile; the need to communicate becomes the necessity of having telephone service; the need to eat becomes a need for a refrigerator, stove, and convenient supermarket (Winner 1977, p. 234).

An understanding of health as a set of tightly controlled prescriptions for exercise and nutrition ignores the meanings and rela-

---

2. An example is public service announcements made on California television recommending friends as a means of procuring health. These commercials were based upon the social science research demonstrating that those who have close friends and rich social networks are healthier (e.g., Berkman and Syme 1979, Cobb 1976).

tionships between the prescription and the person. Scientism becomes the dominant cultural pattern, and the background meaning tends to be that one cannot trust the body, the environment, or one's traditional lifestyle. This technological approach to health is at bottom incoherent because it is not possible to turn life into a series of formulas. Science and technology do not and cannot in principle formalize "all" the answers for health. They can offer guidelines and correctives to traditions and practices, but science and technology lack the integrative meaning system to give one direction, preferences, a sense of salience, and finally a sense of belonging (Bloom 1987, Dreyfus 1979, Schwartz 1986).

Changes in lifestyles and health habits work best when they are integrated into the person's own cultural patterns and traditions. Although it is possible to establish new patterns, it is hard to sustain these patterns if they go against the grain of all of one's normal social patterns. The series of calculated steps to increase health need to be embedded in the person's social context. This is why health promotion programs may be best integrated into families, work, schools, churches, and social clubs (Hatch, Cunningham, Woods, and Snipes 1986). Hatch et al. (1986) present their rationale for introducing physical exercise into the black church:

> The decision to use the Black church as the point of intervention is based upon the awareness of the historical role of the church as advocate, encourager and enabler of actions needed for advancement in the community. Activities as varied as mutual aide societies, political action associations, health and human service committees, day care services, after-school tutoring and drama societies, have been housed in and sponsored by Black churches. The multiple roles played by the Black church were born of necessity, and endure because of the trust and faith that people invest in their pastors, lay leaders and fellow members (p. 11).

The intial results of this program have been promising enough to warrant continued funding by the American Heart Association, and have stimulated requests for participation by additional black churches. Community interventions offer an alternative approach to isolated decontextualized prescriptions that often become a series of broken promises, unattainable "oughts," or one more instance of joyless striving.

Scheper-Hughes and Lock (1987) note that the current culture has become "healthist" and body conscious, "the politically correct body for both sexes is the lean, strong, androgynous, and physically 'fit' form through which the core cultural values of autonomy, toughness, competitiveness, youth, and self-control are readily manifest." Health and "healthy body" have become hot consumer items. This popular press for the healthy body can increase healthy patterns of exercise, but it also brings in its wake obsessive concern over the appearance of the body and may contribute to disorders such as anorexia and bulimia (Scheper-Hughes and Lock 1987).

HEALTH AS A HUMAN POTENTIAL

Health as a basic resilience, an adaptive resource that is present whether one is ill or not, is another current view that is supported by health promotion theorists. It is based on the premise that all people, whatever their degree of health or illness and whatever their circumstances, have the potential for health. And health in this case is not simply a biological condition but also a mental and spiritual one.

This view of health is not limited to health promotion theorists but is also a prevalent lay concept of health (Williams 1983). It is similar to the popularized view that difficulty coping with "stress" causes disease (Lock and Dunk 1987). In this view, health is based on the ability to adapt. Dubos (1959) and Illich (1977), for example, think that the influence of medical science should be curtailed because it impedes people's ability to adapt on their own. Dubos argues that the ideal or utopian theory of health overlooks the human capacity to adapt and flourish in a wide range of circumstances. It is this adaptive capacity that he understands as health rather than a mythical static ideal state.

To a certain extent, general acceptance of this approach to health has been the result of shifting public perceptions of traditional medicine and the medical establishment. Certainly in the past two decades there has been a growing interest in nontraditional forms of intervention, with a resulting burgeoning of approaches to and kinds of diagnoses and therapies. These come under various headings of alternative medicine, holistic health, and "new age" healing (Levin and Coreil 1986). Because nursing has always drawn on its own tradition of healing through care, nursing has been able to develop and incorporate valuable therapeutic interventions derived from these different approaches, such as relaxation techniques (e.g., Bohachick 1984, Di-Motto 1984), visualization (e.g., Achterberg and Lawlis 1980, 1982; Donovan 1980; Gagan 1984) and therapeutic touch (e.g., Krieger 1979, Lionberger 1985).

The limitation of this approach is that its view of what health promotion is places the person in the position of always pursuing, but never attaining, health. The goal of health promotion in this approach is to tap the potential for health in everyone, nondiseased people as well as ill people. But the interest is always in the potential for health, never on an actual healthy condition.

> Health promotion is directed toward *increasing* the level of well-being and self-actualization of a given individual or group. Health promotion focuses on movement toward a positively valenced state of enhanced health and well-being (Pender 1987, p. 57).

In so attending to the "movement toward" health, the notion of a lived condition of health gets lost. Instead, an opposition is set up between the process of realizing a potential and a static condition of health. But since, in fact, people are never in a static condition, these theorists are placed in the position of maintaining that the only way of being healthy is by becoming healthy. The person is placed in the position of always becoming, of always realizing new potentials, only in order to go on realizing new potentials.

> Work for health will be concerned with encouraging normative and positive potentials because these potentials have the effect of opening up possibilities for achieving more potentials, whereas negative potentials reduce the number of possible potentials (Seedhouse 1986, p. 75).

In this view, the burden of health is on the individual. Family, community, work-related, or environmental aspects may facilitate or obstruct the realization of the potential for health, but the potential exists within the person. It is not a relational or meaning-related view of health. It is a personal quality that the person has, and as with all possessions (in our culture), it is the person's responsibility to use it. As a result, the health care provider has the job of eliciting the potential from the person, rather than potentiating a situation that would solicit the person to be healthy or helping the person to develop or reintegrate healthful understandings of the self or the situation. (See Mary Cucci's case study in Chapter Seven as an illustration of helping the person access meanings in order to move toward health.)

When health is seen as a personal possession for which the individual must take responsibility, the role of membership and belonging in a group as health enhancing is misinterpreted. Familial and community ties are not viewed as an integral part of the person's self-understanding but as external resources to be drawn upon. This is what allows some health promotion theorists to recommend developing social supports for the sake of one's health (e.g., Pender 1987). As we have pointed out before, the health-protective aspect of social support is found in the quality of the relationship developed *for its own sake*.

Finally, health viewed as an individual potential and an individual's responsibility weakens our possibilities for community action in the development of health policy. If we think of health as a potential each person must actualize, we are robbed of effective access to shape health policy on a group level, and we lose the perspective of our shared responsibility for the health of everyone in our community. For example, in the city of Oakland, California, children under the age of one year are fourteen times more likely to die before age one than children born to parents living in Piedmont, a wealthy community whose borders abut those of Oakland. This greater risk of mortality has been traced directly to low birth weight and prematurity. The incidence of both of these conditions can be considerably lessened by prenatal care and early intervention in at-risk pregnancies. These known epidemiological facts are useless to us as individuals taking responsibility for our own individual health potential. But as community members who understand that the health of one affects the well-being of all, the facts are highly salient. In this case, a local hospital was prevented from greatly increasing the number of beds in their high-risk obstetrical unit because they were in competition for funds that were going to support store-front prenatal clinics. The hospital was preparing to deal with the problem once the at-risk babies were born. The community action group of nurses and doctors wanted to lower the incidence of high-risk births.

MARK'S STORY FROM THE PERSPECTIVE OF THE FOUR THEORIES OF HEALTH

If we adopt the definition of health as an ideal state, we can say that from the day of his birth, Mark would never be considered healthy. When health is reified as an ideal, unattainable state, courage, strength, and even efforts toward health are not noticed as being "healthy." Under the definition of health as the ability to fulfill social roles, Mark would not be considered healthy because he never took up an independent, adult social role. Under the definition of health as a commodity, Mark would not be considered healthy, because there is no health commodity on earth at this time that could replace his deficits. And even if he could have obtained a cure for his cerebral palsy, would that have given him a sense of wholeness, of positive well-being, of belonging? Under the definition of health as a human potential, Mark would be considered healthy, but only at the point at which he joined the support group and began to "take responsibility for his health" by actively pursuing healthy endeavors such as exercise, making friends, and education. Before that point he would have been considered unhealthy because he was not realizing his potential.

We offer a fifth approach to health in the following section. We argue there that it is possible to think about health as a sense of coherence. From this perspective, it is possible to think of what was healthy in Mark's life, what provided a sense of coherence, and what contributed to breakdown. We can also see how the social group contributes to the health of its members. Part of Mark's health was due to the fact that under his own meanings (which were enabled by his family) he was not disabled. And part of his lack of health was due to societal stigma, which limited his access to a wider social world until his middle age.

HEALTH AS A SENSE OF COHERENCE

Antonovsky's (1979, 1987) view of health is closest to our notion of health because he emphasizes a sense of coherence that comes from belonging to a sociocultural group in which meanings are integrated and lived out as one's own concerns. Antonovsky (1979) defines coherence as:

> . . . a global orientation that expresses the extent to which one has a pervasive, enduring though dynamic feeling of confidence that one's internal and external environments are predictable and that there is a high probability that things will work out as well as can reasonably be expected (p. 10).

Antonovsky's position draws support from the classic research conducted by Durkheim in 1897 (1951). Durkheim found that suicide, although an individual act, is influenced by social context. He found that suicide rates were higher for unmarried than for married people, higher for Protestants than for Catholics, higher for soldiers than for civilians, higher for noncommissioned officers than for enlisted men, higher in times of peace than in times of war, and higher in times of both prosperity and recession than in times of economic stability. Durkheim concluded that the degree to which the individual was integrated into group life determined his or her propensity to commit suicide. Durkheim's methods have been criticized, but his findings have been supported by multiple studies linking social change and social disintegration to suicide as well as to morbidity and other causes of mortality (Antonovsky 1979). Durkheim's (1897, 1951) research is indirectly supported by the well-documented association between being married and longevity (Syme 1986).

Research by Kobasa (1979) and her colleagues (Kobasa, Maddi, and Courington 1981) supports Antonovsky's thesis about social integration and coherence. Kobasa and her colleagues found that the personality style they called "hardy" was more resistant to the impact of the strains presented by life events as measured by the Holmes and Rahe Schedule of Recent Life Events (1967). Kobasa defines hardiness as an interrelated composite of three personal characteristics: " (a) the belief that [people] can control or influence the events of their experience, (b) an ability to feel deeply involved in or committed to the activities of their lives, and (c) the anticipation of change as an exciting challenge to further development" (Kobasa 1979, p. 3).

In a prospective study, Kobasa et al. (1981) found that the personality disposition toward commitment, control, and challenge, (i.e., hardiness) functions as a health-promotion resource. Hardiness, they conclude, protects the individual from illness in the face of stressful life events even in spite of constitutional predisposition to illness. The subjects in this study were predominantly Protestant, white, male, married, and without close ethnic ties. The definition of hardiness can be understood as integrated, engaged participation in Protestant work ethic meanings (Benner 1984b). The hardy subjects experience a sense of coherence in Antonovsky's (1979) terms.

A phenomenological definition of health must incorporate being as well as becoming, must be based on an integrated view of mind/body/ spirit, and must be based on situated possibility rather than on the premise that radical freedom is possible. Since health, like disease, is commonly associated with objective physiological and psychological measures, we choose to use the term *well-being* because it reflects the lived experience of health, just as the term *illness* reflects the lived experience of disease. *Well-being is defined as congruence between one's possiblities and one's actual practices and lived meanings and is based on caring and feeling cared for.* This definition allows for the experience of challenge (positive stress, see Lazarus and Folkman 1984) and involvement even though the situation is difficult. The person is not understood as the rational calculator who stands outside situations and weighs whether or not the costs are worth the effort.

For example, caregiving as a nurse or as a family member is diffi-cult, but it is experienced as a challenge and as a meaningful living out of relational concern (see the discussion of this in Chapter Ten). Caregiving becomes threatening and experienced as a loss when one is unable to provide the care one wants to provide and when one's caregiving is devalued.[3]

In this view, well-being is contextual and relational. Well-being is the exercise and experience of situated possibility. Because well-being is fully embodied, the experience of possibility is not through some form of asceticism or denial of the body (mind over matter). Rather, well-being is a recovery of trust in the incredible powers of the body. Lewis Thomas captures this respect for the capabilities of the body/mind in his essay on autonomy:

> Our smooth-muscle cells are born with complete instructions, in need of no help from us, and they work away on their own schedules, modulating the lumen of blood vessels, moving things through intestines, opening and closing tubules according to the requirements of the entire system. Secre-tory cells elaborate their products in privacy; the heart contracts and relaxes; hormones are sent off to react silently with cell membranes, switching adenyl cyclase, prostaglandin, and other signals on and off; cells communicate with each other by simply touching; organelles send mes-sages to other organelles; all this goes on continually, without ever a personal word from us. When things are going well, as they generally are, it is an infallible mechanism.
>
> But now the autonomy of this interior domain, long regarded as inviolate, is open to question. The experimental psychologists have re-cently found that visceral organs can be taught to do various things, as easily as a boy learns to ride a bicycle, by the instrumental techniques of operant conditioning. . . .
>
> There is already talk of a breakthrough in the prevention and treat-ment of human disease. . . . If a rat can be trained to dilate the blood vessels of one of his ears more than those of the other, as has been reported, what rich experiences of self-control lie just ahead for man? . . .
>
> You can have it.
>
> Not to downgrade it. It is extremely important, I know, and one ought to feel elated by the prospect of taking personal charge, calling the shots, running one's cells around like toy trains. Now that we know that viscera can be taught, the thought comes naturally that we've been neglecting them all these years, and by judicious application of human

3. The Danish philosopher Sören Kierkegaard's description of aspects of human being relates to this view of health, and we refer the interested reader to Rubin (forthcoming).

intelligence these primitive structures can be trained to whatever standards of behavior we wish to set for them.

My trouble, to be quite candid, is a lack of confidence in myself. . . . Nothing would save me and my liver, if I were in charge. For I am, to face the facts squarely, considerably less intelligent than my liver. I am, moreover, constitutionally unable to make hepatic decisions, and I prefer not be obliged to, ever. . . .

On balance, however, I think it best to stay out of this business. Once you began, there would be no end to the responsibilities. I'd rather leave all my automatic functions with as much autonomy as they please, and hope for the best. Imagine having to worry about running leukocytes, keeping track, herding them here and there, listening for signals. After the first flush of pride in owernship, it would be exhausting and debilitating, and there would be no time for anything else. . . . instrumental conditioning of autonomic functions . . . trying to communicate with our internal environment, to meddle, . . . will consume so much of our energy that we will end up even more cut off from things outside, missing the main sources of the sensation of living (Thomas 1972, pp. 90–91).

Lewis Thomas points to the crisis in the control paradigm—that faithless position that seeks as much autonomy as possible and must control as much as possible to feel safe and secure. The problem with the control paradigm is that the premise of full autonomous control over one's destiny, including one's internal operations, is flawed. It overlooks the limits of autonomy and control.

Moving the quest from controlling outside events to controlling inside events does not sidestep the problem of the control paradigm. The quest for control is a never-ending, full-time, effortful job based on bad faith with oneself and one's world. Consequently, the stress-management strategies that hold out the remedy for helplessness and despair as a return of self-control overlook the root cause of the despair—the incoherence of the control paradigm. The background meanings for such a persistent quest for control is that the self and world are badly flawed and need extensive and constant management from the person. Such a position creates fear and distrust in oneself and in others. It is the view of the self as a competitor struggling to survive in spite of a hostile environment. In this technical world of control, one may gain control of one aspect of one's life and win victories, but the victories are always on the background of danger, the threat of loss of control. The *Challenger* disaster was so disquieting not just because of the tragic loss of the brave astronauts. It reminded everyone of the limits of control—of the faultiness of "O" rings. In our most controlled efforts, we confront the limits of control.

In an oppositional, dualistic view of the world, the opposite of control is understood as passivity and helplessness (see Whitbeck 1983). Healing and health may come with the restoration of the illusion of control, but a more coherent and resilient form of health and healing comes from restoring the sense that the world and body are trustworthy and capable. It is possible to trust ourselves and others without incurring crippling dependency or passivity.

The above stance does not preclude the ingenious use of visualization of white cells to attack infection or cancer, or other kinds of visualization that aim to enlist bodily capacities for healing (see Pelletier 1977). However, the metaphor for these exercises needs to be aligned with the powers of the mind/body to heal, and not aligned with the person's ability to control his or her internal environment. The charge to control the cells, a deliberative purely intentional view of the mind's control over the body, sets the person up for feelings of anxiety over the inability to control all of one's bodily operations at once. (Indeed, one does not have the competence to make "hepatic decisions.") Unwittingly, persons are given responsibility for directly controlling their cells, tissues, and organs. This intent to control sets the person up to feel helpless when the limits of control are met. But even more damaging, the "sick" person becomes fully responsible for his or her sickness and now must accept blame for it.

It is possible to alter and influence the internal milieu. One can lower blood pressure through visualization, exercise, relaxation, hypnosis, and coping with anger in new ways (Hartfield 1985). That possibility is based on embodied intelligence and the body's ability to dwell in meanings, not in a mechanical ability to "control" directly the functioning of cells. One cannot move directly from the purely intentional (conceptual level) to the cellular level. Although one can choose to alter, reframe, or move into new meanings and concerns, after this "executive" decision, the actual move is accomplished by the skilled body/mind capacity to dwell in meanings and concerns.

An example of moving from one set of meanings to another is provided by a young man who had received expert nursing care over three months. He returned to tell the nurses who had cared for him that their care had made a profound impact on his life. He entered with the understanding that life is a contract, a social exchange of goods and services, and that you get what you earn. But when he was helpless and had nothing to offer, these nurses had cared for him. This care had changed his understanding of himself and his world. He now lived in a world where it was safe even to be completely helpless and needy. He had no desire to return to the helpless needy place of his invalidism, but he relished his new sense of a more trustworthy, caring world (Benner 1984a). He could be more relaxed in such a world.

In biofeedback circles, faith and trust in the body are called "passive intent" or "passive control," because biofeedback trainers learned early that sheer willpower (e.g., "I *will* go to sleep, I *will* relax or gain peace of mind.") only made sleep and peace more inaccessible. Deliberate willful intents and actions only call attention to the absence of these states. The intent to relax sets up the awareness that one is not relaxed. A performance anxiety then begins, and relaxation eludes the person (Borysenko 1987).

The phenomenological view of the person as embodied offers a new interpretation of bodily skills, emotions, and stress reduction. The self as a collection of basic needs that must be met before higher needs are met (Maslow 1954) is countered by the view that "basic" needs are neither ultimate nor interpretation free (see Lee 1979). Instead, the self is viewed as getting its content and "needs" in relationship to others and to concrete projects. The self both constitutes and is constituted by relationship with others. Both the self and the world are coherent, meaningful, and resourceful. This affirmation does not mean that danger or evil do not exist in the world, it only affirms that possibility, meaning, and coherence also exist. We all participate in it to the extent we choose to, and we are enabled by our relationships and projects.

Nouwen (1986) tells of Jean Vanier's work with handicapped persons:

> Jean Vanier, who has lived for more than twenty years with mentally and physically handicapped people, has become a keen observer of this dynamic of fear [the fear that conjures either too much distance or too much closeness and prevents intimacy]. He saw that these severely handicapped people seem like strangers living in another world, like prisoners caught behind the bars of their own deformation, like sick people who cannot help themselves, like poor and helpless beggars who make no contribution to society. He saw how they evoke fear in the hearts of those who regard themselves as normal: the "regulars," the free, the healthy, the rich, and the successful. He saw how they remind us of another reality to be avoided at all cost.
>
> Jean Vanier realized that as long as these handicapped men and women remain "the others," they become the victims of cold institutions or of suffocating overprotection. He noticed how they are rejected as aliens or clung to as personal property. He understood that either way no

true home exists for them. Their otherness robs them of the free space where they can grow according to their own pace, their own rhythm, and their own, often hidden, gifts. . . .

When Jean Vanier speaks about that intimate place, he often stretches out his arm and cups his hand as if it holds a small, wounded bird. He asks: "What will happen if I open my hand fully?" We say: "The bird will try to flutter its wings, and it will fall and die." Then he asks again: "But what will happen if I close my hand?" We say: "The bird will be crushed and die." Then he smiles and says: "An intimate place is like my cupped hand, neither totally open nor totally closed. It is the space where growth can take place" (pp. 32 and 34).

Health as well-being comes when one engages in sound self-care, cares, and feels cared for—when one trusts the self, the body, and others. Breakdown occurs when that trust is broken. Well-being can be restored. The restoration, however, is not achieved through complete passivity; the young man who discovered the possibility of care had to be open to receive that care (see p. 163). Neither is restoration achieved through sheer autonomous effort. Well-being is relational and contextual; it cannot be viewed solely as an individual achievement, even though individuals have a large measure of choice. Individual choice is always situated in a peopled world.

Restoration and Health Promotion

Restoration and health promotion will be approached from five different vantage points. They are (a) the role of formal beliefs, deliberate choice, and planning in health, (b) the role of emotions, (c) the role of embodied intelligence, (d) the role of meanings and concerns, and (e) the role of the situation. As should be clear from the preceding chapters, these aspects are interrelated and influence each other. The divisions are made here only to facilitate analysis and explication.

FORMAL BELIEFS, DELIBERATE CHOICE, AND PLANNING

Formal beliefs about health, choosing health, and planning for health are powerful allies. They are the long-term change agents for health. Most health education is aimed at this level of functioning. For example, most Americans now have the formal belief that cigarette smoking is harmful. This formal belief has been shaped and changed slowly through much health education on many levels. Because it is now a formal and pervasive belief, the belief itself becomes a force for change and creates tension in our practices that contradict our formal belief. Syme (1986) points out that the cultural practices of continued advertising, easy access, and public acceptance belie our formal belief. Although these cultural practices support continued smoking, the belief in the harmfulness of smoking sets up a tension and creates a force for changing these practices.

Experiencing health as a choice is a powerful first step in making healthy choices, such as proper rest, nutrition, exercise, and recreation. Analytical capacities enable the person to reappraise the situation so that new alternatives are available. Insight therapy is based on this premise. The Health Belief Model (Hochbaum 1958, Kegeles et al. 1965, Rosenstock 1966) and Bandura's Self-Efficacy Model (1977) are examples of research conducted in the area of formal beliefs.

Self-evaluation of abilities, resources, strengths and weaknesses; monitoring and regulating impulses; and formulating realistic plans are essential for health and health promotion. Specific stress-reduction strategies can be counterproductive if they serve only to maintain a person in an unhealthy situation, e.g. overloaded with too many responsibilities or in a destructive relationship. Consequently, stress reduction must be approached with a clear understanding of the person's resources, demands, and constraints. Stress reduction can reduce the distress and facilitate the clear thinking and planning required for reorganizing and restructuring one's demands when no amount of "management" can solve the excessive or faulty demands.

Cognitive-behavioral therapy (Goldfried 1979; Holroyd, Appel, and Andrasik 1983; Lazarus and Folkman 1984; Schwartz 1982) is based upon the notion that the person's beliefs, cognitions, and self-talk are faulty and must be corrected to give the person new patterns of responding to situations. The stress-inoculation training outlined by Meichenbaum (1975, Meichenbaum and Cameron 1983) is a step-by-step preparation for stressful situations. In the education phase, the person is made aware of the ways distressing emotions are created; "self-talk" is examined and made explicit. In the rehearsal phase, alternative self-statements are provided and practiced so that they will be available in the distressing situation. In the application phase, the person practices and evaluates what he or she has learned.

Ellis's (1962, 1975) rational-emotive therapy, an early version of cognitive-behavioral therapy, is based on the changing of irrational beliefs. The person states them formally and then, by holding them up to rational consideration, changes them. An example of an irrational belief that is inherently stressful is: "It is essential to be liked by everyone." By holding up this irrational implicit belief to conscious scrutiny, the person is able to change it.

Beck's (1976) cognitive-behavior therapy takes an approach similar to that of Ellis (1975). Cognitive distortions include

1. *Selective abstraction*—the person focuses on the negative detail and criticism and ignores contradictory, more pertinent evidence.

2. *Arbitrary inference*—the person draws a negative conclusion with no evidence for the conclusion.

3. *Overgeneralization*—the person inappropriately applies the bad consequences of a particular event to other, dissimilar situations.

4. *Magnification*, also called "catastrofication" or "awfulizing" (Borysenko 1987)—the person imagines the worst or elaborates the consequences of an error or negative event.

5. *All or none thinking*—the person views things as all bad or all good or engages in extremely one-sided appraisals with little perspective.

We cannot cover all possible strategies for the use of formal beliefs in the choice of and deliberate planning for health. We selected these for discussion: information seeking, reframing, affirmation, and forgiveness. Time management and assertiveness are not discussed here because they are presented comprehensively elsewhere (Clark 1978, Smythe 1984).

INFORMATION-SEEKING. Information seeking is a major coping strategy especially in a fast-moving, highly technical society. New knowledge is generated daily about health hazards and health promotion. For example, the challenge of the AIDS epidemic is to mount health education efforts fast enough and in the most accessible ways to reach multiple ethnic groups, ages, and socioeconomic levels.

Each person needs access to this information to plan and respond to the challenges and to change. Health newsletters, television programs on health, and newspaper coverage about health are essential to health promotion. A central area of nursing research is health and patient education. Increasingly, nurses are taking a public role in popular presentations of health education in the media, in schools, and in the workplace.

From a phenomenological perspective, information cannot be restricted to oral or written language. Sensorimotor information is also central to coping and to health. Researchers (Johnson 1973, Johnson and Leventhal 1974, Leventhal and Nerenz 1983) have demonstrated that a rehearsal during which the person experiences sensory information matching the actual sounds and sensations experienced in threatening medical procedures decreases distress during the procedure. We posit that the information is grasped best when it is grasped directly by the body. Therefore, the actual perceptual experience of the sensation is the best rehearsal, and this experience gives one the best information about the procedure.

REFRAMING. Reframing a situation requires one to think about one's own current understanding of the situation. By reframing the situation, the person may open up new alternatives. A great deal of psychotherapy is based on the process of reframing. But reframing is also an everyday process. It occurs to the overburdened working mother that her children are no longer dependent toddlers but can help with household chores. The devastated mastectomy patient suddenly sees someone else who is much worse off than she.

Sometimes people can be guided to reframe a situation. At other times, reframing occurs without intent. For example, a man whose wife was an alcoholic reframed his situation one day in the process of being interviewed about daily stress and coping (Wrubel 1985). He was interviewed monthly for one year. During this year, he had very openly told the interviewer about his wife's drinking, but he had also told her that it was a secret he kept from other people. Finally, the interviewer asked him why it was a secret. She expected him to say that he felt ashamed, since he had quite frankly discussed such feelings before. Instead, he was completely speechless. By asking the question, she had reframed the situation for him. He suddenly saw that her drinking did not have to be a secret and that perhaps he was not helping her by keeping it a secret. This man was ripe for reframing because he loved his wife deeply and was always searching for ways to help her.

Humor may be used to reframe a situation. Stretching one's current definition to its extremes, too, may point up fallacies or alternatives. The art of negotiation depends on reframing. For example, when an interpersonal conflict is framed in win-lose terms, it is difficult to resolve. Reframing the situation into a win-win perspective opens up new alternatives. Reframing requires getting in touch with the meanings and concerns that are at stake in the situation. Often these concerns may be met better in other ways. Getting in touch with the concern that is challenged is the first step in reframing the situation.

AFFIRMATION. Positive statements that provide reassurance and encouragement can be chosen and systematically included in one's day (see Borysenko 1987). Affirmations are especially important in dislodging negative thoughts and negative self-talk. The person can become aware of negative scripts learned in childhood: "You don't try hard enough." "You're lazy." The person then deliberately replaces these with new scripts: "I care and I trust my efforts." "I choose not to try too hard, or too little, and I trust my choice." "Today, I have choices and possibilities."

FORGIVENESS. Forgiveness may be explored in both religious and secular contexts. In either context, forgiveness allows the person to let go and move on. Holding grudges is more harmful to the one who holds them than to the people he or she holds them against. Borysenko (1987) writes:

> See people for who they are instead of who you want them to be. Then accept them as they are rather than judging them for who they're not. The more accepting you become of yourself, the more you can see others in the same light (p. 211).

Merleau-Ponty (1962, see Chapter Three, p. 66) explains that some events can become organizing and thus eventually become the very atmosphere we breathe. They are no longer noticed because the way we take up the event becomes the lens through which we see the world. If the event was positive and continues to open up new possibilities, it was fortuitous. If the event was traumatic and closes down options, then therapy is needed to get back to the original event and relive it in new terms. In this way, it loses its privileged status of coloring and organizing perceptions. Guilt and resentment may become the atmosphere of our lives, and superficial statements about letting go and forgiving will not help unless we can somehow return to the original organizing experience and gain a new understanding of it.

THE ROLE OF EMOTIONS

Emotions in the modern Cartesian view of the self are often viewed as disruptive and antithetical to reason and judgment. We have claimed that the human capacity for reason depends on emotion because emotion (feelings) allows the person to dwell in the situation in a precognitive, nonreflective way (Collins 1985, Polanyi 1958). Feelings enable the person to live out meanings and concerns. Feelings create our bonds to the world and are the condition of our possibilities.

Formalism, which views the world as built up element by element in an explicit fashion, has no place for the power of feelings. Feelings have gotten "bad press" by being understood as a threat to rationality, control, and self-possession. But feelings enable us to transcend the limits of formalism (see Benner and Tanner 1987, Dreyfus 1979, Dreyfus and Dreyfus 1986) by giving us direct access to present situations as well as past events and future hopes.

Feelings, in the modern technological view, become a "thing" to be managed and controlled, one more commodity in an instrumental view of the self. Hochschild (1983) calls the understanding of feelings as commodities that must be used to produce services and sell goods the "managed heart." Hochschild paraphrases Rousseau's description of this utilitarian idea of emotion.

> In a social system animated by competition for property, the human personality was metamorphosed into a form of capital. Here it was rational to invest oneself only in properties that would produce the highest return. Personal feeling was a handicap since it distracted the individual from calculating his best interest and might pull him along economically counterproductive paths (p. 185).

The problem with this instrumental takeover of emotion is that one loses touch with the meaning and guidance provided by feelings. When people pretend to feel in ways that they do not as a way of managing themselves and others, their ability to understand and respond to their own and others' feelings diminishes. Estrangement and confusion ensue (Hochschild 1983). Acknowledgment of anger does not need to result in unwarranted action. Indeed, the acknowledgment may allow multiple pathways for expression and action.

By acknowledging and dwelling in the occasions and meanings of our feelings we can gain the skill to rehearse and return to positive feelings such as joy, pride, comfort, and contentment. As opposed to the instrumental approach of managing feelings, this skill makes it possible for us to be managed by our feelings. The experience of positive emotions can enable possibilities that cool calculation cannot. By remembering and reexperiencing positive feelings on new occasions, we are sometimes enabled to change our context or circumstances to ones that foster those feelings, see new possibilities for action in the unchanged circumstances, or simply experience pleasure and see things in a rosier light. This positive ability may provide a respite and offer perspective during a time of negative feelings such as fear or anxiety. This respite may be what one needs to face and understand the source of the negative feelings.

Moving out of an instrumental relationship to emotions allows the person to choose to dwell in feelings, thoughts, and actions that provide a sense of well-being. Negative emotions—when they are not denied or avoided but acknowledged and understood—can show the person what situations, relationships, and meanings cause fear, harm, and threat. Negative emotions such as fear, anger, and anxiety are all about something, or someone that may be current or from the past. Focusing on what the feeling is about—the content—and understanding what it points to allow for choice and growth.

Once again, if one adopts the instrumental control paradigm, the assumption is that a noninstrumental approach to feelings will yield blind passions and loss of freedom. The fear is that the person will be a slave to feelings. Although it is possible to become a slave to feelings (trapped or stuck in a particular way of feeling and perceiving a situation), an instrumental approach to feelings is not the only alternative. In fact, controlling feelings by ignoring, denying, or avoiding them may only give them more power. Acknowledging feelings and allowing them to guide understanding in the situation and the self open up the greatest possibility.

Once acknowledged, feelings are no longer a threat that must be coped with. Instead, they become a guide to a better understanding of the self and the situation. This is because feelings are not "contentless passions" but expressions of lived meanings. Understanding the lived meanings provides the greatest freedom in moving into new possibilities.

Exercises such as guided imagery, dream exploration, and hypnosis all provide a way of allowing feelings to instruct, heal, and create a sense of well-being.

GUIDED IMAGERY. Imagery allows people to imagine themselves in a different place. The imagery calls forth physical responses as the body responds to the visualized situation. Visualizing a place that produced happiness, peace, and comfort recreates emotional/bodily

171

responses similar to those felt in the original situation. Visual images have produced the following physiological changes in the laboratory: changes in heart rate (Green and Green 1977), changes in salivation (White 1978), changes in muscle firing (Luria 1968), and others.

Visualization of an athletic performance can often improve the performance. Visualizing a time of health and contentment can provide guidance and hope for the person who is ill and feeling depleted. Visualization engages bodily and emotional abilities because imagery may involve all sensory modalities, including visual, auditory, olfactory, tactile, and kinesthetic (Achterberg and Lawlis 1982).

Tape-recorded guided images may be developed for the person, using past real experiences that were satisfying and comforting. Tape recording them allows for repeated use and practice with the same event. Listening to the recording may become a ritualized return to a peaceful place.

DREAM EXPLORATION. Exploring dreams can give access to strong feelings that may be covered over or inaccessible during the waking hours. It is widely believed that dreams are a way of dealing with fears and other strong feelings. Borysenko (1987) tells of having clients in the Mind/Body Clinic at Harvard Medical School relive recurring dreams in a relaxed, awake state in order to recover the meanings and possibly reframe the dream.

HYPNOSIS. Hypnosis is best known for its uses in pain management and for achieving a healthful state of complete relaxation. However, hypnosis is also a simple and yet powerful way to access positive emotions. In a hypnotic trance the person can relive the experience of positive emotions like pride or joy, or mood states like confidence and well-being. Once the emotion or mood state is fully felt, the posthypnotic suggestion can be made that the person will continue to feel that positive feeling.

If repeated over time, this process becomes a way of learning about one's own emotions. It is a kind of emotional calisthenics by which the ability to experience positive emotions becomes stronger. Of course, this approach will not work when the emotion, e.g., loss and grief, is not appropriate to the person's understanding. But when a range of different emotional reactions is possible in the situation, the person can be enabled to experience the positive rather than the negative emotion.

Hypnosis has the added usefulness of being self-induced. After a certain amount of training, most people can hypnotize themselves and make their own suggestions.

THE SKILLED BODY AND THE ROLE OF EMBODIED INTELLIGENCE

In Chapters Two and Three it was pointed out that the body has the capacity to respond to meaningful situations. Meanings are actually taken up in our bodily postures and sets to action. For example, a pervasive set to act may be one of flight or retreat, or of relaxation and comfort. In sickness, the body may take up a posture of injury and threat that must be overcome for the restoration of health. The smooth functioning of the habitual body is lost in breakdown and illness, and a major strategy for restoration is the recovery of the habitual body. Placing the person in a situation where the habitual can be elicited may restore a sense of possibility or wellness. For example, an expert nurse had the family of a master piano teacher bring in a lap keyboard early in her convalescence from a stroke to rekindle meaningful embodied habits (Benner 1984a).

Eugene Gendlin (1978) conducted research on embodied intelligence, bodily know-how reflected in felt shifts in tension and feeling tones. He calls this therapeutic technique "focusing":

> When people change, they show it physically. At first this may not be outwardly noticeable, except in the momentary relaxation and easing of a body shift, the better circulation and deeper breathing. But over a longer period, with many shifts on different problems it is definitely noticeable in the face, the carriage, and the whole body. And it can be startling change (p. 27).

Gendlin's research is a good example that "knowing how"—an actual shift in the skilled body in posture, stance, set to act, and tension and attending to the feelings associated with bodily stances—can precede precise formulations of "knowing that"—intellectualized accounts and explanations.

It is possible to read the text of a bodily posture. Judith Ritchie, Ellerton, and Caty (1986) have done this with hospitalized children. Fear of injury and feelings of damage and vulnerability can lead to a "crouching posture," whereas confidence and a sense of strength can lead to fluid motions. Bodily movements may be careful, restrained, or constricted; they may be exaggerated and bold; or they may be natural and smooth. Enriching our descriptive powers of the bodily text could increase our powers of understanding the person's embodied experience of his or her illness.

If the person lives with anxiety and fear for long periods, the tensions of fear and anxiety will be taken up in bodily postures. This is why learning new bodily postures through relaxation exercises, yoga, stretching, walking, running, or swimming may open up new bodily meanings. By taking up new activities, the habitual body is being reinstructed to take a new stance in the world, a more fluid, relaxed, or confident stance. However, a deliberate reframing of the exercise may be required for the person not to carry the anxious, tense stance into the exercise. It is possible, after all, to be a tense, anxious runner. But new bodily stances, activities, and postures can open up new avenues for feelings and new aspects of one's world that may have been buried in postures of tension, fear, and anxiety. The runner may start out tense but, with the rhythm and concentration of the activity, acquire a new stance quite involuntarily or "naturally." Exercise, games, and sports are most beneficial when they are taken up as sources of leisure and enjoyment in their own right rather than as means to "be healthy" or "good." Therefore, the best choice of exercise is always one that can elicit passionate interest and absorption. The game or recreation is freed from an instrumental takeover and is experienced as enjoyable and good in its own right. If the interest is not there in the beginning, it might be developed with increased skill and facility.

Group sports or games set up a world that can provide involvement and engagement apart from outside concerns and distractions (Gadamer 1976). Consequently, participation in team sports may provide the benefit of exercise and sense of participation and community.

The following strategies are all used to promote healing, health, and well-being: breathing, progressive relaxation, massage, therapeutic touch, running, walking, dancing, yoga, martial arts that focus on body-mind coordination, and body therapies. We shall discuss a few of these below to illustrate their use in health promotion.

EXERCISE. According to a systematic review of the literature by Phelps (1987), physical exercise has been consistently associated with decreased risk of hypertension, increased self-esteem, decreased obesity, and decreased postmenopausal osteoporosis. Regular aerobic exercise has been associated with an independent effect in reducing cardiovascular risk. Excessive exercise regimens have been documented to be associated with risks of cardiac arrest, amenorrheic bone loss, and musculoskeletal trauma. Larson and Bruce (1987) summarize their assessment of the benefits and risks of exercise in an aging society as follows:

> In an aging society, preservation of function, postponement of chronic disease, and foreshortening of disability are important health goals. Functional aerobic capacity decreases with age and at relatively constant rates in populations. The rate of this decline is less for active than for sedentary persons. Consequently, "aging" as expressed in the declining functional cardiovascular limits of aerobic metabolism, may be slowed by regular exercise. The cardiovascular benefits of fitness depend not on vigorous training in youth but on habitual exercise. Furthermore the trainability of older men has been well demonstrated and also does not depend on having trained in youth. . . . We are unaware of any definitive evidence that exercise in moderation is more hazardous for the elderly. Risks are clearly associated with more intense exercise and are minimized by exercise of moderate intensity at 70-85% of maximal heart rate, a level that approximates the threshold of fatigue and tachypnea. Regular exercise for 20 to 30 minutes three to four times per week will produce a conditioning effect (p. 356).

The goal here is to choose a program that achieves an aerobic level of conditioning yet is interesting and fits in the person's weekly routine. The best of all worlds is to have the exercise become a source of pleasure and leisure rather than a mere prescription to stave off disease. Borgmann (1984) describes running and walking as focal practices that gather up meanings and rescue the person from the disengagement brought about by instant, convenient packaged approaches to "fitness" created by the separation of means and ends.

RUNNING AND WALKING. Running and walking have become national sports. Borgmann (1984) describes these two health-giving activities as a focal practice:

> Running is simply to move through time and space, step-by-step. But there is a splendor in that simplicity. In a car we move of course much faster, farther, and more comfortably. But we are not moving on our own power and in our own right. We cash in prior labor for present motion. . . . .What I am doing now, driving requires no effort, and little or no skill or discipline. I am a divided person; my achievement lies in the past, my enjoyment in the present. But in the runner, effort and joy are one; the split between means and ends, labor and leisure is healed. . . . This unity of achievement and enjoyment, of competence and consummation, is just one aspect of a central wholeness to which running restores us. Good

running engages mind and body. Here the mind is more than an intelligence that happens to be housed in a body. Rather the mind is the sensitivity and endurance of the body. Hence running in its fullness, as Sheehan (1978) stresses over and over again, is in principle different from exercise designed to procure physical health. The difference between running and physical exercise is strikingly exhibited in one and the same issue of *The New York Times Magazine*. It contains an account by Peter Wood of how, running the New York City Marathon, he took in the city with body and mind, and it has an account by Alexandra Penney of corporate fitness programs where executives, concerned about their Coronary Risk Factor Profile, run nowhere on treadmills or ride stationary bicycles. In another issue, the Magazine shows executives exercising their bodies while busying their dissociated minds with reading (pp. 202–203).

Borgmann's (1984) description of running recovers the exuberance and recreation in running. It is this kind of recovery that is needed for all exercise in order for the activity to be truly recreational to mind, body, and spirit.

THE ROLE OF MEANINGS AND CONCERNS

All meanings and concerns set up conditions of possibility, constraints, and blind spots. There is no perfect set of meanings and concerns that can protect the person from all threat, harm, and loss. Because meanings and concerns set up what coping options are available, there are limits to the coping strategies that are available for anyone. However, by shifting meanings, reinterpreting situations, or taking on new concerns, new coping possibilities can be made available.

Some meanings and concerns may be incoherent, conflicted, or inherently stressful. The coping possibilities in such cases are likewise constricted. The solution to the distress, conflict, threat, or harm caused by inherently stressful meanings is not to detach oneself from meanings and concerns. Rather, it is to examine the source of the conflicts in one's meanings and concerns. One needs always to work within the person's meanings, because the position most bereft of coping options is meaninglessness or anomie. As Benner (1984b) notes:

> When meaning breaks down, coping can no longer be anchored in compelling preferences; therefore, people are confused and in conflict about what they want in any given situation. Problem solving no longer makes sense because they are not sure what the problem is, nor what constitutes

an adequate solution. When people experience pervasive meaningless-ness in their lives, stress is also pervasive. Furthermore, coping options are not readily apparent because all options seem equally plausible (p. 180).

Although stress-reduction strategies aimed at increasing distance and control will not address a sense of meaninglessness and incoher-ence, they may provide the distance and respite needed to regroup and gain a new perspective on one's situation. It is possible to become so focused on one's projects that there is little awareness of the personal toll. The person may actually have meanings and coping strategies that produce or escalate tensions.

As an illustration of the way meanings can shape an unhealthful life, we use the example of a highly successful salesman who participated in a year-long study of work stress (Benner 1984b). This man demon-strates that he acts on the basis of the efficacy of worry.

He believes that goal achievement requires an "all out effort." Therefore he tends to exaggerate the importance of events in order to ensure his "best" effort. Consequently a sales meeting receives the same level of attention and anxiety as trying to make his biggest sale of the year. He spends time psyching himself up, building up all the reasons that "a lot is resting" on the particular test in question. For example, in the eighth month of the study he states: "Well, you always have a certain amount of apprehension. It's like if you are being invited to the White House, same idea. Because these are the people that make or break your future as far as the product is concerned." . . .

He talks about the efficacy of worry for doing well at a sales meeting despite the fact that he has been top salesman for the past two years:

Interviewer: Do you feel like you did a good job?

Sure, and maybe that is what is necessary—getting all those emo-tions stirred up in order to do a good job.

Interviewer: To mobilize your . . .?

To psych yourself up.

Interviewer: You were quite alert, I take it.

You can count on that.

Interviewer: How would others feel in the same situation?

I imagine that a good many of them felt exactly as I did. I don't know of a single person that looks forward in anticipation to a sales meeting. Because they are downers and that is exactly contrary to what they are trying to do. They are trying to psych you up (pp. 78–79).

This is a good example of an instrumental stance toward emotions that has become stylized rather than flexible and attuned to the situation. There is wisdom in going with feelings, admitting the "worry," and using the adrenaline to increase alertness and thus probably improve performance. For instance, sports trainers have begun to recognize that attempts to "relax" and not be anxious before a performance may only make the person more anxious. If athletes cannot control their anxiety, they may come to fear their anxiety and thus increase it. But the salesman whose case is presented above has begun to create anxiety in order to get a performance effect, even when performance may not even be salient or important. He so associates success with anxiety that anxiety is a sought-after state.

This case illustrates how meanings shape how one is in the situation and what options are available and possible for that person. It also illustrates a central challenge for the health care provider whose interest is health promotion. This man's meanings work for him in that the way he is in the situation makes him good at his work as a salesman. Since he is successful at his job, and since the experience of anxiety is laden with the meaning of that success, he has no reason to call those meanings into question. And yet, we have reason to believe that this style of chronic tension is unhealthful. It is unhealthful in itself in that it has become a rigid way of responding to situations. This rigidity increases the chances of breakdown of meaning with concomitant depression and alienation when a slightly different situation arises that does not yield to this way of being. And it is unhealthful in that it increases the chance of physical illness. And being seriously ill is definitely a situation that does not work for someone with this set of meanings.

Given these possible outcomes for this man, what options are available for the health care provider whose aim is health promotion and not just health prevention? This is an extremely difficult question, and one with which health promotion workers struggle daily. There is no simple answer. But since this man did not invent these meanings himself but took them up from the culture in which he lives, one tactic is clearly to work within the culture, and particularly the subculture that promotes the meaning—the workplace. Programs already exist to encourage healthful habits of exercise and diet among workers. Using the meanings of the people in the workplace to help them understand those meanings and their accompanying emotions would be an important added step toward promoting health.

The man discussed above had meanings that are possibly common to people who work in high-pressure sales jobs. His meanings may not be held by many outside that line of work. But there are other cultural meanings that appear to be more general for our culture and have an impact on our health. The instrumental approach to leisure as an antitdote to work stress for the person caught up with overwork is an example of a meaning that can create tensions of its own. As Kerr (1962) points out:

> It is probable that our very awareness of the existence of pleasures that we are either postponing or denying ourselves adds to the tensions induced by unrelieved labor. We feel guilty when we take our pleasure, because there is so much work we might do. We feel guilty when we work so hard, because our lives may depend upon pausing for pleasure. The two guilts are incompatible (p. 41).

The dilemma of incompatible guilts is created by the devaluation of leisure for its own sake. Leisure has become a tool for "health," and the person does not even have the sense that leisure may improve the quality of work. Incoherent and incompatible meanings and concerns as demonstrated above can set up chronic tension and fatigue. An understanding of the meanings and concerns, however, can give the health care provider access to ways to help the person change. Strategies such as consciousness raising, counseling, insight therapy, logotherapy, and religious practices are commonly used to point up and change personal meanings and to create new concerns or reshape old ones.

CONSCIOUSNESS-RAISING. This approach to changing personal meanings has the value of progressing just as fast and as far as the individual can or wants to go. Consciousness raising often occurs in groups devoted to a certain arena of concern, but it can also happen in other contexts, as in a family, in the workplace, or just between friends. The prerequisite for consciousness raising is some sense, however small, that things are not going well. This is the breakdown in background meaning that allows it to be reflected upon. Once one part of background meaning becomes an object of reflection in one situation, it then begins to show up as an object of reflection in other situations.

Yankelovich (1981) provides an example of the consequences of changes in background meanings due to consciousness raising. He reminisces about the interviews and surveys he did in the 1950s. He remembers that most women found questions about why they wanted to get married and have children meaningless and unanswerable. One young woman answered, "Why do you put your pants on in the morning? Why do you walk on two feet instead of one?" (Yankelovich 1981, p.97). That these same questions now make sense is a testament to the power of consciousness raising.

In nursing there has been a similar consciousness raising about "the doctor-nurse game" (Stein 1968). In the past, nurses couched their medical diagnoses in "objective" descriptive language of signs and symptoms. This was to be interpreted by the physician so that the legitimized medical diagnoses could be made. Although this interactional pattern is breaking down due to consciousness raising, there are still subtle and not so subtle remnants. For example, although nurses may now state their opinions in direct terms, physicians may discount or ignore nurses' observations or at least not give them equal weight as the same comments made by other physicians (see Benner 1987).

Consciousness raising works because the largest portion of the person's assumptions remain unchallenged. These unchallenged assumptions and background meanings allow the areas of one's life unaffected by the consciousness raising efforts to continue to function smoothly.

INSIGHT THERAPY. Sometimes meanings become so incoherent as to render the person incapable of living in an interpretable world. And sometimes meanings become so rigidly tied to a past experience or experiences that the person cannot see any new ways of understanding current experience. Insight therapy is useful in these conditions for bringing the person and personal meanings together into a possible present existence that offers options for concerns, actions, and feelings.

RELIGIOUS PRACTICES. Religion is itself a major source of personal meaning in our culture. Religious practices provide traditional forms of reflection on meaning; this reflection can allow for meaning changes or shifts. Devotional practices such as prayer, meditation, and scriptural study are all ways to show up and reflect on meanings. For example, Catholics who say the rosary with focused attention are engaging in a form of meditation that will cause the relaxation response (Borysenko 1987). When meaning breaks down in any part of life, religious practices, if they are part of one's everyday life, can be either reaffirming of old understanding or a source of new understanding. Here, the particularity of one's own religious practices are central. One simply cannot appropriate meanings that are not available to him or her.

THE ROLE OF THE SITUATION

It should be clear by this point that when we speak of situation we are not talking about an environment. An environment is an objectified setting. It can be described in terms of its elements. It may be peopled or not. It is not described in terms of meaning for the person. A situation is what the person inhabits. It is a social world, even if there are no other people present at the time the situation is described. For example, farm workers handling strong pesticides or residents of Love Canal are in a situation because a situation creates constraints of a social order that cannot be understood in environmental terms. It is not simply that the people in these two situations have been exposed to dangerous chemicals (the environmental element). Rather, they are politically, socially, and economically constrained to work with the chemicals (in the case of the farm workers) or prevented from moving away from them (in the case of the Love Canal residents). This fact creates a lived situation, with its concomitant options and possibilities.

People tend to overlook situations and situatedness in our psychological age. The individual is often regarded as the sole source of meaning. Generally a situation is brought in as an object for us to notice, not as a source of meaning, of possibility, or of limit to possibility.

The person is always situated, and the situation both influences and is influenced by the person. For example, the particular coping patterns for tension relief, achievement, and communication that develop in a workplace shape the coping options available for the individual workers. A registry nurse once described her pleasure in being called in to work on one particular unit because the morale was high, the skill levels were advanced, and nurse-doctor tensions were kept creatively in balance. Most people can recall childhood memories of visiting another family that contrasted either positively or negatively with one's own. Perhaps a friend's family seemed to live in a lively jumble of projects and interesting things when one's own family setting was rigidly neat and tidy. Or perhaps another family seemed serene and orderly when one's own was noisy and chaotic. These are situations, and each one offers different possibilities to different people.

The psychoanalytic view of emotions does not accommodate the role of the situation on the person because the person is taken back to the "root" cause in early conflicts (Rorty 1980). Although it may be essential to understand what situations are "loaded" because of personal history, it is equally important to understand the current situation. There are limits to individualistic views of coping, since one's coping options are influenced by group coping patterns, whether of a work group, family, or friends. Thus, the role the situation plays in health is an essential point of departure.

There are various ways to approach the situation to understand its effect. Some useful questions include: What are the situational pulls? What are the coping patterns used by the group? Are the coping patterns used by the group compatible with the individual's preferences? How is the situation defined by the group? Is that definition compatible with the individual's definition?

ASSEMBLING THE ASPECTS: HEALTH PROMOTION AND THE WHOLE PERSON

The person's sense of coherence is crucial to a comprehensive understanding of changing to more healthy lifestyles, making a recovery, undergoing rehabilitation, or coping with major life transitions when the person's world has been radically altered. This sense of coherence includes the whole person—mind, body, personal meanings, concerns, and social context. In the case of changing unhealthy lifestyles, the person must take up new patterns and skills as well as new concerns and meanings. But this change, if successful, usually cannot just be a layering on of new habits and skills. Old ones must be altered and dropped. A reorganization of one's life must take place, and all of this change must take place in the context of many social relationships and well-established work and social patterns.

A deliberate and planned change of health habits in the presence of little social support is extremely difficult because both personal change *and* situational change are required. When a drastic, world-changing alteration occurs, the situation is already altered and the person is solicited to change by the altered situation. The person is left with remnants—concerns, habits, and patterns that are no longer relevant to the changed situation. However, the person can encounter these alterations only as they come up in practical circumstances. The change is encountered in situations where the old habits, assumptions, skills, and customs no longer work or are no longer relevant.

Cognitive-behavioral therapies empirically have been demonstrated to be more effective than either cognitive or behavioral therapy alone (Holroyd, Appel, and Andrasik 1983). The phenomenologist would explain that the combined approach has the advantage of focusing on thinking habits and embodied stylistic patterns. The behavioral approach adds new skills and habits, and the cognitive approach addresses the need for new self-interpretations. Altered self-interpretations, altered behaviors, and altered situations are more powerful in soliciting the ontological capacity to move from former meanings to new ones. However, the phenomenologist would add that a thorough exploration of the person's existing concerns, habits, and skills is needed to understand the predictable issues and barriers to change, along with potential strengths and possibilities offered by the currently held perspectives. This interpretive step assists the person to bridge the gap from past possibilities, concerns, and issues to new ones. Past possibilities and strengths are considered and emphasized because the person has access to the new situation in terms of past meanings, concerns, and skills.

For example, a widow may come to understand survival, with all its grief and loneliness, as a tribute to the past relationship. She may come to feel grateful that the spouse is spared the lonely aftermath of loss, and she may take up new commitments and projects in a way that provides some continuity with the past world (Frankl 1963, Rubin, forthcoming). But such perspectives can come only with time, as through grief work, the person takes in the loss and change and encounters new situations. Helping relationships are guided by the stage of the grief and the issues encountered by the grieving person. It is common to find a change in posture and embodiment as the person takes up new ways of being in the world as a result of a major life change. Bodily orientation and perceptions actually change with ways of being in the world (Gendlin 1978).

In sum, we can say that a view of health based on a phenomenological approach offers the health care provider a wide range of possible interventions. Since the person is an integrated being, change in any one area will bring about a change in others. It is a truism, but not one to be taken lightly, that a change in how one thinks about something or in one's understanding will affect how one feels. Or to use the language of this chapter, a change in formal beliefs or in personal meanings will affect emotions. Likewise, a shift in emotional outlook opens new ways of thinking about things. Emotions also affect body tone and bodily expressiveness. And the reverse is also true; changes in bodily states

183

affect emotions. The role of the situation should not be overlooked, since changes in situation also affect all of these aspects.

The integrated nature of human beings is a tremendous advantage to a health care provider whose main concern is health promotion. There is, of course, no ready formula for which intervention to use when since this view of health is not a medicalized one. But an awareness of the person's understanding and the person's own way of being in the world can give the health care provider clues to which kind of intervention would fit with that person's meanings. The health care provider does not necessarily have to introduce a comprehensive plan that involves major life changes all at once. Such changes are effortful and difficult to maintain anyway. But knowing that a change in one aspect will affect all the others gives the health care provider an advantage. It is much easier to bring about a permanent change in one area at a time than it is to change many areas at once.

The Assessment of Coping

Health promotion is a broad field and encompasses many possible areas of help and intervention. The aim of the chapter so far has been to provide a phenomenological perspective of health promotion by discussing health under the various aspects of the person. Now we turn to an area of particular interest to health care providers, that of assessing coping.

CARTESIANISM AND THE ASSESSMENT OF COPING

If health care providers are to make assessments of the need for intervention in stressful situations and judgments about what intervention would best help a person, they need to know the effects of different coping choices in the lives of people. But this aspect of the field of stress and coping, like all other aspects, has been affected by Cartesianism.

The practice of science since the seventeenth century has consisted of unitizing and generalizing (Guignon 1983). The major strategy for gaining "truth" has been objectification through decontextualization. Unfortunately, this single-minded strategy, although successful in many arenas where content is not so important, fails in circumstances where content shapes the event. Decontextualized accounts cannot adequately address human action because the relationship of the person *in* the situation and the *content* of the situation are overlooked. This perspective is echoed by Evelyn Fox Keller (1985):

> My argument is not simply that the dream of a completely objective science is in principle unrealizable, but that it contains precisely what it rejects: the vivid traces of a reflected self image. The objectivist illusion reflects back an image of self as autonomous and objectified: an image of individuals unto themselves, severed from the outside world of other objects (animate as well as inanimate) and simultaneously from their own subjectivity. It is the investment in impersonality, the claim to have escaped the influence of desires, wishes, and beliefs—perhaps even more than the sense of actual accomplishment—that constitutes the special arrogance, even bravura, of modern man, and at the same time reveals his peculiar subjectivity (p. 70).

The goal of Heideggerian phenomenology is to overcome the subjective-objective opposition. The person is no longer viewed as private subject, and objectivity is no longer viewed as the decontextual and the general. Consensus becomes the basis for validating findings.

Haan's (1977) hierarchical model of coping is an example of a purely Cartesian approach. Haan's coping model cannot be used to evaluate coping in relationship to the situation because the model determines from the start what good coping is, regardless of the situation. "Good coping" is defined just as thinking and action that match "reality" regardless of how the person weathers or alters the circumstance. When the person's apprehension distorts reality, his or her activity is called a defense or, worse yet, fragmentation. For example, Haan describes the generic process of selective awareness as concentration when it is coping, denial when it is defensive, and distraction and fixation when it is fragmentation. In the Haan model, the effect or the outcome of the activity is irrelevant. All coping is good, because reality is not distorted. All defenses are bad, because reality is distorted.

In this view, emotion has no content on its own and is defined as an "interruption" or force that must be diverted, restrained, or transformed. This view of emotion as a contentless signal and interruption is held by psychodynamic and cognitive theorists. The definitions are abstract, general, and given without consideration for the situation and the way the person is in the situation.

Another approach, which is not so clearly Cartesian in its explanation, views whatever works as coping and whatever does not work as not coping (for an example of this approach, see Pearlin and Schooler 1978). This approach to what coping is matches the popular, cultural ideas of coping. For example, when situations are felt to be overwhelming and dealing with them is beyond individuals' resources, people say, "I can't cope!" This view reflects our cultural background meaning of instrumentality that imbues much of our self-understanding with the sense that we can and must control ourselves and our life situations. This cultural meaning does not allow for the common life experience of situations that are beyond remedy. These are the situations that no human action can change, situations in which coping possibilities are limited to whether or how people can experience their despair, grief, distress, sorrow, resentment, rage, anger, or frustration. And yet, in spite of the popular view, these various experiences of emotion are ways of coping too, because they are ways of interpreting and integrating (or reinterpreting and reintegrating) an understanding of the situation.

An attempt has been made by some working in the field to break away from the good coping/bad coping approach by distinguishing between coping activity and coping effectiveness (Lazarus and Folkman 1984, Wrubel, Benner, and Lazarus 1981). This distinction allows the researcher to describe everything the person does in stressful circumstances and then note what effect those activities had. However, even this distinction does not fully break away from the Cartesian-based view of what it is to be a person, because the assessment of coping effectiveness still typically is based on an ahistorical, decontextualized view of the individual that has produced in all the helping professions a pathological view of the person.

THE PATHOLOGY MODEL OF COPING

In the pathological view, coping activity is judged to be effective or ineffective, coping or defensive, coping or not coping, and so on. Whatever the terms used, there is always a dichotomy of good and bad. The assumption is that an objective reality exists and that someone outside the situation (e.g., the researcher who studies coping) has a clearer view that allows for the right/wrong judgment to be made. But the right/wrong judgment denies the personal meanings that might make the person's actions *right* for him or her even if they are not *good* for him or her.

In so rejecting and misunderstanding personal meanings, the pathological approach limits the possibility of helping, because meanings are what make sense of what the person is doing. They may not work to get the person well, but that does not mean that they are not working in another way for the person. This approach is negatively reductionistic because it reduces the person to a label. It cuts the helper off from possible ways of helping and the person off from his or her possibilities. One cannot, just because one is ill, develop a whole new set of conditions for possibility. For health care providers to condemn an ill person's coping as wrong and uphold their understanding of the illness and of the cure as right limits both their understanding of what is going on and their ability to help. Personal meanings determine what coping options are available to the person, but they do not prohibit possibility. If helpers can become attuned to the patient's personal meanings, they can recognize the patient's conditions for possibility. Sometimes they can help create new conditions for possibility by interpreting, coaching, and training the patient to acquire new skills, or by simply caring about the patient.

The pathological model puts helpers in a superior position and those they help in an inferior position. To be helped or be in need of help means that one is incompetent, wrong, hapless, helpless, or stupid. For example, the hypertensive man who takes his medicine only when he thinks his blood pressure is elevated would be judged as noncompliant under the pathological approach. That is a limiting, one-dimensional view of the person. It leaves no room for understanding the meaning of the illness for the man, his experience of taking the medication or the meaning of being on medication, or the meaning of being a patient.

For example, an eighty-seven-year-old woman was hospitalized briefly after a minor stroke. Upon being interviewed, she said she was taking her hypertensive medication only when she "felt she needed it." She had been observing this practice for some years in spite of several lectures from her physician on the necessity of compliance. The woman lived alone, although she had children who offered to share their homes with her. She valued her independence above all else, and her greatest concern was not dying, but becoming either physically or mentally incompetent and thus unable to care for herself. Taking her hypertensive medication was interpreted in the light of this concern. When she took her medication, she often felt dizzy, uncertain on her feet, and very slowed down. She felt that she could not care for herself when she felt like this and that she might fall and break her hip and end up in a nursing home. When she did not take her medication, she felt much more energetic and functional. But she was concerned that she might have a debilitating stroke and would not die. Laboratory studies showed that she was not metabolizing her medications and that she was in a near toxic state. A decision was made to take her off all medications, and, in her words, "let nature take its course."

Thus, the pathological approach produces categories and labels for patients that limit the health care providers' understanding and shut down possibilities for interventions. And in so categorizing and labeling, the pathological model puts out of consideration the temporality that is so essentially human, because an avoidance of personal meanings is a denial of the individual's history. In the instance cited above, what was labeled as noncompliance was actually the patient's lived understanding of herself. She had been independent her entire life, beginning at age eight, when she worked in a fruit-packing plant to help support her widowed mother. She could not at age eighty-seven envision ending her life physically or mentally incompetent.

The Cartesian, pathological approach is at base an objectification of the person. The objective stance is what affords the view of an individual as other, as an objectified presence to be judged, rated, or evaluated. But personal background meanings and shared cultural understandings cannot be understood as objects; they must interpreted as they are lived out in a life.

In the Cartesian-pathological view of the person, there is no room for personal meaning except as private and idiosyncratic. Thus, its description of the coping process is not an account of how meaning works; it is devoid of any specific content of how meaning is lived out in life. In approaches to coping that reflect this pathological view of the person, the coping process has become an abstract, generalized account of life situations. Diagnostic models that focus on deficits fall into the pathology model. This is particularly evident in the nursing diagnostic label "ineffective coping."

A PHENOMENOLOGICAL APPROACH TO THE ASSESSMENT OF COPING

The phenomenological alternative to the pathological approach can be demonstrated using examples drawn from a study of personal background meanings and interpersonal concerns (Wrubel 1985). Here, we illustrate the role of personal concern in defining the meaning of illness and in delimiting the range of coping. In these two cases, the ill person was a family member.

In the first case, a middle-aged woman's interpersonal concern was described as "engaged care." In one interview, she describes the time when her son suffered a severe concussion in a skateboarding accident. He was cared for at home, and for several days there was the possibility that he might require surgery to relieve pressure on the brain. He could not bear the slightest sound or the faintest light. She covered the bedroom windows with blankets, and she, her two other children, and her husband tip-toed around and whispered. She attended to him almost constantly, taking minimal time out to care for the other family members. He recovered without requiring surgery.

In the second case, another middle-aged woman's interpersonal concern was described as "self-care in balance with care for others." She had a very demanding husband who allowed her little time for her own pursuits. When he had to cancel a business trip because of an illness, she was concerned about his health, but she was equally upset about canceling the plans she had made for herself.

Interpersonal concern, that is, the concern that defined how the family member mattered to each woman, affected how the situation was understood by each one and what was to be done. (It should be noted that situational aspects themselves contributed to their understanding, since the illness in the first case was more serious.) In the first case, the concern of engaged care ruled out the possibility of concern about the self. What the second woman understood as stressful the first understood as coping. Canceling plans was not a disappointment but a way of feeling she was doing all she could for her son by staying with him.

We need to acknowledge that there are culturally preferred ways of being in the world. In our culture we admire the person who has an interpersonal concern of engaged care. Magazines report and television programs dramatize true-life accounts of people who care for others in this way. But we must not confuse culturally preferred ways of being in the world with morally right ways of being in the world. The second woman took excellent care of her husband during his illness. Being concerned for herself did not mean that she was not also concerned for her husband.

We have a long tradition of idealism handed down from fifth-century B.C. Greece. In this tradition, the ideal is an abstract and eternal idea of the perfect good. All things in the temporal world are measured against the ideal. In this way, all things are measured on a single continuum and are placed on the continuum according to their deficiencies.

The phenomenological approach to stress and coping is not a

deficit view. In this approach, it is important to understand the meanings at work for people in their own terms: how they experience their concerns and what options those concerns open up or close off. Once the individual's possibilities are understood in their own terms, it is possible to make an evaluation. But this is not the same as setting up a criterion first. The deficit view would rate the second woman in a quantitative way as less committed to her husband than the first woman was to her son. But greater understanding of her life and her coping was gained by seeing her not as less committed than the first woman, but as concerned in a different way.

If health care providers are to understand when and where interventions are needed, they must first understand a person's meanings in that person's own terms. In a deficit approach, the second woman might be judged not involved enough with her husband, or not involved in the right way. But also, in the deficit approach, the first woman's need for help might be overlooked. Since we typically admire people with engaged care and describe them as "brave," "strong," and "selfless," we often overlook the fact that the lived experience of engaged care is not that one is being selfless but that one is doing the only thing possible. No other options show up for this person. When such a person has cared for a terminally ill person, feelings of guilt that she or he has not done enough arise. Reassurances, especially from health care professionals, that all that could have been done was done, can alleviate much distress. Chesla (1988), using Wrubel's (1985) definition of interpersonal concerns, has identified four different forms of interpersonal concerns in family coping with caring for a schizophrenic member: engaged care; self-care in tension with the care of the other; concern as specialized management; and care from a distance. Each form of care sets up its own possibilities and coping options and precludes others. Chesla (1988) effectively demonstrates that understanding family coping from the perspective of the families' interpersonal concerns offers a better understanding and more options for assisting the family than a deficit or pathological perspective and provides validation and extension of the theoretical perspective taken in this book.

REFERENCES

Achterberg J, Lawlis GF: *Bridges of the Body-Mind: Behavioral Approaches to Health Care.* Champaign, Ill.: Institute for Personality and Ability Testing, 1980.

Achterberg J, Lawlis F: Imagery and health intervention. Topics Clin Nurs 3(4):55, 1982.

Antonovsky A: *Unraveling the Mystery of Health, How People Manage Stress and Stay Well.* San Francisco: Jossey-Bass, 1987.

Antonovsky A: *Health, Stress and Coping.* San Francisco: Jossey-Bass, 1979.

Antonovsky A: Social class, life expectancy, and overall mortality. Milbank Memorial Fund Q 45:31, 1967.

Bandura A: Self-efficacy: Toward a unifying theory of behavioral change. Psychol Rev 84:191, 1977.

Beck AT: *Cognitive Therapy and the Emotional Disorders.* New York: International Universities Press, 1976.

Benner P: *From Novice to Expert, Excellence and Power in Clinical Nursing Practice.* Menlo Park, Calif.: Addison-Wesley, 1984a.

Benner P: *Stress and Satisfaction on the Job: Work Meanings and Coping of Mid-Career Men. New* York: Praeger Scientific Press, 1984b.

Benner P: A dialogue with excellence. Am J Nurs 87:1556 (in press).

Benner P, Tanner C: Clinical judgment: How expert nurses use intuition. Am J Nurs 87:23, 1987.

Berkman L, Syme SL: Social networks, host resistance, and mortality: A nine year follow-up study of Alameda County residents. Amer J of Epidem 94:105, 1979.

Bloom A: *The Closing of the American Mind.* New York: Simon & Schuster, 1987.

Bohachick P: Progressive relaxation training in cardiac rehabilitation: Effect on psychologic variables. Nurs Res 33:283, 1984.

Borgmann A: *Technology and the Character of Contempory Life.* Chicago: University of Chicago Press, 1984.

Borysenko J, with Rothstein L: *Minding the Body, Mending the Mind.* Reading, Mass: Addison-Wesley, 1987.

Chesla CA: Parents' Caring Practices and Coping with Schizophrenic Offspring, An Interpretive Study. Unpublished doctoral dissertation, University of California, San Francisco, 1988.

Clark CC: *Assertive Skills for Nurses.* New York: Contemporary Pub. Co., 1978.

Cobb, S: Social support as a moderator of life stress. Psychosom Med 38:300, 1976.

Collins CE: *The Last Dogma of Empircism.* Unpublished doctoral dissertation, University of California at Berkeley, 1985.

DiMotto JW: Relaxation. Am J of Nurs 84:754, 1984.

Donovan MI: Relaxation with guided imagery: A useful technique. Cancer Nurs 3:27, 1980.

Dreyfus H: *Being-in-the-World: A Commentary on Heidegger's Being and Time, Division I.* Cambridge, Mass.: MIT Press, in press.

Dreyfus HL: *What Computers Can't Do. The Limits of Artificial Intelligence.* rev. ed. New York: Harper & Row, 1979.

Dreyfus HL, Dreyfus SE, with Athanasiou T: *Mind Over Machine: The Power of Human Intuition and Expertise in the Era of the Computer.* New York: The Free Press, 1986.

Dubos R: *The Mirage of Health.* New York: Harper & Row, 1959.

Durkheim E: *Suicide: A Study in Sociology.* Spaulding JA, Simpson G (trans). New York: The Free Press, 1951. Originally published 1897.

Ellis A: *How to Live with a "Neurotic" at Home and at Work.* New York: Crowne, 1975.

Ellis A: *Reason and Emotion in Psychotherapy.* New York: Lyle Stuart, 1962.

Foucault M: *The Birth of the Clinic.* Sheridan Smith AM (trans) London: Tavistock, 1973.

Frankl V: *Man's Search for Meaning.* New York: Washington Square Press. 1963.

Gadamer H-G: *Truth and Method*. Barden G, Cumming J (eds and trans). New York: Seabury, 1976.

Gagan JM: Imagery: An overview with suggested application for nursing. Perspect Psychiatr Care, 22:20, 1984.

Gendlin ET: *Focusing*. New York: Bantam Books, 1978.

Goldfried MR: Anxiety reduction through cognitive-behavioral intervention. In Kendall PC, Hollon SD (eds): *Cognitive-Behavioral Interventions: Theory, Research, and Procedures*, pp. 117–152. New York: Academic Press, 1979.

Green A, Green E: *Beyond Biofeedback*. New York: Delta Dell, 1977.

Guignon C: *Heidegger and the Problem of Knowledge*. Indianapolis, Indiana: Hackett Publ Co., 1983.

Haan N: *Coping and Defending: Processes of Self-Environment Organization*. New York: Academic Press, 1977.

Hartfield M: Appraisal of anger situations and subsequent coping responses in hypertensive and normotensive adults: A comparison. Unpublished doctoral dissertation, University of California at San Francisco, 1985.

Hatch JW, Cunningham AC, Woods WW, Snipes FC: The fitness through churches project: Description of a community-based cardiovascular health promotion intervention. Hygie 5:9, 1986.

Hochbaum GM: Public participation in medical screening programs: A socio-psychological study. Public Health Service Publication no. 572. Washington, D.C.: U.S. Government Printing Office, 1958.

Hochschild AR, *The Managed Heart*. Berkeley: University of California Press, 1983.

Holmes TH, Rahe RH: The social readjustment rating scale. J Psychosom Res 11:213, 1967.

Holroyd KA, Appel MA, Andrasik F: A cognitive-behavioral approach to psychophysiological disorders. In D Meichenbaum and ME Jaremko (eds.) *Stress Reduction and Prevention*. New York: Plenum, 1983.

Illich I: *Limits to Medicine*. London: Pelican Books, 1977.

Johnson JE: Effects of accurate expectations about sensations on the sensory and distress components of pain. J Person Social Psychol 27:261, 1973.

Johnson JE, Leventhal H: Effects of accurate expectations and behavioral instructions on reactions during a noxious medical examination. J Person Social Psychol, 29:710, 1974.

Journal of Public Health Policy. What is health promotion? J Pub Health Policy. Summer:147, 1986.

Kegeles SS, Kirscht JP, Haefner DP, et al: Survey of beliefs about cancer detection and taking Papanicolaou tests. Pub Health Rep 80:815, 1965.

Keller EF: *Reflections on Gender and Science*. New Haven, Conn.: Yale University Press, 1985.

Kerr W: *The Decline of Pleasure*. New York: Simon & Schuster, 1962.

Kobasa SC: Stressful life events, personality and health: An inquiry into hardiness. J Person Social Psychol 37:1, 1979.

Kobasa SC, Maddi SR, Courington S: Personality and constitution as mediators in the stress-illness relationship. J Health Social Behavior 22:368, 1981.

Krieger D: *The Therapeutic Touch: How to Use Your Hands to Help or Heal*. Englewood Cliffs, NJ: Prentice-Hall, 1979.

Larson EB, Bruce RA: Health benefits of exercise in an aging society. Arch Intern Med 147:353, 1987.

Lazarus R, Folkman S: *Stress Appraisal and Coping.* New York: Springer, 1984.

Lee DC: Is social competence independent of cultural context? Am Psychol 34:795, 1979.

Leventhal H, Nerenz DR: A model for stress research with some implications for the control of stress disorders. In Meichenbaum D, Jaremko M (eds): *Stress Prevention and Management: A Cognitive Behavioral Approach.* New York: Plenum, 1983.

Levin JS, Coreil J: "New Age" healing in the U.S. Social Sci Med 23:889, 1986.

Lionberger HJ: An interpretive study of nurses' practice of therapeutic touch. Unpublished doctoral dissertation, University of California at San Francisco, 1985.

Lock M, Dunk P: My nerves are broken: The communication of suffering in a Greek-Canadian community. In Coburn D, D'Arcy C, New P, Torrence G (eds): *Health in Canadian Society: Sociological Perspectives,* 1987.

Luria A: *The Mind of a Mnemonist.* New York: Basic Books, 1968.

Maslow AH: *Motivation and Personality.* New York: Harper and Row, 1954.

McKeown T: The Role of Medicine: Dream, Mirage or Nemesis (2nd ed). Princeton, New Jersey: Princeton Univ. Press, 1979.

Meichenbaum D: A self-instructional approach to stress management: A proposal for stress inoculation training. In Spielberger CD, Sarason IG (eds): *Stress and Anxiety,* vol. 2. New York: Wiley, 1975.

Meichenbaum D, Cameron R: Stress inoculation training: Toward a general paradigm for training coping skills. In Meichenbaum D, Jaremko ME (eds): *Stress Reduction and Prevention.* New York: Plenum, 1983.

Merleau-Ponty M: *Phenomenology of Perception.* Smith C (trans). London: Routledge & Kegan Paul, 1962.

Nightingale F: *Notes on Nursing: What It Is and What It Is Not.* Edinburgh, New York: Churchill Livingstone, 1980.

Nouwen HJM: *Lifesigns.* Garden City, New York: Doubleday, 1986.

Parsons T: Definitions of health and illness in the light of American values and social structure. In Caplan AL, Englehardt HT Jr, McCartney JJ (eds): *Concepts of Health and Disease: Interdisciplinary Perspectives.* Reading, Mass.: Addison-Wesley, 1981.

Pearlin LI, Schooler C: The structure of coping. J Health Social Behav 19:2, 1978.

Pelletier KR: *Mind as Healer, Mind as Slayer: a Holistic Approach to Preventing Stress Disorders.* New York: Delacorte Press, 1977.

Pender NJ: *Health Promotion in Nursing Practice.* Norwalk, Conn.: Appleton and Lange, 1987.

Phelps JR: Physical activity and health maintenance—Exactly what is known? West J Med 146:200, 1987.

Polanyi M: *Personal Knowledge.* London: Routledge & Kegan Paul, 1958.

Ritchie JA, Ellerton ML, Caty S: Children's coping, innovative methods in research design. Paper presented at International Research Conference, Edmonton, Alberta, May 1986.

Rorty AO: *Explaining Emotions.* Berkeley: University of California Press, 1980.

Rosenstock IM: Why people use health services. Milbank Memorial Fund Q 44:94, 1966.

Rubin J: *Too Much of Nothing: Modern Culture and the Self in Kierkegaard's Thought.* Forthcoming.

Scheper-Hughes N, Lock MM: The mindful body: A prolegomenon to future work in medical anthropology. Med Anthropol Q 1:6, 1987.

Schwartz GE: Testing the biophysical model: The ultimate challenge facing behavioral medicine? J Consult Clin Psychol 50:1040, 1982.

Schwartz B: *The Battles for Human Nature.* New York: W. W. Norton, 1986.

Seedhouse D: *Health: The Foundations for Achievement.* Chichester, England: Wiley, 1986.

Sheehan G: *Running and Being: The Total Experience.* New York: Warner Books, 1978.

Smythe EM: *Surviving Nursing.* Menlo Park, Calif.: Addison-Wesley, 1984.

Stein LI: "The doctor-nurse game." Am J Nurs 68:101–105, Jan 1968.

Syme LS: Strategies for health promotion. Prevent Med 15:492, 1986.

Thomas L: Notes of a biology watcher: Autonomy. New Eng J Med 287:90, 1972.

Thomas L: Notes of a biology watcher. New Eng J Med 293:1245, 1975.

Whitbeck C: A different reality: Feminist ontology. In Gould CC (ed): *Beyond Domination: New Perspectives on Women and Philosophy,* pp. 64–88. Totowa, N.J.: Roman and Allan Held, 1984.

White KD: Salivation: The significance of imagery in its voluntary control. Psychophysiology 15(3):196, 1978.

Williams R: Concepts of health: An analysis of lay logic. Sociology 17:185, 1983.

Winner L: *Autonomous Technology: Technics-Out-of-Control As a Theme in Political Thought.* Cambridge, Mass.: MIT Press, 1977.

Wrubel J: Personal Meanings and Coping Processes. Unpublished doctoral dissertation, University of California, San Francisco, 1985.

Wrubel J, Benner P, Lazarus RS: Social competence from the perspective of stress and coping. In Wine J, Smye M (eds): *Social Competence,* pp. 61–99. New York: Guilford, 1981.

Yankelovich D: *New Rules in American Life: Searching for Self-Fulfillment in a World Turned Upside Down.* New York: Random House, 1981.

CHAPTER SIX

Coping with Symptoms

She had never talked about what the symptoms meant to her. She had never said: "This means that I can't . . . even get out of bed without calling for help." When we finished I said something like: "Rheumatoid arthritis really has not been nice to you." She burst into tears, and her daughter did also, and I sat there, very close to losing it myself. She said: "You know, no one has ever talked about it as a personal thing before, no one's ever talked to me as if this were a thing that mattered, a personal event. *Clare Hastings, RN, MS*

What Is a Symptom?

SYMPTOMS AS A LIVED HUMAN RESPONSE

Symptoms are experienced differently by the patient and are studied differently by the health care worker, depending on the situation. In the case of an acute or a new illness, symptoms function as an empirical guide to diagnosing and treating underlying disease. In chronic illness, symptoms usually function as a signal for an understood but persistent problem. Because the symptom signals a familiar problem in chronic illness, the symptom takes on meanings related to the implications of the impending illness on the person's life. The symptom is no longer just empirical evidence of an underlying disorder, it now may give the person permission to take needed rest, be an ominous sign of impending disruption, or even raise feelings about the person's strength and self-worth. This chapter is concerned with the role of symptoms in chronic illness, but to explicate this role fully, we must first discuss a more basic question: What is a symptom?

Nowhere is Cartesian dualism more entrenched, and nowhere are the limitations of that dualism more obvious, than in the realm of symptomatology. According to the Cartesian model, the mind is the receiver and interpreter of impressions from the body. Thus, a symptom is viewed as the mind's subjective interpretation of the body's real disease experience. The health care worker's task here is to discern what is really going on from the patient's account of his or her symptom. Furthermore, the separate and nonphysical mind may go so far astray in its subjective appraisal as to create bodily symptoms. This means that the health care worker must be ever on the lookout for symptoms that are "merely" psychosomatic and do not reflect underlying disease.

There are a number of serious problems with understanding symptoms in terms of a mind-body split. These problems disappear when the person is thought of as a whole and the body is itself regarded as a knower. First, under the Cartesian model it is not possible to appreciate and take advantage of the basic interpretive skills by which diagnoses are made. The Cartesian view of the private subject creating private meanings overlooks the role of common background meanings and practices that create the diagnostician's ability to notice the most relevant symptoms. Blois (1980, 1983) has called this the role of commonsense understanding in making a diagnosis. The ability to attend selectively, which is often (and wrongly) given the pejorative label *subjective,* is actually a necessary requisite for making accurate diagnoses. The alternative to attending to the most appropriate lines of inquiry is to rely on a checklist of *all* possible questions, much as a computerized diagnostic system does. The problem with computerized approaches is that they subject the user to long lists of irrelevant questions (Schwartz, Patil, and Szolovits 1987).

Second, the role of an individual's history is either ignored or underestimated in the assessment process when the health care worker's focus is on the issue of whether the symptoms are "real" or not. The individual's understanding of his or her symptoms is shaped by past experiences, and that understanding must be grasped by the health care worker if treatment is to be acceptable to the patient and thus effective.

Finally, the practice of regarding symptoms as legitimate only if they are the result of disease means that the patient requires a license for suffering. Suffering that the health care worker assesses as resulting from an "imaginary" illness is not accorded the same concern as that resulting from a pathologic condition. Because the nursing perspective is concerned with illness as well as disease and with human responses as human responses (ANA Policy Statement 1980), any symptom can be heard and attended to in its own right and not just as a means to diagnose pathology. Unfortunately, nurses can be caught up in the quest for accurate diagnosis and see symptoms only as a sign or cause for determining underlying pathology. Such a view prevents remedial nursing action, as is illustrated in the following example.

A mother brought her five-year-old son into the hospital. She was extremely anxious over the possibility that her son might have a hemorrhage as a result of a tonsillectomy performed on an outpatient basis. The child was admitted despite reservations that the admission was not really warranted. Thus far, the bleeding had been in the high normal range, but the mother was extremely anxious. She called for the nurses to check each time her son spit out small amounts of blood. The nurses repeatedly answered the call light, thinking that the only intervention was a medical intervention *should* the child develop a hemorrhage. After about the tenth call, late in the afternoon, a nurse responded once again, this time feeling a bit skeptical. She found a major postoperative hemorrhage. She immediately notified the physician and prepared the child to return to surgery for control of the hemorrhage. This story could be repeated with many different complaints, symptoms, and fears.

The point is to question what might have happened had the nurse attended to the symptom of anxiety rather than to the possibility of bleeding. What if the nurse had responded to the mother's fear and anxiety and spent time with the mother and child to reduce their anxiety? The nurse overlooked the significance of anxiety as a human response and focused on the diagnostic significance of excessive bleeding. The nursing value is to attend to pain and suffering as a worthy end in itself. In this situation, as in many, such nursing interventions could have had a profound medical significance.

Research on the relationship between emotional distress and platelet aggregation suggests that suboptimal clotting occurs in the presence of emotional distress (Haft and Arkel 1976; Haft et al. 1982; Buxton et al. 1982). However, even if attentiveness to the fear of the mother and child had not prevented the hemorrhage, the nursing intervention of listening to the mother's concerns would have been significant in its own right. Listening, validating, coaching, and reassuring the mother and child are all ways of attending to the human response. Such attending would have established a climate of respect and care prior to any emergency.

A similar example with a nursing focus on human responses is provided by Nancy Karthas, a nurse from Children's Hospital, Boston. In this instance a nine-year-old girl with rheumatoid arthritis was brought into the emergency room by her parents. The nurse thought the child looked extremely ill and persuaded the resident to order additional diagnostic checks to look for electrolyte imbalance and liver involvement. The nurse thought the little girl needed to be admitted to the intensive care unit even though the resident had initially planned to admit her to an intermediate care unit. The resident ordered additional tests and a nasogastric tube stat.

Emergency Caring

Nancy Karthas, RN, BSN
Children's Hospital, Boston

It was change of shift, I was working evenings and had just taken report on my team. One patient in particular was worrisome to me. Karen had come in with a chief complaint of "vomiting blood." Her condition was complicated by arthritis for the past three years, and she took Ascriptin daily. Thus far, her treatment in the emergency department included an initial check of vital signs (which were normal except for a temperature of 40 C), blood work, and physical exam. Upon entering the room, I found the patient to be pale, listless, and experiencing mild abdominal pain.

The physician came in and stated that he wanted to pass a nasogastric tube to help determine the site of bleeding. I negotiated privately with the physician for a ten-minute delay to establish my relationship with Karen and her family. I suggested that more complete lab work be done to check for possible liver involvement. I also told him that I thought Karen may need to be admitted to ICU. During this period I was able to gain Karen's trust and establish a rapport with her family that I knew would be important. I explained the equipment and procedure to Karen and enlisted her cooperation by involving her directly. I gave her a "job" to do, which was to swallow when I told her to. I negotiated for Karen's mother to be able to stay, as she was a source of great support. Prior to insertion of the nasogastric tube, I had Karen supinate her arms and hold my fingers. This gave Karen a feeling of control when in reality it gave me a better control of her arms, should that become necessary.

Insertion went smoothly, with Karen's cooperation. Initial aspirate was bloody, but it cleared easily and the nasogastric tube was removed. Her fever remained elevated. Both aspirin and Tylenol were contraindicated due to her potential for bleeding and liver involvement. Sponging worked initially, but her fever spiked between tepid baths. Her lab studies came back grossly abnormal, with her prothrombin time being greater than 100. The decision was made to give vitamin K IV. Because of the dangers associated with intravenous administration of vitamin K, prior to administration, I placed Karen on a cardiac and respiratory monitor, had emergency equipment and drugs at bedside, and an infusion pump to assure accuracy of administration. I explained to Karen and her parents that these were only precautionary measures. I monitored her closely and the infusion was completed without incident.

The resident explained to the mother that her daughter was gravely ill and would have to be admitted to the intensive care unit because of the complexity of her illness, the presence of acute liver involvement, intractable fever, and her abnormal lab studies. She would need the close monitoring of the ICU. I checked with the mother and found that she was extremely anxious and that she had understood that her daughter was dying. I said: "You know, your daughter is very ill, but we can give her the help she needs in the intensive care unit. I think that you need to talk to the resident again, because I think you heard that your daughter was dying. I do not think that is the case." I clarified the mother's fears and understanding and then filled the resident in so that he could reassure the mother. This was accomplished so that the mother was no longer so frightened.

While Karen was getting settled in at the ICU, I spent time with the parents, offering support to a family who until this evening did not fully understand the complexity and gravity of Karen's illness. I followed Karen's rocky course through the ICU, which involved eventual multisystem failure, followed by a slow recovery period and eventual discharge home. Karen and her parents thanked me for the care and support I had given to them.

In three instances in the above exemplar, the nurse's attention to human responses to illness may have been lifesaving, though they are worthy in their own right because they maintain human dignity. Her recognition that the little girl was very ill upon initial assessment led to the suggestion of additional laboratory work and early planning for admission to the intensive care unit. This was an "early warning" based upon Nancy Karthas's clinical recognition of Karen's human responses. The vital signs alone did not point to the gravity of the situation. The additional laboratory work provided a confirmation of Karthas' judgment. By astutely working with the little girl and achieving a nontraumatic insertion of the nasogastric tube, Nancy Karthas no doubt minimized Karen's alarm or fright response. By intervening with the parents, allaying their anxiety, and coaching the physician in decreasing their fear, she prevented the parents from conveying panic and fear to the little girl. In both cases, an exaggerated stress response could have been extremely dangerous to Karen by further compromising her fragile physiological status.

Symptoms belong to the lived experience of the illness rather than being a precise map to underlying disease. Peterson, Sturdevant, and Frankl (1977) provided one of the more dramatic demonstrations of this human reality in their study of the effectiveness of high doses of antacids for peptic ulcers. Each patient underwent endoscopy at the beginning of the study and at the completion of the four-week study period. Of those who received high doses of antacids, 78% showed a higher healing rate, whereas in the placebo group only 45% showed healing. However a concurrent assessment of the symptom experience demonstrated that both the placebo and antacid groups had reduced their symptom distress only by 20%. Degree of healing was not necessarily related to symptoms. Some patients whose ulcers had healed continued to have pain, and some whose ulcers persisted had decreased pain. The authors noted that the loss of symptoms did not predict the ulcer healing or even decrease in ulcer size (Peterson, Sturdevant, Frankl 1977).

Because symptoms are expressions of the lived experience, they are related to the person's meanings and social transactions. Symptoms of a chronic illness come to be a familiar way of being in the world. They are also imbued with meaningful responses to situations. It would have been a worthy follow-up to the research of Peterson et al. to investigate under what circumstances the symptoms continued and what the quality of the pain was like. Symptoms of pain may become a form of expression (see Polhemus 1975, 1978). It is not surprising that new physical states may not be readily experienced as new bodily and social possibilities. We take up the problems of separating mind and body and taking a suspicious approach to symptoms, counting them as significant only if they point to "real" disease, again and at greater length in the following pages as we examine other issues relating to coping with symptoms.

The rest of this part of this chapter is organized into the following sections: how symptoms lead people to seek medical help, the role of symptoms in the process of medical diagnosis, symptoms as part of a life context, and symptom expression as communication. The second part of the chapter deals with the role of symptoms in chronic illness and the role of meaning in coping with symptoms.

SYMPTOMS AND THE REQUEST FOR MEDICAL HELP

A person engaged in an activity does not notice bodily sensations because they are not the focus of attention. However, in the presence of a disruptive symptom such as pain or nausea, internal sensations become the focus of attention, and awareness of the sensations is heightened. The sensations themselves may be elaborated with focused attention. Even as the person's attention becomes focused on the bodily sensation of the symptom, he or she begins to interpret it and to form his or her own diagnosis. For example, nausea could be possibly understood as the result of pregnancy, something one ate, or a "stomach flu." If none of these diagnoses applies, or if the symptom persists in severity over time, the person would then probably consult a physician. The point here is not to elaborate on the somewhat complicated question of under what conditions who seeks medical help. Rather, it is to indicate that patients arrive in doctors' offices with a diagnosis in mind.

Social epidemiology, a relatively new field of great interest to nurses, systematically studies the psychosocial determinants of the following: (a) illness or disease onset (incidence of new events), (b) course of illness or disease (exacerbations, repeat events), and (c) outcome of disease process and/or degree of recovery (Berkman 1981, Kasl 1977). This field is adding to our understanding of the conditions under which people seek medical help and how symptoms are understood in that process.

THE PROCESS OF MEDICAL DIAGNOSIS

Although they operate from a different knowledge base, both patient and doctor probably make diagnoses in the same way. Tentative hypotheses about the underlying cause of the symptoms organize perceptions about the symptoms (Bursztajn, Feinbloom, Hamm, and Brodsky 1981; Elstein, Shulman, and Sprafka 1978). Salient symptoms are noticed more and nonsalient symptoms or symptoms inconsistent with the hypothesized diagnosis are overlooked or discounted (Feinstein 1967). Under the Cartesian assumptions of the mind-body split, this selective attention is considered a subjective handicap. However, it is clear from the process of clinical diagnosis that the human capacity for a sense of relevance is required for active problem solving (Benner and Tanner, 1987). This very ability to attend selectively—this capacity for bias—makes human problem solving superior in open-ended unstructured situations. Human problem solvers, unlike passive computers, use history actively so that the current situation is understood through a web of perspectives of past similar and dissimilar sensations or patterns. This "subjective handicap," although fallible, does allow for recognition of patterns for ambiguous, underdetermined information, an absolute prerequisite for forming clinical diagnoses. The Cartesian perspective, in fact, handicaps arrival at an understanding of how embodied perceptual abilities work.

If we adopt the Cartesian perspective, we are suspicious that symptoms are "all in the mind," as if it were possible to stand completely outside of the self and one's history to get the "true" picture. Neither patient nor health care worker can have an unbiased, "true" picture. Both rely on their own history and the current understandings of the body and bodily symptoms. This historical situatedness is the very condition for any active problem solving and at the same time sets up limits to what meanings and interpretations are available. Preunderstanding and history allow the expert diagnostic specialist called in for a consultation to ask relatively few questions and come up with a plan for a differential diagnosis. The beginning medical student, by contrast, follows a very long structured history protocol covering all the bases. The presenting symptoms and history are not sufficiently meaningful to allow the beginner to narrow the range of questions asked. Through experience, the expert diagnostician learns to ask the questions in the right region, choosing those that will yield fruitful information for the differential diagnosis. By comparison, the beginning medical student or expert computerized diagnostic system has to go through very long lists of questions, with the negative responses yielding little direction or productive lines of questioning (Blois 1980, 1983). The medical student is in a similar situation as the expert computerized diagnostic system. The presenting symptoms and recent and past history allow expert diagnosticians to hone in on an accurate region; they are not reduced to purveying the entire Merck Manual for potential diagnoses.

The health professional making a medical diagnosis relies on a historical situatedness and a developed perceptual skill that together are commonly called "experience." Because this skill is embodied and results from a historical/contextual relationship, it completely contradicts all the Cartesian notions on which modern science is based. For example, the reliance on decontexualization for objectivity, the development of a brute data language free of "subjectivity" or "interpretation," the separation of the knower from the known, and the assumption that the causal force must be mechanistic and not teleological are all assumptions of the Cartesian view of science. (See Chapter Two, pp. 33–35 for a full discussion of these Cartesian assumptions related to empiricism.) Hence, in the absence of a generally acceptable and understandable term, real diagnostic skill is often called an art.

The art of diagnosis refers mainly to the capacity for skillfully grasping the significance of reported symptoms and physiological indicators. It can also include the ability to interpret the patient's own self-understanding and the influence of that self-understanding on the patient's reporting of symptoms, although this ability is rarer among clinicians. In fact, prior assumptions about the patient are commonly known to affect a diagnostician's judgment of the severity of symptoms. For example, the stereotypical assumption that women tend to overrate the severity of pain might prevent a diagnostician from understanding a stoical woman, causing the physician to underrate the severity of her pain.

Historical situatedness is the case for the diagnosing health care worker and the diagnosing patient alike. Because neither has exhausted the practical and theoretical knowledge available or overcome all constraints to understanding the underdetermined clinical situation, neither one should claim a completely privileged position, even when a "definitive diagnosis" has been reached. Language that reflects a Cartesian, technological understanding of the body, such as "psychological overlay," "purely mental," and "purely physical," blocks recognition of the relationships between the mind and the body. Once a person is defined as "ill," the emotional responses to the illness influence the disease process for better or for worse. Therefore, attention to separating out "physical" and "psychological" causation and influence, by definition, prevents identification of relational or synthetic terms that would indicate the mutual constituting influence of personal and cultural meanings and physical sensations.

SYMPTOMS AS PART OF THE LIFE CONTEXT

Symptoms are always experienced as meaningful, and that meaning is shaped by prior history and by the current context. Here, the seventeenth-century limitations of meaning must be expanded from merely pointing and naming functions to include the expressive and constitutive roles of meaning. Charles Taylor (1985) points out that scientific theories of meaning have been limited to pointing and labeling functions, which he terms the "designative theories of meaning." Pointing and labeling functions work for identifying and describing objects but fall short of the full range of functioning of meaning for persons, the expressive and constitutive functions of meaning. Meanings are what makes sense of the world to the person. Because they are the way things are for a person, they also open the way to the way things could be. In short, meanings set up the very conditions of possibility.

A symptom, then, can never be experienced in isolation. It will always be understood in terms of past and current life. One well-known example of this is the "medical student's syndrome" (Hunter, Lohrenz, and Schwartzman 1964; Woods, Natterson, and Silverman 1966). The context of student doctors' and nurses' lives is illness of all kinds, and they tend to interpret every symptom in terms of the diseases they have studied. Thus a headache becomes a brain tumor; a stomachache becomes a case of roundworm. Very common physiological occurrences, which would ordinarily remain in the background, move into the foreground and become the focus of attention because of current experience. Fortunately medical student's syndrome is short-lived and does not develop into long-term hypochondriasis. Increased knowledge about the disease, decreased anxiety, and general acknowledgment of the tendency to overinterpret symptoms when learning about new diseases seem to short-circuit the syndrome (Woods et al. 1966).

The medical student's syndrome is so typical that it is a joke. But the usual way in which life history and context inform one's understanding of symptoms is not often funny. For example, people in acute grief over a loved one who has suffered an extended illness typically experience their own physical symptoms in terms of their recent experience. In the context of a recent loss, the person's own mortality is a very real issue. Understanding the context is no excuse for overlooking or discounting the symptom. When the issue is diagnostic, all prudent steps toward diagnosis must be followed. But the teaching and coaching of the patient about the diagnostic procedures and the interpretation of the results can and should incorporate a sensitivity to excessive worry and sense of vulnerability that is common in acute grief (Parkes 1972).

Pellegrino (1982), discussing the moral basis for a healing relationship, describes illness as an assault on one's context and captures the way in which illness interrupts:

> Illness forces a change in existential states. It thrusts man into contact with the reality of the via dolorosa that eventually all must traverse. It is only in part defined medically as a concrete organic or psychosocial aberration. It is the perception of the change in existential states that forms the central experience of illness—the perception of impairment

and the need to be made whole again—to be cured, healed, or cared for. ... The ill person becomes homo patiens—a patient—a person *bearing* a burden of distress, pain, or anxiety; a person set apart; a person wounded in specific ways. . . . For the emotionally ill person the rupture of ontological unity may be more subtle and deeper. The psyche or spirit is interposed as an impediment between the self and its intents and purposes as well as the unity of the self and body. . . . Genuine healing must be based on an authentic perception of the experience of illness in *this* person. It must aim at a repair of the particular assaults that illness makes on the humanity of the one who is ill (pp. 157–158, 160).

To be healed is to reestablish a normal relationship with one's world, one's context.

SYMPTOM EXPRESSION AS COMMUNICATION

The Cartesian perspective sets up a question about the reality of symptoms. Do they point to "real" disease? The legitimacy of the symptom depends on the underlying problem. This perspective sets up a climate of doubt that interferes with acceptance of the person's symptom expression. As Scheper-Hughes and Lock (1987) point out, it is an extremely materialistic view of the body initiated by Aristotle, continued by Hippocrates, and finally established as the biomedical view of the separation of mind, body, and spirit by Descartes. Scheper-Hughes and Lock (1987) describe a typical medical conference:

In halting sentences the patient explained before the class of two hundred that her husband was an alcoholic who occasionally beat her, that she had been virtually housebound for the past five years looking after her senile and incontinent mother-in-law, and that she worries constantly about her teenage son who is flunking out of high school. Although the woman's story elicited considerable sympathy from the students, many grew restless with the line of clinical questioning, and one finally interrupted the professor to demand "But what is the *real* cause of the headaches?"

The medical student, like many of her classmates, interpreted the stream of social information as extraneous and irrelevant to the *real* biomedical diagnosis. She wanted information on the neurochemical changes which she understood as constituting the true causal explanation. This kind of radically materialist thinking, characteristic of clinical biomedicine, is the product of a Western epistemology extending as far back as Aristotle's starkly biological view of the human soul in *De Anima* (p. 9).

If an alternative perspective is taken, this climate of doubt and question of legitimacy can be avoided altogether. For example, pain management in the past was often framed under the Cartesian suspicion: "Was the pain real, severe enough for pain medication, or was the symptom expression only a sign of impending addiction?" This whole climate of suspicion has been replaced by increasing the patient's control over various self-care pain relief strategies or through receiving pain medication either through "patient-controlled dosing" or through establishing a schedule of regularly timed administration of medication so that the patient does not have to wait for the pain to escalate to legitimize the use of pain medication. This shift is basically an interpretive one. The patient is no longer required to experience severe pain to "earn" pain relief.

Symptom expression as a means of communication has been discussed extensively in the literature of illness behavior and health psychology (Mechanic 1978, Pennebaker 1982). Several studies found that people under stress are more likely to experience symptoms and are more likely to search for help (see Mechanic and Volkart 1961; Tessler, Mechanic, and Dimond 1976). But the associations between stress and illness and help seeking are not uniform for all groups. In a study of the use of health services by 512 young families, Roghmann and Haggerty (1972) found that the patterns of stress, illness, and help seeking were different for mothers and other family members. Stress indices were based on a diary kept by the mother of upsetting events that occurred in the family. The researchers found that the combination of family stress with illness increased by 50% the likelihood of seeking medical contact. Stress alone without illness increased the chances for help seeking about 80%. This pattern held true for all family members except mothers. When the mother was ill, family stress *decreased* the likelihood that she would utilize medical care.

This research highlights the debate over how best to allocate medical care. There has been concern voiced over how to distinguish the "worried well" (Garfield 1970), that is, those for whom stress and not illness is the reason for the medical contact, from the actually ill. But as Roghmann and Haggerty (1975) point out, the issue should not be how to screen out those who seek medical help because of current life distress, but how best to help them.

Nurses sometimes get engaged in a struggle with patients who express symptoms to convey distress or gain desired benefits. This climate of secondary gain or manipulation through symptom expression sets up yet another climate of suspicion in the expression of symptoms. Who has not had the childhood experience of enjoying the mother's solicitous care after a minor injury, and upon another occasion exaggerated yet another injury to procure the longed-for attention? The astute mother attempts to make her attentiveness generous enough so that the child does not require injury to gain attention. But the secondary gains of injury and pain persist in minor and major ways throughout life. For example, teammates on a high school football or basketball team may encourage one another to lie still for a moment after injury to gain the attention of the officials and the sympathy of the crowd.

A chronic illness may set up a familial and social pattern of solicitation and reward that extends or entrenches the illness behavior even though the person is unaware of the relationship between the side benefits and the symptom expression. This is why pain clinics have found success in setting up new social and familial responses to pain. These new responses break the cycle of pain expression. This can be quite effective even when the person in pain sets up the new conditions for relating to the chronic pain. From the phenomenological perspective, what is involved is a retraining of bodily responses to meaningful situations. The situation is altered in ways that offer new bodily responses.

Mechanic (1978) points out that illness behavior is often a way of coping with pain or problems that are not easily expressed directly because of social constraints. In psychology, this is called somatization. Because the body is culturally understood and expressed, different cultures yield different physical expressions of distress (Kleinman 1982, Kleinman and White 1982, Kleinman and Good 1985). The secondary gain or cultural learning hypotheses about symptoms do not necessarily have to lead to a discussion of the "legitimacy" of the symptom once it is understood that secondary gains and cultural learning are not deliberate conscious choices. This is where the addition of the middle term for embodied intelligence, a term that includes habits, skills, and practices (see the discussion in Chapter Three), is crucial for changing the understanding of illness behavior in a way that does not lead to useless "blame-the-victim" approaches that have such negative moral overtones.

Even on an "unconscious" level, the person does not typically set out to manipulate others through illness behavior. Instead, the person is caught in a web of behavior patterns and learned bodily responses to meaningful situations that he or she does not notice or comprehend. The same cultural and habitual body that opens up fluid and flexible action also creates the possibility of unwittingly overlearning bodily responses to stressful situations and the possibility of unwittingly responding in ways that yield pleasant responses. The embodied intelligence and cultural learning view of "secondary gains" takes away the moral overtones and allows people to restructure their situations to ensure new cultural learning and new habitual bodily responses.

From the phenomenological perspective, symptoms can be taken seriously, and the body is no longer viewed as merely an extension of the mind's intents. The body is understood to have an intentionality, the kind of intentionality inherent in bodily responses to meaningful situations (Collins 1985, Merleau-Ponty 1962). The body is no longer an alien object that is subject to the mind's will. It is understood as an equally legitimate expression of the person's way of being in the world. Suspicion and blame are no longer issues.

Role of Symptoms in Chronic Illness

For a person who is not already ill, a symptom is an interruption, a break in the usual smoothly functioning body. For a person with a chronic illness, symptoms take on a different meaning. There are two main ways in which symptoms play a role in chronic illness. New symptoms or reappearing symptoms can signal the failure of management efforts and/or the progress of the disease, and persistent symptoms in chronic illness can take on a life of their own.

The chronically ill patient who develops new symptoms or whose formerly controlled symptoms reappear faces a difficult coping challenge. Through careful management, a chronically ill person can achieve an adaptation to his or her illness that in some ways resembles the smooth running bodily experience of the healthy person. Self-monitoring and medications become part of the mundane, ordinary experience of daily life, that is, they, and the illness they are managing, become part of the background for the person.

Mechanic (1978) notes that the way people come to understand and conceptualize their experiential change in the course of a chronic illness is one of the most neglected areas in the study of coping and help seeking. In the study of coping in a healthy population, we refer to the skillful adaptive learning that occurs over time as the acquisition of a "cushion of experience" (Benner 1984b, Wrubel 1985). People gain a web of perspectives and a host of routinized responses that offer a flexible understanding of a situation so that recurring illness episodes may come to be much less stressful over time. It is intriguing to consider why, or under what circumstances, recurring episodes of illness become less stressful and why in some cases recurring episodes become *more* stressful over time. Instead of the expected habituation, the reverse occurs, and the person experiences increasing panic and fear (see Dirks, Kleiger, and Evans 1978).

COPING WITH SYMPTOMS

Coping with symptoms in an era of technological self-understanding means that symptoms are a sign of technological failure or breakdown. The body-machine is broken and needs to be fixed. The technological promise of disenburdenment and pain-free existence through science and technology is currently being questioned. When the technological fix is readily available, this interpretation is not troublesome. However, when there is no easy fix and the symptom persists and must be coped with, the person may find the technological and biomedical language ill suited to describe the persistent experience of pain, fatigue, weakness, or dizziness. Virginia Woolf notices that literature does not easily come to the rescue in providing a language for illness:

> English, which can express the thoughts of Hamlet and the tragedy of Lear, has no words for the shiver and the headache. It has all grown one way. The merest schoolgirl, when she falls in love, has Shakespeare or Keats to speak her mind for her; but let a sufferer try to describe a pain in his head to a doctor and language at once runs dry. There is nothing ready made for him. He is forced to coin words himself, and, taking his pain in one hand, and a lump of pure sound in the other (as perhaps the people of Babel did in the beginning), so to crush them together that a brand new word in the end drops out. Probably it will be something laughable. For who of English birth can take liberties with the language? To us it is a sacred thing and therefore doomed to die, unless the Americans, whose genius is so much happier in the making of new words than in the disposition of the old, will come to our help and set the springs aflow. Yet, it is not only a new language that we need, more primitive, more sensual, more obscene, but a new hierarchy of passions; love must be deposed in favour of a temperature of 104; jealousy give place to the pangs of sciatica; sleeplessness play the part of villain, and the hero become a white liquid with a sweet taste—that mighty Prince with the moth's eyes and the feathered feet, one of whose names is Chloral (Woolf 1948, pp. 11–12).

Virginia Woolf describes the world-changing character of illness, but she also describes the impoverished meanings and language for suffering in a technological era. In illness, the person is reduced to objectified biomedical language to depict anguish and suffering that occur in a world of broken meanings and disrupted projects and dreams. It is not accidental that the "cure" is chloral hydrate or some other numbing potion in Woolf's account, because that too is the modern conception of pain relief and illness behavior.

Language, meanings, social practices, and social relationships are the major resource for coping. Meaninglessness is the position most bereft of coping (Benner, Roskies, and Lazarus 1980; Benner 1984b). This was the great tragedy for the returning Viet Nam veteran. Unlike the veterans of earlier wars, they had no language, no readily available meanings, no agreed-upon social practices for the returning soldier. The result was disturbed social relationships rife with disagreements about the cause and the results of the war. In stark contrast to the Viet Nam veteran's experience are the experiences of the returning World War II veterans and the meanings and social practices surrounding widowhood.

Illness in a technological age falls into a chasm of impoverished language, social meanings, and practices. On one hand, this has liberated us from superstitions about disease being caused by possession of evil spirits or being a punishment for sin. The biomedical explanation and language work best as a coping resource when there is a quick biomedical cure for a disease. However, with the liberation comes the loss of meaning terms and self-understanding related to pain and suffering. The impoverished meanings may decrease the embodied capacity to dwell in meanings and actualize bodily resources as in an enhanced immune response or as in the release of endorphins. Alternative therapies have been developed that use elements of the immune system in symbolic ways. T cells or white cells are visualized as powerful resources that attack infection or cancer cells. Nurses under the direction of Delores Krieger (1975, 1979) have developed therapeutic touch that creates healing symbolism based on metaphors from physics. The major metaphor of therapeutic touch is physical exchange of energy (Lionberger 1985, 1986). These alternative therapies may be viewed as attempts to empower the patient to recapture the symbolic healing powers of the body.

Like placebos (Cousins 1979, Wadden 1984, McCaffrey and Blanchard 1985) these alternative therapies work only if there is authentic faith in their efficacy. Authentic faith means the body's ability to dwell in the meanings. It is not enough to "pretend" that white cells are efficacious or that a drug will work. Once a patient discovers that the "efficacious drug" is a placebo, the placebo loses its power. Faith in a technological age is hard to come by because the ultimate authority rests in scientific knowledge and absolute clarity and certainty. Visualizing microscopic pictures of the cells of the body and imbuing them with symbolic power is an ingenious modern response to exercise bodily intentionality and embodied powers of healing.

The technological promise is to rid the human race of poverty and disease, thus any disease nullifies the promise. The call for an "objective" stance toward disease and illness cuts the person off from the lived experience of illness, even though being objective may offer temporary comfort and stem the tide of panic.

The language of symptoms—for example, dizziness, pain, tinnitus, angina, fatigue, dyspnea, itching, hunger, and thirst—has been plagued with the problem of "interior" versus "exterior" Cartesian thinking. The root metaphor is the opposition of "inside" versus "outside" (Pennebaker 1982, Schrag 1982). Consequently the discourse is typically on the private and the public experience of a symptom such as pain. The Cartesian subject is seen as a private knower, possessing private idiosyncratic thinking, and most perceptions are turned into rational, adjudicated concepts. The discourse is divided into "sensations" and "pain behavior." Sensations come from the interior, and the quest is for descriptions of pure sensations of "dull," "heavy," "sharp," "gnawing," and so on. Pain behavior is external, and the quest is for reliable public descriptions of "grimacing," "drawn expression," "paleness," "tight lips," "irritability," and so on (Schrag 1982).

The problem with this perspective is that it is far from the lived experience of most symptoms because pain, itching, and dizziness are not experienced by one sense organ, nor are they pure sensation unencumbered by concern, situation, embodiment, and temporality. Sensation and "feeling tone" (the emotional response) cannot really be separated. The nursing language of human response and a phenomenological and existential perspective based on the works of Heidegger (1982, Dreyfus in press) and Merleau-Ponty (1962) can recover the lived experience of symptoms and open up a discourse on coping with symptoms as they are lived. This can be done without discounting the value of clear descriptions that give clues to underlying pathology or anatomical physiological changes. Coping with symptoms is now discussed in relation to the role of cultural meanings and concern, embodiment, situation, and temporality. Finally, the expertise of patients and parents of children who have chronic illnesses will be examined.

THE ROLE OF CULTURAL MEANINGS AND CONCERN

Symptoms are never experienced as isolated, meaningless phenomena, even though the current language and self-understanding related to symptoms is shaped by a biomedical self-understanding that seeks to strip symptoms of meanings. Consequently even the person on the street attempts to describe symptoms objectively without feelings or theoretical constructions, despite the fact that the symptom is laden with meaning and feelings (Engelhardt 1982). Symptoms can seldom if ever be separated into pure sensation and pure emotional responses; the sensation is shaped by the emotion and the emotion is shaped by the sensation. The constructions of biomedical science and anatomical, physiological self-understanding now shape (constitute) the way people describe and experience symptoms. For example, pain associated with treatment in cancer is not as distressing as pain associated with signs of recurrence (Coyle and Foley 1985). The "pain" of childbirth is constituted by cultural and personal meanings. It may be experienced as discomfort, and concentration and distraction can turn the work of labor into an "athletic" experience during which "pain" is reinterpreted and not experienced as such. This example can be contrasted with the pain experienced by a person with kidney stones, which is supposedly similar to that of childbirth. The woman unfortunate enough to have had a kidney stone soon after a childbirth experience that she managed by distraction, concentration, and athletic metaphors, will find that these simply are not available for the experience of "kidney stone" because the cultural meanings are different (Benner 1985).

With chronic illnesses, the persistent symptoms take on a life of their own. For example, in a study of patients with chronic dyspnea, the symptom, shortness of breath, was totalizing in distinctly different ways for two groups of patients. For one group of patients, the symptom was totalizing in that the symptom came to define their very existence. All activities were experienced as relative and in relation to dyspnea. Even in the absence of overt dyspnea, activities were colored by its threat. Dyspnea itself becomes a major concern and a world-defining experience. These patients need to rekindle memories of what their lives were like before dyspnea to overcome the engulfing nature of the symptom.

A similar analogy can be drawn by patients with chronic pain. When the chronic pain becomes totalizing, the patient's entire life is given over to the experience of pain, or warding it off, preventing it, or intervening in it. The interventions offered in the successful pain clinics typically attempt to restructure people's experience so that they do not get all their social and personal definition from the pain experience.

For the second group of patients, dyspnea became totalizing in just the opposite way. Their concern was to "defeat" and "overcome" their handicap of dyspnea. These patients exerted enormous efforts toward living their lives in spite of the dyspnea. They undertook strenuous sports activities and hazardous occupations as a means of not letting dyspnea take over their lives. However, in the effortful negation and quest for mastery over the symptom through "overcoming" it, the patient ran the risk of making the symptom more prevalent. This was the case for the research scientist who continued to work in a laboratory with rats for over fifteen years despite being violently allergic to them. Militant overcompensation sometimes causes the person to make unreasonable demands of his or her physical energy and stamina.

In this study of patients with dyspnea there seemed to be a middle ground. Some patients accepted the symptom but at the same time did not let it take over or define them as a person. This middle ground has many variations and is recognizable in patients who neither are engulfed by the symptom nor set up unrealistic activities to prove mastery over the symptom. It is as if the person takes this stance: "My dyspnea sets limits. But I am more than those limits, and I can work around the limits to express my intents and desires." For example, a housewife who no longer could do much of her housework still drew great pleasure and meaning from arranging flowers for her house. This simple practice was within her severe activity limits, but it gave her a sense of contribution and continuity with her former role as homemaker.

EMBODIMENT OF SYMPTOMS

Symptoms are never completely clear. The nature of bodily sensations and bodily understanding is ambiguous. This is not a mere handicap, it is actually an ingenious gift of being embodied. Vague information can be sensed and attended to. This allows an orienting response even when what one is attending to is unclear. With chronic illness, symptoms come to be more clearly defined. However, circumstances may change gradually over time, making old interpretations obsolete or at least less informed. For example, an expert nurse described working with a patient in a coronary care unit who had severe congestive heart failure. His energy was very low, and his cardiac output had been very low for approximately six months with very little successful medical intervention. He was brought into the coronary care unit to receive experimental drugs. His cardiac output had improved dramatically in response. All of his vital signs had improved, his color was better, his lungs were clearer, and he showed few signs of dyspnea, yet his facial expression and bodily posture had not changed. It was just as difficult for him and he required the same amount of assistance to move from the bed to the chair as had been the case earlier. His expert nurse noticed his response and reflected back to him the way his posture appeared to her. She said: "Do you know how much energy you are expending on keeping this tense position?" She coached him to change his posture, take some deep breaths, and assess how he was feeling. He found that he did in fact feel better; he did have more energy. He began attending to his environment. He found it easy to move to his chair. Before the nurse's suggestion, he had simply not yet changed his self-understanding or interpretation of his condition to match his new circumstances. He had been sitting in bed, somewhat fearful, waiting for the other shoe to drop. With her expert coaching and prompting, he was able to change his understanding of himself and his condition. He had been laboring under his self-understanding for the past six months. It is understandable that it would take some reevaluation and interpretation to sense his new energy. This example should not be misconstrued as an example of "the power of positive thinking" (a Cartesian understanding) because it was not just his thinking that gave him a new sense of possibility, he had a new physiological environment and capability.

One of the major contributions that nurses make to their patients who require a long convalescence and rehabilitation is to reflect and document even the smallest increments of improvement. Patients often overlook improvement because their standard of comparison tends to be their old fully capable state. Therefore, careful reflection of even the smallest increments of improvement offers hope and a sense of progress. This process of documenting progress and holding out the next possibility in recovery pushes back the experience of institutionalization and loss of a familiar world full of projects and concerns. Indeed, we have much to learn about the recovery process itself. Oliver Sacks' (1984) description of his own recovery from a severe leg injury serves as an eloquent reminder of the uneven process of recovery (see Chapter three, p. 65). Sacks understands first hand the necessity of expert coaching for recovery. Expert nurses who have taken care of many patients with similar recovery trajectories can provide the patient with a rough timetable and even hints about recovering sensations that they have learned from observing and coaching other patients. The expert nurses provide the "imagination" necessary for hope (see also Benner 1984a).

We also have much to learn from studying the different perceptions of embodiment during various recovery trajectories. We have very little study and knowledge about the cultural body and the meanings attached to symptoms experienced in different parts of the body. There is anecdotal evidence that symptoms related to the genitals may be particularly laden with significance, and there are fairly extensive accounts of the meanings associated with the breast in Western culture (Bard and Sutherland 1955). Social tensions and conflict seem to be reflected in the prevalence of diseases. Gastrointestinal diseases such as ulcers have sharply declined in the United States (Susser and Stein 1962, Vogt and Johnson 1979); however, eating disorders seem to be on the rise. Crawford (1985) offers the cultural explanation that the two extremes of binging and purging in bulimia and excessive exercising in anorexia reflect the current contradictory cultural injunctions that women be self-disciplined, controlled, and fit and at the same time be fun-loving, self-indulgent, and hedonistic consumers. Crawford (1985) points out that since it is impossible to be both hedonistic and self-controlled at the same time, the eating disorders take the pattern of binging alternating with jogging, purging, and the taking of diuretics. This relationship to food, exercise, and body can also be interpreted as a manifestation of a technological self-understanding. Eating is unrelated to hunger and appetite, and control is highly valued, as are ease and disenburdenment (Borgmann 1984). Drugs and exercise are the quick technological fix to a disturbed and rather alienated, disembodied approach to eating, rest, and exercise. The self is literally viewed as raw material void of patterns and rhythms of its own. Consequently, it must be shaped, mastered, and controlled by calculating energy input and output.

Ischemic heart disease also seems to be on the decline (Stallones 1980), but there is no clear, unequivocal relationship between this decline and the major known risks for heart disease. Heart disease has the most clearly documented relationship to social turmoil, speed, overload, rapid change, and hostility (Review Panel on Coronary-Prone

Behavior and Coronary Heart Disease 1981). The study presents ischemic heart disease as an embodied result of hurried, tense, controlling, and alienated ways of being in the world. The modern way of being in the world seems to take its toll on the cardiovascular system over time. This epidemiological evidence (Stallones 1980) raises the question of whether the modern person is changing his or her way of being in the world and thus his or her embodiment.

THE ROLE OF THE SITUATION

Symptoms are situated. This has been discussed above in terms of whether the symptom is new or recurrent. Here the discussion is expanded to consider the response to the symptom in relation to the person's current situation. Does the symptom occur in the context of an impending birth, of a highly valued business transaction, or of grieving? It seems a statement of the obvious to call attention to the role of the person's situation in his or her perception of and coping with symptoms. Yet the anecdote about the medical student's search for the "real" cause of the woman's headaches apart from her situation demonstrates that the situation is all but overlooked in the Cartesian view of perceptions.

In Chapter Seven, the experience of symptoms in persons with cancer is considered in terms of the prediagnostic, diagnostic, treatment, and palliative phases of medical and nursing care. The adaptive demands and significance of symptoms vary in relation to the biomedical definition of the situation. Similarly, angina and other symptoms of disease hold different meanings during prediagnostic, treatment, and palliative care.

THE ROLE OF TEMPORALITY

The way one experiences time, projected from the past and thrown into the future (Dreyfus in press, Heidegger 1982) shapes the illness experience and the perception of symptoms. In turn, symptoms such as pain, weakness, fatigue, and hunger shape one's sense of time. Schrag (1982) gives a phenomenological description of temporality for the person in pain:

> In experiencing particularly intense pain we speak of every moment's seeming like an eternity. The "now" of pain appears to be endless. It is precisely the *living through* pain that becomes the uppermost concern. Indeed, we wonder how we will live through it; we wonder when it will stop; we may even despair in the face of the possibility of its never

stopping. In all this we see illustrated a peculiar fabric of temporality, a time span of concern, comprehended not as a succession of discrete, homogeneous, instantaneous nows but as a stagnating present with breadth and thickness that moves ever so slowly toward a hoped-for liberated future (p. 122).

Symptoms typically disrupt one's normal sense of time. The future can be foreshortened to the immediate future, as in the next hour or the next few days or weeks. The present can take on a great immediacy, and this change in temporality may for some be experienced as a new possibility to live fully in the now in a way that was not possible prior to illness, when they were caught up in excessive planning for the future or excessive reflection on the past. The change in temporality brought about by illness is relative to the person's past experience of temporality. Consequently, prescriptions for how people *should* experience their temporality, their basic way of being in the world, miss the point.

In the case of chronic illness, symptoms may give rise to fears experienced during past episodes of illness and actually exacerbate the current symptoms. Likewise a symptom experienced on the eve of a performance or other important event may be minimized or exaggerated by the person's self-understanding and coping with the anticipated event.

PRACTICAL KNOWLEDGE EMBEDDED IN PATIENT EXPERTISE

Over time, many if not most patients or parents of sick children can become experts in their assessment of their disease and in their self-care. Two studies (Carrieri and Janson-Bjerklie 1986, Popell 1983) and a parents' guide for children with asthma (Plaut 1984) suggest that the greatest fear of the expert patient is that this expert knowledge will be discounted and less-than-expert interventions will be given in a new medical care setting or by a new physician. Parents of asthmatic children talk about learning how to phrase their assessments and recommendations for treatment in neutral, nonmedical language (see excerpt below). This is not unlike the doctor-nurse game (Stein 1968) in which nurses are supposed to carefully avoid drawing any medical conclusions, but the occasion to describe the symptoms would never have arisen if the nurse or patient did not have a diagnosis in mind.

The expectation that patients remain naive over the course of long-term experience with an illness blocks enlightened health care. Parents and patients can be coached to carry with them brief history and preferred treatment approaches by their doctor, but ultimately the solution lies in acknowledging the expertise that patients gain in understanding and treating their illness over time. This is not to say that even the expert patient's assessment will *always* be correct but rather to insist that the patient's or parents' assessment be seriously respected by those considering the diagnosis and course of treatment. This lesson for all health care workers is painfully illustrated in Gail Hall's description of a Thanksgiving weekend that was turned into a disaster by lack of medical acceptance of her expertise about her daughter's asthma. Excerpted below is Ms Hall's own description, which was originally published in Plaut's (1984) excellent manual for parents who have children with asthma:

> The decision to visit my brother in New York for the Thanksgiving holiday was in some ways a difficult one and some ways easy. I remembered our last visit to New York when six-year-old Emily had an asthma reaction to my brother's cats. . . . I planned for trouble as best I could.
>
> [Emily did get a full-blown asthma attack in response to the environment. Ms Hall describes her encounter at the emergency room:]
>
> I brought Emily in and after the usual insurance procedures I told the nurse that Emily was having trouble with asthma, that I thought she needed an injection, that we had been there before, that she took theophylline, a 200 mg tablet twice a day and that she used a metaproterenol inhaler, but was no longer useful to us because she was unable to hold her breath.
>
> The nurse spoke with the intern or resident and he came over and asked me what I thought the problem was. I repeated what I had said to the nurse and added that, given Emily's previous experience with asthma, the situation warranted an injection of adrenaline. "I think she needs a shot because the oral medication we've been using is no longer working," I said. "I think you need to calm down," was his response.
>
> I had entered the emergency room aware that I had to play a low key role because I knew some physicians found it difficult to deal with parents who have a lot of information, and, God help them, an opinion. I understood that it was important to avoid acting as if I were going to be the one to make a decision. Instead, it was my role to simply feed information, and very slowly at that. I understood it was important not to irritate the people who had the drug my kid needed. In retrospect, I see that I should have followed this insight more closely and not suggested the shot. At any rate, I was not prepared for the level of hostility that I met, partly because it was not there on my last visit, and partly because I'm never prepared for hostility.
>
> We had to wait another fifteen minutes for the physician who was on

duty. . . . He finally came over and listened very briefly to Emily's chest. His diagnosis was, "This isn't an asthma attack." As he walked away with an air of disdain, he remarked over his shoulder, "She's hyperventilating."

I was amazed that he did not notice her retractions or that her inhale/exhale ratio was reversed, two signs of real trouble breathing. They occur with asthma but not with hyperventilation. I knew why he said she wasn't having an asthma attack. It was because she wasn't wheezing. But wheezing isn't necessary to an asthma attack; in fact, you can only wheeze if some air goes through the windpipes. Emily wasn't wheezing because many of her windpipes were completely closed (pp. 109–112).

The physician finally did give Emily an injection, but the "disaster" continued through the night. Another two trips to the emergency room were required and an overnight stay in a motel. Ms Hall's request for hospitalization was denied. The side effects of three adrenaline shots in one night were discounted by the attending physicians. Emily's own physician, Dr. Plaut, responded (Plaut 1983) by supplying Emily and Ms Hall with a letter explaining their level of knowledge and the usual best treatment course for Emily in an acute episode of asthma, and more instruction and preparation so they could avoid the emergency room even during out-of-town visits. But this is only a partial solution that cannot take the place of educating health providers to take seriously the knowledge of patients and parents about their own chronic illness.

Experiential knowledge gained as a result of living with a chronic illness is a form of practical knowledge (see Benner 1984a for a full discussion of aspects of practical knowledge). This experienced know-how

1. May reside in a skilled bodily response to symptoms. For example, the patient who learns to relax or use self-hypnosis early in a pain experience may diminish or block a full-blown pain response.

2. May concern knowledge of bodily states. For example, some diabetics become expert in detecting low and high blood sugar from bodily sensations (Cox, Gonder-Frederick, Pohl, and Pennebaker 1983).

3. May be complex skills related to the accurate recognition of activity patterns that lead to vulnerability or precipitation of an illness, and thus improved management is achieved.

4. May reside in knowledge concerning particular responses to dosage and sequencing of frequently taken medications.

5. May reside in knowledge concerning tolerances and intolerances for foods under treatment or illness conditions.

6. May reside in skilled bodily knowledge related to bodily movement and exercise tolerance relative to specific illnesses and injuries.

All of these kinds of practical knowledge gained through experience are likely to be more advanced and particular than any theoretical account based on the usual or underlying isolatable mechanisms, structures, and interactions.

We have much to learn by studying the practical knowledge of expert patients. In many instances, a systematic study of this practical knowledge will lead to new theories, or at least an increased understanding of the illness experience and the possibilities for recovery at different points in the illness.

REFERENCES

American Nurses' Association. ANA policy statement. Kansas City, MO.: The Association, 1980.

Bard M, Sutherland AM: Psychological impact of cancer and its treatment: Adaptation to mastectomy. Cancer 8:656, 1955.

Benner P: *From Novice to Expert: Excellence and Power in Clinical Nursing Practice.* Menlo Park, Calif.: Addison-Wesley, 1984a.

Benner P: Quality of life: A phenomenological perspective on explanation, prediction, and understanding in nursing science. Adv Nurs Sci 8:1, 1985.

Benner P: *Stress and Satisfaction on the Job.* New York: Praeger Scientific Press, 1984b.

Benner P, Roskies E, Lazarus RS: Stress and coping under extreme conditions. Dimsdale JE, (ed.). *Survivors, Victims, and Perpetrators: Essays on the Nazi Holocaust.* Washington, D.C.: Hemisphere, 1980.

Benner P, Tanner C: Clinical judgment: How expert nurses use intuition. Am J Nurs 87:23, 1987.

Berkman L, Syme SL: Social networks, host resistance, and mortality. A nine-year follow-up of Alameda County residents. Amer J of Epidem 94:105, 1979.

Blois MS: Clinical judgment and computers. New Eng J Med 303:192, 1980.

Blois MS: Conceptual issues in computer-aided diagnosis and the hierarchical nature of medical knowledge. J Med Philosophy 8:29, 1983.

Borgmann A: *Technology and the Character of Contemporary Life.* Chicago: University of Chicago Press, 1984.

Bursztajn H, Feinbloom RI, Hamm RM, Brodsky A: *Medical Choices, Medical Chances: How Patients, Families and Physicians Can Cope with Uncertainty.* New York: Delacorte Press. 1981.

Carrieri VK, Janson-Bjerklie S: Strategies patients use to manage the sensation of dyspnea. West J Nurs Res 8:284, 1986.

Collins CE: The last dogma of empiricism. Unpublished dissertation, University of California at Berkeley, 1985.

Cousins N: *Anatomy of an Illness as Perceived by the Patient: Reflections on Healing and Regeneration.* New York: Norton, 1979.

Coyle N, Foley K: Pain in patients with cancer: Profile of patients and common pain syndromes. Semin Onco Nurs 1:93, 1985.

Cox DJ, Gonder-Frederick L, Pohl S, Pennebaker, JW: Reliability of symptom-blood glucose relationships among insulin-dependent adult diabetics. Psychosom Med 45:357, 1983.

Crawford R: A cultural account of health: Self control, release, and the social body. In McKinlay J (ed): *Issues in the Political Economy of Health Care.* London: Tavistock, 1985.

Dirks JF, Kleiger JH, Evans NW: Asthma symptom checklist, panic-fear, and length of hospitalization in asthma. J of Asthma Res 515:95, 1978.

Dreyfus HL: *Being-in-the-World: A Commentary on Heidegger's Being and Time, Division I.* Cambridge, Mass.: MIT Press, in press.

Elstein A, Shulman L, Sprafka S: *Medical Problem-Solving: An Analysis of Clinical Reasoning.* Cambridge, Mass.: Harvard University Press, 1978.

Engelhardt HT Jr: Illnesses, diseases, and sickness. In Kestenbaum V (ed): *The Humanity of the Ill: Phenomenological Perspectives.* Knoxville, Tenn.: University of Tennessee Press, 1982.

Feinstein AR: *Clinical Judgment.* Baltimore: Williams and Wilkins, 1967.

Garfield S: The delivery of medical care. Sci Amer 222:15, 1970.

Haft JI, Arkel YS: Effect of emotional stress on platelet aggregation in humans. Chest 70:501, 1976.

Heidegger M: *The Basic Problems of Phenomenology.* Hofstadter A (trans). Bloomington: Indiana University Press, 1982.

Hunter RCA, Lohrenz JG, Schwartzman AE: Nosophobia and hypochondriasis in medical students. J Nerv & Mental Dis 139:147, 1964.

Kasl SV: Contributions of social epidemiology to studies in psychosomatic medicine. In Kasl SV, Reichsman R (eds): *Advances in Psychosomatic Medicine,* vol 9, pp. 160–223. Basel, Switzerland, Karger. 1977.

Kleinman A: Neurasthenia and depression: A study of somatization and culture in China. Culture Med Psychiatry. 6:117, 1982.

Kleinman A, Good B (eds): *Culture and Depression: Studies in the Anthropology and Cross-Cultural Psychiatry of Affect and Disorder.* Berkeley: University of California Press, 1985.

Kleinman A, White GM: The role of cultural explanations in "somatization" and "psychologization." Social Sci Med 16:1519, 1982.

Krieger D: *The Therapeutic Touch: How to Use Your Hands to Help or Heal.* Englewood Cliffs, N.J.: Prentice-Hall, 1979.

Krieger D: Therapeutic touch: The imprimatur of nursing. Am J Nurs 75:784, 1975.

Lionberger HJ: An interpretive study of nurses' practice of therapeutic touch. Doctoral dissertation, University of California at San Francisco, School of Nursing, 1985.

Lionberger HJ: Therapeutic touch: A healing modality or a caring strategy? In Chinn PL (ed): *Nursing Research Methodology: Issues and Implementation.* Rockville, Md.: Aspen Publishers, 1986.

McCaffrey RJ, Blanchard EB: Stress management approaches to the treatment of essential hypertension. Ann Behav Med 7:5, 1985.

Mechanic D: *Medical Sociology,* 2d ed. New York: The Free Press, 1978.

Mechanic D, Volkart EH: Stress, illness behavior and the sick role. Am Sociol Rev 26:51, 1961.

Merleau-Ponty M: *Phenomenology of Perception.* New Jersey: The Humanities Press, 1962.

Parkes CM: *Bereavement.* New York: International Universities Press, 1972.

Pellegrino E: Being ill and being healed: Some reflections on the grounding of medical morality. In *The Humanity of the Ill.* Knoxville: University of Tennessee Press, 1982.

Pennebaker JW: *The Psychology of Physical Symptoms.* New York: Springer-Verlag, 1982.

Peterson WL, Sturdevant RA, Frankl HD, et al.: Healing of duodenal ulcer with an antacid regimen. N Eng J Med 297:341, 1977.

Plaut TF: *Children with Asthma: A Manual for Parents.* Amherst, Mass.: Pedipress, 1984.

Polhemus T (ed): *The Body Reader.* New York: Pantheon, 1978.

Polhemus T: Social bodies. In Polhemus T (ed): *The Body as a Medium of Expression,* pp. 13–35. New York: Dutton, 1975.

Popell CL: An interpretive study of stress and coping among parents of school-age developmentally disabled children. Unpublished doctoral dissertation, The Wright Institute, Berkeley, California, 1983.

Review Panel on Coronary-Prone Behavior and Coronary Heart Disease. Coronary-prone behavior and coronary heart disease: A critical review. Circulation 63:1199, 1981.

Roghmann KJ, Haggerty RJ: Family stress and the use of health services. Intrnatl J Epidem 1:279, 1972.

Roghmann KJ, Haggerty RJ: The stress model for illness behavior. In Haggerty RJ, Roghmann KJ, Pless IB (eds): *Child Health and the Community.* New York: John Wiley & Sons, 1975.

Sacks O: *A Leg to Stand On.* New York: Simon & Schuster, 1984.

Scheper-Hughes N, Lock MM: The mindful body: A prolegomenon to future work in medical anthropology. Med Anthropol Q 1:6, 1987.

Schrag CO: Being in pain. In Kestenbaum V (ed): *The Humanity of the Ill: Phenomenological Perspectives,* pp. 101–124. Knoxville: University of Tennessee Press, 1982.

Schwartz WB, Patil RS, and Szolovits, P: Sounding board. Artificial intelligence in medicine where do we stand? JAMA 316:685, 1987.

Stallones RA: The rise and fall of ischemic heart disease. Sci Am 243:53, 1980.

Stein L: The doctor-nurse game. Am J Nurs 68:101, 1968.

Susser M, Stein Z: Civilization and peptic ulcer. Lancet 1:115, 1962.

Taylor C: Philosophical Papers, vols 1 and 2. Cambridge, England: Cambridge University Press, 1985.

Tessler R, Mechanic D, Dimond M: The effect of psychological distress on physician utilization: A prospective study. J Health Social Behav 17:353, 1976.

Vogt TM, Johnson RE: Recent changes in the incidence of peptic ulcer. Amer J Epid 110:353, 1979.

Wadden TA: Relaxation therapy for essential hypertension: Specific or nonspecific effects. J Psychosom Res 28:53, 1984.

Woods SM, Natterson J, Silverman J: Medical student's disease: Hypochondriasis in medical education. J Med Ed 41:785, 1966.

Woolf V: On being ill. *The Moment and Other Essays,* p. 9. New York: Harcourt, 1948.

Wrubel J: Personal meanings and coping processes. Unpublished doctoral dissertation, University of California at San Francisco, 1985.

CHAPTER SEVEN

Coping with a Coronary Illness

I am reading his body and his tones, and I am reading his exhausted-looking face, and I commented to him about that: "You look as if you need a friend. You look as if something is wrong." *Mary Cucci, RN*

In Chapters Seven, Eight, and Nine, stress and coping are examined in relation to the specific disease processes and illness experiences of coronary heart disease, cancer, and neurological injury. These diseases are the three top causes of death and disability of adults in the United States. At least one of these illnesses will be experienced directly by most Americans or indirectly by their family members.

We selected coronary heart disease, cancer, and neurological injury not only because of their prevalence but also because they illustrate the divergent social definitions and stress-and-coping issues of three life-threatening and life quality–threatening illnesses. We do not intend, nor is it a reasonable project to address, all the particulars of each *disease*. But each *illness* does bring with it common, shared meanings, meanings that arise out of cultural understandings of the illness and ways the disease is often felt and experienced as an illness by the individual. Coronary heart disease, though often life threatening, is less feared than cancer and less associated with stigma than neurological injury. Consequently, the coping issues faced by people with those illnesses do not arise for coronary patients. However, assault on the heart is symbolically an assault on life and the core of being. A heart attack can threaten the person's identity and whole life situation (Wiklund, Sanne, Vedin, and Wilhemsson 1985).

Thus, each disease poses its own threats and has its own social definition, its own particular resources, and its own constraints that are set up by different treatment and recovery patterns. All of these aspects of the disease, along with the person's own history, context, and concerns, shape the illness experience. Understanding these relationships between the illness and disease is essential to understanding stress and coping related to any illness. We will explore the meanings of the illnesses and some aspects of the illness experience to address the questions central to understanding stress and coping with illness: "What is the nature of the stress?" and "What are the actual coping demands, resources, and constraints?"

Because our focus of interest is on the relation between personal/cultural meanings and coping, and because the occurrence of coronary illness is associated with a unique set of meanings, we focus in this chapter on the psychosocial risk factors and purposely omit other known risk factors such as hypertension, smoking, family history, sedentary lifestyles, aging, presence of diabetes mellitus, and obesity. We first describe morbidity and mortality rates of the illness. Then we present the major theoretical perspectives explaining predisposition to coronary disease due to psychosocial factors. In the next two sections, we describe and compare two major intervention programs, Freidman and Ulmer's program (1984) for the person who already has coronary heart disease (CHD), and Roskies's program (1987) for healthy type A individuals. Finally we discuss stress and coping in cardiac rehabilitation.

Morbidity and Mortality Rates of Coronary Heart Disease

Coronary heart disease has been referred to as a high-status illness incurred as a result of overwork, diligence, and success (Chesney, Black, Chadwick, and Rosenman 1981). In fact, the coronary prone personality is viewed as having overadapted to the modern Western self-understanding (Roskies 1987). Interestingly, from a psychosocial perspective, CHD is a disease of the last century in modern Western civilization. The mortality rates from CHD, after being relatively stable for the previous twenty years, rose sharply in the early 1920s and continued to rise, reaching a peak in the 1950s and 1960s (Stallones 1980). Others have noted that stigma is increasingly being attached to coronary disease in the wake of the push for individuals to take more responsibility for their health (Helman 1987).

Blue-collar men are at greatest risk for CHD, white-collar men are second, and women are third. However, despite the fact that blue-collar male workers are at 43% higher risk of dying from heart disease (Hennekens 1987), the predominant focus of the research and intervention has been on white-collar male workers, a bias that calls for a reshifting of research focus. Coronary heart disease rates are still higher in men than women after statistics are corrected for alcohol consumption, marital status, personality type, smoking, and working status (Friedman, Dales, and Ury 1979; Haynes and Feinleib 1980; Talbott et al. 1977).

Ischemic heart disease has been the single greatest cause of death in the United States for more than thirty years. However, the mortality rates for CHD have begun to decline since the mid-1960s. According to Stallones (1980), the explanation for this decline is far from clear:

> Four major variables are known to be associated with the risk of ischemic heart disease in individuals. Among the four, hypertension does not fit the trend of the mortality from ischemic heart disease at all; physical activity fits only the rising curve, serum cholesterol fits only the falling curve and only cigarette smoking fits both. In no case is the fit as precise as one would like. This raises doubt that any one of the factors is a fully satisfactory explanation for the variation in mortality (p. 59).

The decline in mortality cannot easily be attributed to improved treatment of coronary heart disease because it is doubtful that these treatments have had an equal effect on males and females and whites and nonwhites across a broad age span or that the lowered trend would have occurred in California ten years before the decline began in the rest of the country (Stallones 1980). This decline in mortality rates from ischemic heart disease remains a mystery and raises questions about changing lifestyles that cannot be answered at this time.

The Association of Type A Behavior and Coronary Heart Disease

Friedman and Rosenman (1959) call the personality style that has been shown to be associated with the incidence of CHD the type A behavior pattern. Although there continues to be a great deal of controversy (see Ragland and Brand 1988, Dimsdale 1988) over the validity of the association between type A personality and coronary disease, considerable evidence supports this association (Review Panel on Coronary-Prone Behavior and Coronary Heart Disease 1981). Links between personality style and coronary disease were noted as early as

225

the end of the last century. In 1892, Osler described the coronary patient as a "keen and ambitious man . . . whose engines are set at full speed ahead." By the 1960s, empirical studies had found that the person with the type A behavior pattern was six times more likely to have severe atherosclerosis than the person with the more relaxed type B pattern (Friedman and Rosenman 1974).

The type A behavioral style has been described by Friedman and Rosenman (1959) as:

> . . . an action-emotion complex that can be observed in any person who is aggressively involved in a chronic, incessant struggle to achieve more and more in less and less time, and if required to do so, against the opposing efforts of other things or other persons. It is not psychosis or a complex of worries or fears or phobias or obsessions, but a socially acceptable— indeed often praised—form of conflict. Persons possessing this pattern also are quite prone to exhibit a free-floating but extraordinarily well-rationalized hostility (1974, p. 67).

Less controversy exists about the protective nature of the type B pattern than about the definitive aspects of the type A pattern that leads to coronary artery disease (Miller, Lack, and Asroff 1985). While the global type A behavior pattern includes both coronary prone and noncoronary prone behavior, the type B classification appears to identify accurately noncoronary prone behavior (Blumenthal, Williams, Kong, Schaneberg, and Thompson 1978; Chesney, Black, Chadwick, and Rosenman 1981; Krantz, Sanmarco, Selvester, and Matthews 1979; MacDougall, Dembroski, and Musante 1979). Currently, efforts are underway to understand the type B pattern in its own right (Chesney, Black, Chadwick, and Rosenman 1981).

Although the type A behavior pattern has now been established as a risk factor for CHD, it remains to be discovered what it *is* theoretically and how it works physiologically. Research in individual reactivity is providing promising new insights. Laboratory studies have demonstrated that, while type A and type B subjects do not differ in their baseline physiological measures, the type A behavior pattern is associated with greater elevations in blood pressure, heart rate, cortisol, epinephrine, and norepinephrine in response to certain kinds of threatening or challenging situations (Dembroski 1978, Williams et al. 1982, Glass et al. 1983, Krantz and Manuck 1984). People with the type A behavior pattern may be said to be more physiologically reactive than type B's in situations that evoke type A concerns, for example, situations that are competitive, time-dependent, and uncontrollable (Glass et al. 1983).

Type A individuals who show the strongest behavioral reactions to the Structured Interview (the interview designed by Friedman and Rosenman to assess the type A or type B behavior pattern) also show the greatest physiological response. It is not surprising that the Structured Interview demonstrates this relationship, since it acts as a challenge. By contrast, Roskies (1987) reports that about half the studies using the Jenkins Activity Scale, which does not provide a challenge nor elicit behavioral style, fail to demonstrate the relationship between laboratory stress, behavioral pattern, and physiological response.

Genetic and other biologic factors may also predispose the person to hyper-reactivity regardless of the behavioral classification (Kahn et al. 1980, Obrist 1981, Glass et al. 1983). Kahn et al. (1980), in a study of diastolic blood pressure during coronary artery bypass surgery, found that patients with type A behavior characteristics manifested significantly greater autonomic hyperactivity than type B patients even under general anesthesia. The relationship may be set up by a bodily predisposition (the inborn complex), or by physiological changes that occur as a result of the habitual, skilled bodily responses, or through a complex relationship between the two (Kahn et al. 1980). It is plausible to think that the body constitutes situational responses, and is further constituted (shaped or altered) by the responses to situations over time. This line of research is promising and needs to be extended by more longitudinal, naturalistic studies.

During the last five years, research efforts have focused on the specific aspects of this behavioral style that are linked with the actual disease. This is the classical empirical strategy of isolating the "elemental" cause or causes as definitively as possible. For example, Dembroski et al. (1985) state:

> . . . it is clear that some aspects of the TABP are probably more important than others in mediating an association between globally defined TABP and CHD endpoints. Thus, an important task is to isolate the specific components of the multidimensional TABP that are consistently related to CHD (p. 220).

If it is possible to separate out some quite particular behaviors that are highly associated with a type A rating, then a simple but highly predictive measure of those at risk for coronary disease could be developed. For example, a rapid and emphatic speech style is part of the type A pattern, but some researchers think that the particularly predictive feature is the degree of explosiveness of speech. They are trying to develop an assessment for explosiveness of speech separate from the other stylistic elements of speech and separate from the content of what is said.

Other researchers have been taking a different approach. Rather than trying to increase the predictive power of the type A pattern by searching for isolatable elements, they have tried to understand just what that pattern is and how it works in day-to-day life. The following section is devoted to an examination of five approaches to a theoretical understanding of type A behavior pattern. These approaches are presented because we believe that in the case of the coronary-prone behavior pattern, the success of the search for traits, or isolatable elements, will be limited because the type A behavior pattern is transactional and a manifestation of an ontological stance. By "transactional" we mean that the behavioral style is elicited by transactions with particular situational demands. And by "ontological stance" we mean that the type A pattern derives from the way the individual takes up cultural background meanings. These meanings become a basic way of being in the world and relating to others. If these explanations of the type A pattern are correct, then identifying isolated "elements" predictive of the disease will not further our understanding of how the type A pattern is lived out. Nor will the elements alone suggest how particular meanings and concerns set up the type A behavior pattern.

The current theoretical constructs for the type A behavior pattern may be divided into five major categories: (a) overadjustment to the modern Western culture exemplified by a technological self-understanding, the Protestant work ethic, and utilitarian individualism; (b) a pattern of vacillation from extreme efforts to control the environment to its opposite extreme of learned helplessness and giving up; (c) an interactional view using the person-environment fit model that suggests that type A behavior is elicited by environments that do not match the person's style and interests; (d) hostility and chronic anger; and (e) self-involvement. Each one of these explanatory views is discussed below and followed by a synthesis from a phenomenological perspective.

OVERADJUSTMENT TO MODERN CULTURE

One recurrent plausible explanation for type A behavior is that it is an overadjustment to the modern Western culture (Benner 1984,

Cohen 1978, Marmot and Syme 1976, Cohen et al. 1979, Cohen and Reed 1985, Roskies 1987, Helman 1987). The composite picture of the type A worker is one who works hard and long under constant deadline pressures and extreme work overload, experiences time as an adversary, finds leisure and relaxation stressful (indeed, often chooses strenuous or busy recreation), constantly competes with internal high standards, experiences work and achievement more in terms of quantity than quality, and prefers work that he or she can control.

These American work meanings stem from two major traditions, the Protestant work ethic (Berger, Berger, and Kellner 1974; Glock and Bellah 1976; Gouldner 1971; Weber 1958; Yankelovich 1981) and utilitarian individualism (Bellah et al. 1985, Gouldner 1971, Tipton 1982). In a study of work meanings of mid-career men, Benner (1984) found tensions between the "duty-to-duty" meanings of the Protestant work ethic and the "duty-to self-fulfillment," which is the more recent variation of the utilitarian tradition (see also Yankelovich 1981). In both of these traditions, personal worth is demonstrated through acquisition, gain, and winning. Success is a sign of God's election in the work ethic tradition. In the utilitarian tradition, success is a sign of personal worth and fosters self-esteem. Both traditions share a goal-oriented structure of meaning, so that striving toward a goal can be more important in both traditions than actual goal achievement (Benner 1984):

> The duty to duty, the penchant for activity, the future-oriented structure of meaning, and the experience of time as an adversary are background meanings that go hand-in-hand in the utilitarian and protestant work ethic traditions. When any of these meanings become the ascendent meaning of work, a means-ends displacement occurs (see Merton 1968). The individual substitutes a commitment to a certain way of going about his or her work for a commitment to the work itself. While a commitment to the means or way of getting one's work done can supply the motivation and perseverance needed to get the job done, it cannot supply the joy or sense of reward in the actual concrete content of the work itself. . . .
>
> The person who does his duty for duty's sake can feel morally upright but is denied the fulfillment of having his particular talents, interests, and abilities solicited by work. When others do not sanction or value duty for duty's sake, he loses out on his feeling of being upright and exemplary. . . . The person who has an adversarial relation to time use can feel trapped in excessive demands on himself. . . . A future-oriented structure of meaning proves troublesome for the person who has reached his major goals (pp. 67–68).

The type A worker operates from a "control" paradigm and seeks increasing control and rationalization of his or her environment (Glass 1977). This picture also fits the cultural press for increased rationalization and control prevalent in the Enlightenment tradition and the current technological age (see Bellah et al. 1985, Borgmann 1984, Dreyfus and Rabinow 1982, Heidegger 1962, Shils 1981, Helman, 1987). The extreme form of the modern technological perspective causes the person to understand the self and the environment as raw material to be shaped and controlled by the individual (see the discussion on p. 51). The way this shows up is illustrated in an interview excerpted from Benner (1984):

> It has got to be perfect. I don't know how many times my mother said to me: "Anything worth doing is worth doing well." And it stuck! It didn't matter whether it was in my professional career or in my singing. I was seldom happy with a performance because I demanded more of myself. Same thing is true on the job. You have got to be number one. There is no other place (p. 79).

The quest for autonomy and control can interfere with a sense of interdependence and connectedness. The individual becomes hyperresponsible and cannot trust that others will behave responsibly unless he or she controls or shapes their behavior. From an ethic of utilitarian individualism, the most one can expect from anyone else is an enlightened self-interest. Thus, one's own interests are safe only as long as they coincide with another's. Such a self-understanding easily leads to mistrust, vigilance, and anger over infringements.

Evidence for the link between acculturation to Western culture and CHD comes from Marmot and Syme's study (1976) of Japanese in Japan, Hawaii, and the United States. They found that there was a systematic increase in coronary disease among Japanese living in Hawaii and California. The steepest increase was seen among those Japanese who dropped their traditional Japanese culture and took on American cultural practices (Marmot and Syme 1976).

Understanding excessive aggressiveness, hostility, and competitive individualism as an extreme form of adapting to the Protestant work ethic, utilitarian individualism, and technological self-understanding does not explain why the type B person does not take up this extreme cultural stance. One explanation for the variation in the way these traditions are taken up lies not only in the other options for self-understanding and practices that are available from diverse ethnic groups in the culture but also from many remaining forms of community such as the biblical and republican traditions evident in American life (Bellah et al. 1985).

VACILLATION FROM EFFORTFUL CONTROL TO LEARNED HELPLESSNESS

A second explanation for the type A behavior pattern, based upon Glass's empirical findings (1977), draws on Seligman's learned helplessness theory (Seligman 1975). Seligman's theory is based primarily on animal research. Animals failed to avoid electric shock when possible because of having been conditioned to a "no avoidance" situation (Overmeier and Seligman 1967, Seligman and Maier 1967). Seligman (1975) developed the concept of learned helplessness to account for depression; however the model has not held up consistently in experiments with people (Cutrona 1983, Dobson and Shaw 1981).

Glass (1977) found that type A people have a high need for control and exert great effort to control situations. When control is impossible, however, they give up and experience extreme apathy. According to Glass, type A behavior is based on the Western notion that it is possible to control one's environment, but when type A people are confronted with the limits of control they have an extreme response of giving up. Glass concludes that it is this vacillation between high mobilization and hyporeactivity that damages the coronary arteries.

AN INTERACTIONAL PERSPECTIVE—THE PERSON-ENVIRONMENT FIT

The person-environment fit model examines the relationship between personal dispositions and the environmental match or fit (Campbell 1973; Caplan 1971; French and Caplan 1972; Harrison 1976, 1978; Thoresen and Ohman 1987). In a study of the relationships between work environment and blood pressure of type A and type B men, no significant main effect associations were found with work environment and CHD risk factors except for comfort (Chesney, Sevelius, Black, Ward, Swan, and Rosenman 1981). Workers who described their work environments as comfortable had a lower mean systolic blood pressure (128.19 mm Hg) than those who described their work environment as uncomfortable (mean systolic blood pressure 133.06 mm Hg). However, on three work environment variables—peer cohesion, autonomy, and physical comfort—there were significant type A-B behavior pattern interaction effects. The type A men fared better in environments with high autonomy and high peer cohesion, and they were indifferent to physical comfort. By contrast, the type B men fared better (had lower blood pressure) in environments that did not stress autonomy, where peer cohesion was low, and that were comfortable. Chesney, Sevelius, Black, Ward, Swan, and Rosenman (1981) explain these differences in terms of person-environment fit. The type A person prefers autonomy and because of extroversion fares better in a cohesive group. By contrast, the type B person is more introverted and is less stressed by groups whose cohesiveness is low and in environments where there is little demand for autonomy. Type B people are more sensitive to their environmental comfort, whereas type A people tend not to notice physical discomfort, including fatigue (Carver, Coleman, and Glass 1976; Weidner and Matthews 1978).

The person-environment fit model is an attempt to capture the interactional nature of the type A behavior pattern, which is not usually conceptualized as a personality trait but rather as an interaction between susceptible individuals and challenging environments (Matthews 1982).

CHRONIC HOSTILITY AND ANGER

Chronic anger and hostility have always been a part of the type A behavior construct (Friedman and Ulmer 1984). However, Williams, Barefoot, and Shekelle (1985) report that chronic anger and hostility appeared to be independent of the components of the type A behavior pattern. Researchers (Barefoot, Dahlstrom, and Williams 1983; Williams et al. 1980) have found that a hostility subscale derived from the MMPI correlates more strongly with arteriographically documented coronary atherosclerosis than the more global assessment of the type A behavior pattern. Hostility by this subscale as defined by Cook and Medley (1954, as cited by Williams et al. 1980, p. 541) is characterized by a person "who has little confidence in his fellow man. He sees people as dishonest, unsocial, immoral, ugly and mean, and believes that they should be made to suffer for their sins . . . hostility amounts to chronic hate and anger."

Further emphasis on the clinical link between chronic anger and hostility was given by a reanalysis of the original Friedman and Rosenman Western Collaborative Group Study (WGCS) conducted by Spielberger (reported by Roskies 1987). Spielberger conducted a principal components analysis. He found that one major factor, described as the anger-hostility factor, accounted for over 65% of the variance.

Rapid psychomotor movement, a high drive level, and job involvement were not predictive of coronary disease.

Dembroski (1978) defines a potential for hostility evident in the structured interview to assess type A behavior when:

> Responses are argumentative, repeatedly and unnecessarily qualified, pointlessly challenging of the interviewer. The voice characteristics suggest boredom, condescension, or surliness. Subject's answers to specific questions suggest impatience and irritability when faced with obstacles and the tendency to make harsh generalizations. Extreme levels of hostility may be accompanied by obscenity and the use of emotion laden words (p. 103).

Matthews et al. (1977), in a reanalysis of the WCGS, found that only seven items discriminated those who had coronary disease from their age-matched healthy controls. Three of the seven items directly dealt with self-reported competitiveness and the remaining three dealt with items that demonstrate a potential for hostility as described above.

Dembroski et al. (1985), in a study of 131 patients (98 men and 33 women) who underwent diagnostic coronary angiography at Duke University Medical Center, found that two factors, potential for hostility and anger in (a style of coping with anger by keeping the anger to oneself), were consistent predictors of disease endpoints. Furthermore, they found that increases in potential for hostility were associated with increased disease only for patients who coped with anger by holding it in. They caution that this is the first indication of this interaction and that further replication is warranted. Hostility was conceptualized in this study as:

> . . . a relatively stable predisposition in a variety of circumstances to experience varying degrees and combinations of anger, irritation, disgust, annoyance, contempt, resentment, and the like that may or may not be associated with overt behavior directed against the source of frustration (Dembroski et al. 1985).

Mary Hartfield (1985) studied anger appraisals and coping responses in thirty white adult normotensives and thirty white adult hypertensives between the ages of 35 and 55. She found that the two groups did not differ on anger frequency or negative emotional feeling about the anger situation. However, the groups differed in the way they experienced their anger:

Hypertensives experienced their anger more intensely, for a longer duration, felt more physical symptoms during the anger episode and inhibited expressing their anger. They used more distancing, self-controlling and escape-avoidance behaviors in coping with their anger than normotensives. They were bothered more by the daily hassles of living than normotensives. In contrast, normotensives were more likely to confront the situation and seek social support when involved in an anger situation (p. 84).

In an interpretive analysis of this same data set, Hartfield (1985) found that violations of codes of conduct and threats to the self (e.g., "loss of face," humiliation, and threats to self-esteem) were the most common themes in the anger episodes. The appraisal and coping pattern that had the most negative effects (more expressive reactions and physical symptoms) involved an appraisal of personal threat (regardless of the cause) with an inability to deal effectively with the situation and an internalization of feelings. Sixteen hypertensives and only three normotensives exhibited this appraisal and coping pattern. Hartfield's (1985) work has promising implications for interventions that focus on teaching people to understand their anger appraisal and coping patterns and to learn new patterns when the pattern is particularly troublesome.

Roskies (1987) points out that the isolation of the importance of hostility for the pathogenesis of coronary disease has implications for intervention programs aimed at the portion of the type A behavior pattern that is damaging to health. But she warns against overlooking the evidence from questionnaires such as the JAS (Jenkins 1978), the Framingham (Haynes, Levine, Scotch, Feinleib, and Kannel 1978), and the Bortner (1969), which have also shown hard-driving work involvement, speed, and impatience to also be predictive of CHD.

SELF-INVOLVEMENT

Self-involvement has been measured by counting the number of times the person uses the first person pronoun or directly refers to the self. In a study of college psychology students (twenty-three type A people and twenty-two type B people), Scherwitz, Berton, and Leventhal (1978) found that type A people were more self-involved than type B people were as reflected by the number of times the personal pronouns *I*, *me*, or *my* were used in the structured interview and in their expression of anger and distress. The number of self-references by type A people correlated with their speech characteristics, anger and distress intensity, blood pressure, heart rate, and finger pulse amplitude. These authors reason that self-involved individuals would also be self-aware (not to be confused with insightful). Lovallo and Pishkin (1980) replicated the results of Scherwitz et al. that type A people who made frequent self-references show higher resting systolic blood pressure and greater cutaneous vasoconstriction.

Scherwitz et al. (1978, 1983) point to research by Scheier and Carver (1974) indicating that when individuals are made more self-aware through the use of mirrors, the number of emotional reactions to slides that induce feelings of attraction, repulsion, elation, or depression are increased. Also, Carver (1974) found that subjects in the presence of a mirror give more electric shocks to an experimental accomplice who provoked them. Increased self-awareness may increase responsiveness to challenge, the hallmark of type A behavior.

Scherwitz et al. (1983) assessed 150 men referred for angiographic study or coronary bypass surgery for type A behavior using the structured interview, two questionnaire measures, and the number of self-references (I, me, my) made during the structured interview. They found that the self-references emerged as an independent correlate of the extent of coronary artery disease and that the other standard instruments were not correlated with the degree of coronary heart disease as measured by the number of occluded arteries, the index of disease severity, the number of myocardial infarctions, and the results of the exercise stress test. A separate analysis was conducted to rule out the possibility that the severity of the illness itself caused increased self-involvment, however, this analysis revealed a stronger correlation with self-referencing with those who had no previous myocardial infarctions. The authors speculate that self-involvement contributes to and is increased by anger and repression.

SYNTHESIS OF THE TYPE A BEHAVIOR PATTERN EXPLANATIONS

From a phenomenological perspective, all of the above explanations are interrelated. Precision, in terms of isolating the exact weight of each of the contributing causes, may only cloud our understanding of the lived meanings of type A behavior pattern, i.e., the way of being in the world that contributes to the type A behavior pattern. Each of these empirically derived aspects of the type A behavior pattern reflects a particular whole way of understanding the self and the world that is embodied.

The person does not take up type A meanings formally and explicitly. For this reason, it is inaccurate to think of this cultural pattern as being one of explicitly adopted formal beliefs. Instead, this behavior pattern is embedded in cultural practices, skills, expectations, social norms, and the cultural body. For example, the logic of the quest for control is based on the technological self-understanding that things do not work well on their own and that both situations and self are raw material that must be directed and controlled by the individual. However, control in the practical world is tenuous and constantly thwarted. If control is a central personal concern, then chronic agitation over the limits of control may well lead to generalized hostility and irritation. Also, the quest for control limits relationships with others to contractual agreements that end in chronic negotiations about getting and giving (see Yankelovich 1981).

The modern technological self-understanding is extremely individualistic and clouds the understanding of the self as member participant. This way of being in the world naturally spawns self-preoccupation and self-protection. From the phenomenological perspective of the type A behavior pattern as a way of being in the world (a system of interrelated meanings), empirical findings of self-involvement are a consequence of understanding the self as a private, separate compilation of needs that must be chosen and met by the individual (Maslow 1943).

Radley (1984) calls attention to the problem of narrowing the concept of the type A behavior pattern in the service of greater predictive utility. He notes that the earlier success of Rosenman and Friedman came not from precise psychological constructs but from close attention to the clinical presentation of coronary patients. Radley points up that the psychological aspects of coronary patients are *embodied* and *embedded* in a social milieu. He argues:

> To separate mind from body ("behavior pattern" from "cardiac function") in one's conceptualization is to create a juxtaposition of mentalism and physicalism by restricting mind within behaviour (or personality) and reifying the body (p. 1229).

Radley (1984) goes on to suggest that the body be understood as a "distribution of muscular tonicity in view of future action." Such characteristic body expressions as tension, impatience, and fatigue must be understood in terms of what the body is straining toward—the aims, goals, concerns, and meanings of the person. This is similar to Merleau-Ponty's (1962) notion of the body as "intentional tissue."

Radley suggests that coronary heart disease patients set up symmetrical social relationships of struggle and competition in which they live out their intolerance for dependency or inactivity. When challenged (and challenge becomes easier and more frequent as all others are viewed as idealized others and competitors in opposition to the self), type A people respond with passionate, obsessive activity in order to feel in control. This overactivity may continue until the person collapses with exhaustion. It is the oscillation between extreme activity and passivity that is believed to create the damage to the arteries (Glass 1977).

The passion for overactivity in work should not be confused with work where the person is involved and attuned to the requirements of the task (Radley 1984). The overactivity of the type A person is of a frenzied, unrealistic quality. It is an overinternalization of the quest to acquire and achieve more and more in less and less time. Friedman and Ulmer (1984) aptly cite Alexis de Tocqueville's (1945) interpretation of this common American meaning:

> He who has set his heart exclusively upon the pursuit of worldly welfare is always in a hurry, for he has but a limited time at his disposal to reach it, to grasp it and to enjoy it. . . . Besides the good things which he possesses, he every instant fancies a thousand others which death will prevent him from trying if he does not try them soon (p. 145).

The four major conceptualizations of the type A behavior pattern reflect an embodied and socially embedded web of meanings and self-understanding. They do not conflict with one another but rather depict a whole way of being in the world. Left unanswered is the question of why some people in the culture are seemingly immune from this highly individualistic, competitive, hostile, hurried way of being in the world.

Coronary heart disease is primarily a man's disease. Although the incidence of coronary disease among women is on the rise, the rate still does not approach the rate for men. Second, the behavioral qualities exemplified by the type A behavior pattern are accepted, even valued, qualities in men in our culture. We commonly believe (although research does not support this belief) that this type of man is successful in work. These aspects of how the type A behavior pattern is regarded all reflect cultural meanings, meanings that have ceased to work well for us and that we have come to reflect on as an entire community. The women's movement has, over the past decade, uncovered and interpreted many of our shared cultural meanings that have given men status and denigrated women. American business has recently been involved in interpreting its own meanings, especially those relating to competition versus cooperation. Cultural comparisons with the Japanese have led to attempts to develop new management practices in our own businesses.

These are all necessary and worthy efforts to find new possibilities, new ways of interpreting our cultural meanings in daily life. But the nature of cultural background meaning—namely, that it is the light that illuminates the world and not a thing in itself and that it is lived out in daily practices that are usually not reflected upon—means that changing practices in one area will not automatically change all the others. This, then, is the challenge for health care promotion today: to bring the entire community to reflect on our positive regard for those common understandings and practices that support type A behavior. Change cannot occur until we recognize that the type A pattern is a culturally promoted way of being and not strictly an individual choice. A positive regard for speed, aggression, and extreme individualism creates an unhealthy tension between individual and group life. Only a cultural dialogue about these self-understandings and practices can resolve this tension and effect change. Although this challenge has not yet been taken up as an effort to change cultural meanings in the entire community, health care researchers have taken on the task of changing the practices of type A men themselves.

Helman (1987) concludes that the type A behavior pattern is a culture-bound syndrome because it symbolizes "core meanings and behavioral norms of the community" (p. 975). The debate is a moral one between right and wrong behavior: between the societal press for acquisition of capital, competitiveness, efficiency, and speed and the conflict that these behaviors engender in smaller social groupings. Helman (1987) claims that the type A behavior pattern, as a culture-bound illness, plays a role in expressing and resolving social conflict between the societal press for the type A behavior and the social conflict engendered by it. He identifies the following polar opposites in the moral debate: hostile versus friendly; competitive versus non-competitive; impatient versus patient; work oriented versus family-oriented; obsessed with time versus indifferent to time; modern versus

238

traditional; and masculine versus feminine. Helman (1987) points out that seeing the type A coronary heart disease as a culture-bound syndrome does not make it less true or real, nor less valuable in predicting and preventing coronary heart disease.

From a phenomenological perspective, all diseases and illnesses have a cultural aspect, since cultural meanings are taken up and lived out in daily habits, skills, and social patterns, and are finally embodied. However, in a scientific approach, underlying moral debates about illnesses are covered over in the quest to objectify the contributing variables and control for them without interfering in values or personal perferences. But, as Helman (1987) points out, the quest for objectivity fails and the cultural debate about preferred ways of living and being in the world show up in the characterization of the illness, in the prescribed treatments, and in the characterization of the patients themselves.

The debate over appropriate interventions has heated up even more since Ragland and Brand's (1988) study of the survival patterns of 257 male patients with CHD from the initial 8.5-year phase of the Western Collaborative Group Study (Rosenman, Brand, Sholtz, and Friedman 1976). This study demonstrated that the mortality rate associated with the 160 type A patients was unexpectedly lower than the mortality rate of type B patients (19.1 per 1000 for type A patients, and 31.7 per 1000 for type B patients, $p = .04$). Ragland and Brand conclude that type A behavior does not indicate an adverse prognosis for type A people with CHD.

Dimsdale (1988), in commenting on Ragland and Brand's study, reflects the passion of the cultural and scientific debate about the type A personality:

> First, there has been far too much fervor on both sides of the argument. Disappointed protagonists have been all too ready to dismiss summarily the findings of studies contradicting theirs, instead of asking what such contradictory findings may mean. Dispassionate efforts to replicate findings are uncommon in this field (p. 111).

Reforming versus Transforming the Type A Behavior Pattern

Two major intervention programs have been researched: Friedman and Ulmer's San Francisco Recurrent Coronary Prevention

239

Project (1984), a clinical trial designed for patients who had already suffered one heart attack, and the Montreal Type A Intervention Project designed by Ethel Roskies (1987), a clinical trial designed to alter type A behavior in healthy type A managers. These two intervention programs make an interesting comparison because one aims at preventing a recurrence of heart attack and one aims at preventing the first attack and also because the assumptions underlying the programs differ markedly. Friedman and Ulmer (1984) take the stance that the type A behavior pattern is maladjusted and ill advised, and that old beliefs, goals, and ways of living have to be radically altered. Roskies (1987), by contrast, views the type A person as a successful coper whose coping efforts are too expensive personally. Therefore, the intervention program is aimed at helping the type A person to live out the same meanings and pursue the same goals more efficiently using less personal energy in the process. Friedman and Ulmer take an insight-oriented counseling approach, and Roskies takes a cognitive-behavioral stress-management approach.

The Friedman and Ulmer program undermines and challenges the control paradigm, the technological self-understanding, and encourages the participants to abandon quantitative language and to enrich their lives with metaphorical thinking, literature, and, if accessible to the person, religious faith. Friedman and Ulmer (1985) are careful to avoid the instrumental trap of suggesting religion to change type A behavior. Instead, they recommend a rediscovery and reappropriation of religious faith as a possible alternative self-understanding if such a reappropriation is compatible with the person's history and beliefs.

Friedman and Ulmer (1984) recommend that the type A person replace old beliefs with new ones. They outline the following major beliefs that the person must change: "My sense of time urgency has helped me gain social and economic success" (the belief that the person cannot do anything about his or her sense of time urgency). "My covert insecurity is too deep-seated to change." They recommend: "Pay attention to things worth being." They clearly evaluate type A behavior as negative and urge their participants to repair their damaged personalities:

> Just as your sense of time urgency makes you feel you can't spare the time for memory, it makes you feel that you are too rushed to take part in the lives of your friends or your family, even to be truly interested in them . . . your sense of time urgency is progressively expunging all color and complexity from your thinking and your speech, as "how much" and "how

many" take over. Figures of speech, similes, metaphors—all these wither and die. In a very real sense you more and more begin to resemble a binary computer (p. 185).

Friedman and Ulmer (1984) are challenging the modern self-understanding of the individual as isolated, increasingly acquisitive, and competitive. They encourage participants to focus on memorable events, and to enhance their language with qualities and metaphors in order to recover the self as member and participant. Their program seeks to create transformation at the ontological level, the level of being and self-understanding.

Groups who underwent Friedman and Ulmer's counseling program plus traditional medical advice had significantly fewer recurrences of myocardial infarction than control groups who received only traditional medical advice (avoid vegetable or animal fat, strenuous physical exercise, and high altitudes). In the group receiving type A behavioral counseling plus the traditional medical advice, the recurrence of myocardial infarction was reduced by almost 50%, as compared to 7.2% to 13.2% in subjects who received only cardiologic counseling (Friedman et al. 1984, Freidman and Ulmer 1984).

The Roskies program, in contrast to the Friedman and Ulmer program, does not challenge the control paradigm but rather strives to make the participants more effective in operating *within* the control paradigm. The goal of the program is not ontological, having to do with being, but rather epistemological, having to do with knowlege and skills:

> First, and perhaps most important, this model is as much a recognition of health as a diagnosis of illness; in emphasizing the task accomplishments of type A's, this model makes a clear distinction between the healthy type A, whose general mastery of the environment is demonstrated by the ability to fulfill multiple and complex social roles, and "sick" individuals unable to manage basic environmental demands. . . .
>
> A second advantage of this model is that it does not threaten cherished goals but simply seeks to improve the methods used to reach these goals. Stress management for healthy type A's is not an attempt to reconstruct the individual in the image of the "healthy personality," or even to refashion him or her according to the tastes and preferences of the therapist. For instance, if a given type A values occupational achievement more than personal relationships, then the purpose of the intervention is not to alter that preference in favor of closer family ties. Similarly, one would not seek to change a life-style based on serial sexual conquests into

one committed to monogamy, or to advocate quiet walks in the woods to a devotee of gambling at Las Vegas. Instead, the scope of the program is limited to showing individuals how to use resources more efficiently in pursuing existing goals and commitments (pp. 50–51).

Roskies' program turns the control quest inward. Her stance is the classic therapeutic stance that avoids any discourse on the notion of what end or good is worth pursuing and focuses on means and efficiency (see MacIntyre 1981):

> The rationale for modifying self-talk is a simple one: We seek to modify our thinking, not because certain thoughts are wrong, or irrational, but simply because they are unproductive. By now the notion of efficient use of energy should be well implanted in a group. Unproductive thinking, by definition, is that which leads to inefficient use of time (p. 148).

Healthy type A people in the Montreal Type A Intervention Project (Roskies 1987) were taught how to use relaxation techniques, how to recognize physical signs of tension and fatigue, how to control behavioral and cognitive responses to stress, and how to develop stress resistance through planning for rest and recuperation. This program was superior in reducing behavioral reactivity as measured by the Structured Interview in healthy type A managers than aerobic exercise and weight-training programs.

Although the underlying assumptions of these two programs differ markedly, both may actually alter self-understanding. The new skills of relaxation and self-talk in the Roskies (1987) program may well change the person's way of being in situations without deliberate attention to values and beliefs. If the phenomenological view that meanings are embodied is accepted, then focus on changing bodily habits through relaxation, exercise, and attention to bodily responses would produce changes in meaning. Support for this hypothesis is provided by two studies demonstrating that beta blockers decrease cardiovascular reactivity and the intensity of the type A behavior pattern (Krantz, Baum, and Singer 1983; Schmieder, Friedrich, Neus, Rudel, and Von Eiff 1983).

Roskies' program was designed for healthy type A people, and the long-term effectiveness of the program in diminishing recurring myocardial infarctions is yet unstudied. The divergence of these two programs may reflect the difference in situation and life experience of the person who has had a heart attack versus the healthy type A person. It may be easier for the person who has succumbed to a myocardial infarction to reexamine basic assumptions and thus be motivated from a sense of crisis to engage in more profound change as a result of the chaos and unfreezing of old patterns (Wiklund, Sanne, Vedin, and Wilhelmsson 1985).

These two treatment programs engage in a cultural dialogue about the notion of good and social acceptibility embedded in the meanings inherent in type A behavior patterns. The Friedman and Ulmer (1984) interpretation is that the type A behavior pattern is culturally, socially, and personally undesirable, whereas Roskies' assumption is that the type A pattern is a successful but inefficient coping pattern and that the therapist cannot make judgments on the soundness of the underlying values. The divergent appraisals of the type A behavior reflected in these two programs point to a cultural dialogue about preferred ways of being. In our program success at the expense of health, relaxation, and close social ties is deemed culturally unworthy, and, in the second program speed, efficiency, and maximizing one's potential through individual coping effort is valued.

Coping and Rehabilitation Following a Heart Attack

A heart attack is sudden, shocking, and life threatening. A small myocardial infarction may be healed within six to eight weeks; however, large infarctions may require three to six months for a firm scar to develop (Hackett et al. 1986). Although a great proportion of patients physically recover from the *disease* with a "firm scar," the *illness* may be more tenacious. Many patients may consider themselves more damaged than warranted by the physical signs of recovery. Also, many patients recover only to have a "high incidence of emotional disturbance, pessimism, self-reported symptoms, avoidance behaviour, and sexual decline" and the belief that they are severely impaired during convalescence and even one year after (Gulledge 1979; Wiklund, Sanne, Vedin, and Wilhelmsson 1985).

The type A behavior pattern includes the use of activity as a protection against anxiety and loss of control. Consequently, it is not surprising that a convalescence period of forced inactivity would commonly bring anxiety, depression, weakness, fear of sexual arousal, and disturbed sleep (Gulledge 1979). Frankenhaeuser, Lundberg, and Forsman (1980) found that type A persons were equally aroused by inactivity and work, whereas type B persons were more aroused by work than inactivity as measured by catecholamine and cortisol excretion and heart rate. Frankenhaeuser et al. (1980) concluded that type A people may suffer health risks because of their inability to cope with inactivity and that it is stressful to deprive the type A person of work. The problem of inactivity during convalescence for the coronary patient has strong implications for the development of comprehensive rehabilitation programs that deal with psychological distress, social support systems, exercise, and sexual counseling.

Excessive fear coupled with overprotection by significant others can excessively restrict the recovering patient's activities. Extreme inactivity can lead to physical deconditioning with its sequelae of tachycardia, orthostatic hypotension, shortness of breath, and weakness. These in turn lead the patient to conclude that his or her cardiac impairment is indeed severe (Gulledge 1979, Wenger 1973). This pattern of overprotection and inactivity may become totalizing so that the person's primary way of being in the world and relating to others is that of "cardiac invalid" (Gulledge 1979). The longer this pattern is left unchallenged, the more difficult it will be for the patient and his or her social network to change this social definition of the illness.

The role of family and social network in mortality and quality of life has begun to receive increasing attention (Chandra et al. 1983, Lynch 1977, Ruberman et al. 1984). In a study of the impact of marital status on survival after a heart attack, Chandra et al. (1983) found that the adjusted hospital case fatality rate was 19.7%, whereas for unmarried males it was 26.7% (p = 0.05). The results were similar for women, with the case fatality rate for married females at 23.3% and 37.4% for unmarried females (p = 0.05). A ten-year follow up of 888 heart attack patients also showed a significantly better survival rate for the married compared to the unmarried males and females (Chandra et al. 1983). Ruberman et al. (1984) found that patients classified as being socially isolated and as having a high degree of life stress had more than four times the risk of death than the men with low levels of both stress and isolation.

A World Health Organization report underlines the importance of family support for recovery, indicating that strong family support that is reasonable and not overprotective is the key to limiting cardiac impairment. The spouse, which is more often the wife, may suffer as much psychological disturbance as the husband (Croog, Levine, and Lurie 1968). Crawshaw (1974) provides a vivid description:

It has been said that the patient may recover from his coronary but that his wife may not. She has often seen her husband when he looked near to death, she may have been warned that he could die. . . . She has the same fears, lack of knowledge and misconceptions as her husband. . . . Months after the infarct many wives report that they lie awake listening to their husband's breathing to make sure that he is still alive. . . . She may also collapse under the strain of anxiety, become sick, depressed, develop chest pains. . . . Alternatively, wives may take over decision-making and bread-winning roles and become highly overprotective; this may increase the patient's feelings of helplessness and despondency (p. 258).

The situations of the patient and spouse are markedly different but can be equally trying in their own ways. The spouse may be less able to engage in denial initially because she or he observes the patient's distress directly but cannnot directly apprehend relief from pain or a sense of returning strength. If the patient has many high-risk behaviors, such as smoking and overwork, the spouse may feel trapped by a need to change the spouse's dangerous behavior and frustrated by the spouse's continued high-risk behaviors. Thus, the disease may affect only one, but the illness can be experienced by close loved ones. The patient education and rehabilitation efforts have to be aimed at the patient and significant others.

Just as there is controversy surrounding the role of type A behavior in the etiology of coronary artery disease, so is there controversy about the importance of changing type A behavior for recovery and recurrence (Ragland and Brand 1988, Case et al. 1985). Case et al. (1985) studied 866 patients in a variety of community and university hospitals from one to three years following a heart attack and found that type A behavior as measured by the Jenkins Activity Survey did not increase the mortality risk. The physiological factors of low ejection fraction (less than .40), ventricular ectopy (greater than 10 beats per hour), pulmonary rales that were more than bibasilar at entry, and New York Heart Association Class II to IV before enrollment were the only ones that contributed to a significant and independent mortality risk. This study suffers from the known weakness of the Jenkins Activity Survey in predicting clinically relevant events and in the variability of enrollment in the study from one to three years. Nevertheless, it adds to the controversy over what aspects should be included in a comprehensive rehabilitation program for patients having had a heart attack.

The consensus is that the rehabilitation program for the patient should be comprehensive, that is, it should include information and support groups for significant others, counseling or other approaches to altering the stressful aspects of the type A behavior pattern, a stress-management component, sexual counseling, a physical reconditioning program, early counseling and planning for return to work, and modification of high-risk behaviors such as smoking and obesity (Wenger, Almeida-Feo, and Rosenthal 1985; Hackett 1986; Halhuber 1986). The demands for change are great, and they may be made against a background of fear, anxiety, and depression.

The heart attack confronts the patient with the possibility of dying and with the limits of control. However, all the treatments for heart attack assume that the disease is controllable. These treatments include angioplasty, pharmocological strategies, coronary artery bypass surgery, stress management and lifestyle change, or all of the above. Unlike the patient with cancer, the coronary patient is typically treated with the hope of improvement even in the extreme end stages of heart disease. The assumption is that the disease can be controlled, even if the solution turns out to be a heart transplant. This view that heart disease is controllable radically alters patient, family, and health care workers' understanding of the disease and the possible coping options available. Unlike cancer patients, the heart patient and family may have little perception of the plausibility and reasonableness of limiting intrusive therapies when the quality of life has diminished beyond a tolerable level (see the paradigm case, p. 247).

The patient who experiences the illness as breakdown may be excessively reflective and fearful about resuming life. It is as if patients are placed in a double bind. They are told that they have the keys to controlling their health. They must modulate their diet, exercise, and emotional response and yet to recover their sense of health, they must learn to be spontaneous and enjoy life without excessive fear. It is little wonder that patients find these adjustment demands challenging and that many become ill from fear and inactivity.

Family members can come to feel responsible for "keeping the patient alive." The sense of responsibility for the compliance and health status of the cardiac patient has been reported to cause friction, fustration, anger, depression, and anxiety for patient and family members (Croog and Fitzgerald 1978; Mayou, Roster, and Williamson 1978). Research in this area has shown that teaching cardiopulmonary resuscitation (CPR) can increase the family's depression and anxiety and retard psychological adjustment. Control groups that did not receive CPR training experienced decreased anxiety and depression and increased psychosocial adjustment over time (Dracup et al. 1986). The symbolism of formal classes on CPR may have increased the families' sense that such a cardiac catastrophe was just around the corner. The authors reasoned that CPR should be taught but with counseling, debriefing, and follow-up to lessen the impact on patients and families. Clearly, the prospects for recovered spontaneity and sense of wholeness for patient and family are better with a well-paced rehabilitation program that deals with one area of change at a time and includes information and support for significant others.

Coping with the myocardial infarction begins at its onset for better or worse. If the patient cannot believe the warning signals, he or she may imperil his or her health by delaying medical attention. With each episode, the adaptive demand is for rest and recovery within the limits of the functional capacity of the heart. The nurse can play a key role in coaching the patient through the ordeal of the initial assault, rehabilitation, and possible recurring illnesses. In each case, the question of the limits of control, the desire for controlling the disease, and the desire for a resumption of work and love set up the stress and coping issues (Blumenthal, 1982). This is eloquently illustrated in the following exemplar of expert coaching by Mary Cucci.

PARADIGM
A Dialogue with Technology, a Case of Expert Coaching
Mary Cucci[1]
University of California San Francisco Hospital

Mr. Jones is a sixty-year-old gentleman who four months prior to this hospitalization had an automatic cardiac defibrillator implanted to convert malignant ventricular tachycardia and prevent cardiac arrest. He also had a more recent diagnosis of lung cancer for which he had begun radiation therapy. He had a five year history of arrhythmia and had suffered two previous cardiac arrests. Mr. Jones was admitted to the telemetry unit for evaluation of his arrhythmia because the defibrillator had fired four times in one week. The night of his admission, he was transferred to the coronary care unit because he had been "automatically" defibrillated twenty times in the period of an hour before an intravenous medication could control the rhythm.

I first met Mr. Jones the morning after his admission to the CCU. The

---

1. This paradigm case was published in a slightly abridged form in *The American Journal of Nursing* 87:1170–1172, September, 1987.

nurse on the previous shift told me about the terror he had been through. He had screamed with the repeated defibrillation, had required a significant amount of sedation, and had been rambling and panicky until the sedation took effect.

As I entered the room, his face was drawn and he looked fatigued. His eyes focused on me, but the rest of his body seemed frozen in the bed. His body was limp, and his muscles looked wasted as if he had lost considerable weight. We had a brief, quiet conversation of introduction. I told him that I was very interested in his comfort and that it was important that he call for whatever he needed, no matter how small it seemed. I told him that I understood that he had been through a great deal. I asked him gently if he would tell me how he felt about it. He replied:

"How would you feel? It was a nightmare." As he continued to speak, his face began to reflect his pain and anxiety. His eyes began to tear. His voice was tremulous and frail. His questions and statements reflected his intelligence: "What am I going to do now? I thought this (the implanted defibrillator) was the last answer. What if it happened again? I couldn't stand that." I answered his questions as clearly and simply as I could. I told him that I would help him find some answers, and that I was going to help him through this. I shared my impressions of him, that he appeared overwhelmed, with a million thoughts running through his mind at once, and that he seemed as if he felt out of control. He said: "Yes, that is how I feel." He seemed surprised that somehow I understood. He also talked about feeling betrayed by the device that was supposed to be the answer. He talked about his fear of it happening again. I discussed Mr. Jones's distress with the physicians and encouraged them to discuss the possibility of turning off the defibrillator while he was in the CCU. By two in the afternoon, with Mr. Jones's approval, the defibrillator was turned off and Mr. Jones's expression appeared more relaxed. I encouraged him to rest.

I learned more about Mr. Jones throughout the day. Questions about family, work, his interests, and medical history invariably ended with some tearful reflection of the loss he felt. "It isn't fair," he stated. I listened, and told him that I felt that everything he was feeling was normal. I told him that this period could be considered one of the most important times of his life. He said that he had never experienced anything like this before. Despite his history of cardiac arrests and resuscitations and his diagnosis of lung cancer, he stated that he never had believed that he was going to die. He had always felt that there was some answer, some option that gave him hope. Days later, he illustrated his coping style further when he told me that in his work he had always followed a diagram or set of plans. He always had a plan, and what was driving him crazy was that now he did not have any good option. He couldn't formulate his plan. He stated: "This time everything has been taken away." I reminded him that not *everything* had been taken away. His wife, his main support, sat by his side through most of this hospitalization. She was still there, I reminded him, and he had said many times: "If it wasn't for her, I don't know what I would do." I also told him that I thought he might benefit from talking to someone else who would help him think through all the issues he had raised, the future, his fears, his family, his life plan. I referred him to our psychiatric nurse specialist who counseled many people facing the same types of questions. He said, "I like talking to you. You've helped me." I told him that I would continue to be available, but I thought he could use someone outside to help him systematically think through the issues he was facing. He agreed, and the clinical nurse specialist began a supportive relationship that lasted throughout his hospital stay.

Later that morning he brought up the issue of whether he ever wanted the defibrillator turned back on. He said: "I don't want to die, but I also don't want to be out in the garden and have the defibrillator fire repeatedly like it did the other night. I would be totally helpless. What if my wife were there? I couldn't ask her to turn it off. I would be totally helpless." He was tearful. He then began to address a major moral issue for him: He asked me if I thought turning the defibrillator off was committing suicide. "Do I have the right to turn it off?" he wanted to know. I told him that I felt that was something no one could decide or judge for him, and that my perception of facing the possibility of death was that you truly do it on your own. He persisted, and I shared my opinion with him, that is, that the device was meant to be a life extender and not intended to create pain, especially emotional pain. I then asked him if he would like me to contact someone in the chaplain's service that would be helpful in addressing these moral issues. He agreed.

Despite the emotional and intellectual intensity he displayed, Mr. Jones moved minimally in the bed. This intense man appeared trapped in a frozen shell. Some of it was due to the debilitation of his weight loss and recent illnesses, but as I began talking to him about moving more and maintaining and building his physical strength, I began to realize that he was afraid to move. He admitted it. Apparently, several of his tachycardias had occurred during exertion. This time I persisted and after an explanation of the importance of moving his arms, legs, and body gently around in bed, he began to make some progress. Suddenly he was aware of every premature heartbeat he had. I told him when he was right and when he was wrong. We watched the monitor together. We set up a plan for increased mobility and negotiated each limit. I stayed with him through each new step. It was like watching somebody wake up physically, but the process was slower and more obviously sequential. It was the mental hurdle we were really facing. I challenged him to meet the goals we set. I distracted him with conversation. He watched the clock ferociously and met his goal with not a minute extra given. He began moving more in bed without thinking about it. More of his body participated as he continued to talk of the intense emotional issues he faced. I teased him, cajoled him, and danced with him as he transferred to the chair. I challenged him more each day and ignored his fake whine when he half-heartedly pleaded abuse. It became a joke. He learned to monitor his pulse to guide his activity progression. This was a long, slow process of building belief in himself. I told him throughout that I knew it was difficult, that I admired his strength, and that I knew he could do it.

I encouraged his family to create distractions. The room became lighter and brighter and more personal as a few of his treasures arrived and he began to play cards with his son. A few old and close friends came by. He could still look very forlorn, but you would notice a smile more often in response to a joke from one of the nurses or to us singing him a lullaby as he tried to settle in for a nap. Some silliness and distraction mixed with the psychological support he received from his family, physician, and the nurses, and the steady physical progress he made helped bring him back to a better balance. I knew he was making progress when I discovered him and his wife cuddled up taking a nap one day.

He left the CCU having decided not to turn his defibrillator back on. The chaplain had helped him to resolve his moral questions. He failed the first drug trial after coming to the CCU, requiring a single defibrillation. He had passed out and was unaware of any physical pain. After trials with a new antiarrhythmic failed, the only choice was amiodarone (Cordarone), a drug that had worked for him in the past but had caused pulmonary toxicity. The goal was to buy some time. The side effect was reversible with withdrawal of the medication and had shown up after months on the medication. He agreed to risk the pulmonary toxicity and maybe have a better chance of avoiding the arrhythmia. He was discharged home three weeks after his admission and continued his radiation treatments.

Several months after discharge, Mr. Jones and his wife returned to the CCU to say hello. We greeted each other with hugs and smiles. He had gained weight and I teased him about his pot belly. Eight months after discharge he is still doing well and reports to his physician that he is feeling better and better.

COMMENTARY

This is a stunning example of the moral and personal dilemmas created when a medical therapy fails and when the illusion of limitless "cures" is removed. This exemplar also demonstrates expert coaching. Mary Cucci notices that Mr. Jones is terrified and reflects and clarifies his feelings. She reads his body language. She notices that Mr. Jones appears "frozen" in bed. She clarifies with him that he is afraid to move because it may trigger his tachycardia again. She selects an approach that matches his own coping style, they set a goal and create a plan for his recovery. She uses humor and even dances with him as he transfers to the chair. She makes him notice his progress and monitor his abilities. She enlists the family to solicit his participation in life again. She draws on the chaplain and the psychiatric nurse specialist to augment her own care. She interprets the patient's fears and understanding to the physicians. Mr. Jones has become a prisoner in his own body. His world has shrunk, and he is a classic case of the effects of being institutionalized. Illness robs one of perspective and shrinks both the familiar world and the world of possibility. Mary Cucci demonstrates expertise in world conserving and world restoring, as well as expertise in assisting someone to imagine the next step. We can learn much from such expert nursing practice on the nature of the shrinking world of illness, the personal consequences of institutionalization, and the nature of recovery.

REFERENCES

Barefoot JC, Dahlstrom WG, Williams RB: Hostility, CHD incidence, and total mortality: A 25-year follow-up study of 255 physicians. Psychosom Med 45(1):59, 1983.

Bellah RN, Madsen R, Sullivan WM, Swidler A, Tipton S: *Habits of the Heart, Individualism and Commitment in American Life.* Berkeley: University of California Press, 1985.

Benner P: *Stress and Satisfaction on the Job.* New York: Praeger Scientific Press, 1984.

Berger P, Berger B, Kellner H: *The Homeless Mind.* New York: Vintage Books, 1974.

Blumenthal J, Williams RB, Kong Y, Schaneberg SM, Thompson LW: Type A behavior pattern and coronary atherosclerosis. Circulation 58:634, 1978.

Blumenthal JA, Williams RS, Wallace AG, Williams RB Jr, Needles TL: Physiological and psychological variables predict compliance to prescribed exercise therapy in patients recovering from myocardial infarction. Psychosom Med 44(6):519, 1982.

Borgmann A: *Technology and the Character of Contemporary Life.* Chicago: University of Chicago Press, 1984.

Bortner RW: A short rating scale as a potential measure of pattern A behavior. J Chron Dis 22:87, 1969.

Buring JE, Evans DA, Fiore M, Rosner B, Hennekens CH: Occupation and risk of death from coronary disease. JAMA 258:791, 1987.

Campbell DB: A program to reduce coronary heart disease risk by altering job stresses. Doctoral dissertation, University of Michigan, 1973.

Caplan RD: Organizational stress and individual strain: A social psychological study of risk factors in coronary heart disease among administrators, engineers, and scientists. Doctoral dissertation, University of Michigan, 1971.

Carver CS, The facilitation of aggression as a function of self-awareness and attitudes toward punishment. J Exper Soc Psych. 10:365, 1974.

Carver CS, Coleman AE, Glass DC: The coronary-prone behavior pattern and the suppression of fatigue on a treadmill test. J Person Social Psychol 33:460, 1976.

Case RB, Heller SS, Case NB, Moss AJ, The multicenter post-infarction research group. New Engl J Med 312(12):737, 1985.

Chandra V, Szklo M, Goldberg R, Tonascia J: The impact of marital status on survival after an acute myocardial infarction: A population-based study. Amer J Epidem 117:320, 1983.

Chesney MA, Black GW, Chadwick JH, Rosenman RH: Psychological correlates of the type A behavior pattern. J Behav Med 4:217, 1981.

Chesney MA, Sevelius G, Black GW, Ward MM, Swan GE, Rosenman RH: Work environment, type A behavior, and coronary heart disease risk factors. J Occupat Med 23:551, 1981.

Cohen JB: The influence of culture on coronary-prone behavior. In Dembroski TM, Weiss SM, Shields JL, Haynes SG, Feinleib M (eds): Coronary-prone behavior, pp. 243–252. New York: Springer-Verlag, 1978.

Cohen JB, Reed D: The type A behavior pattern and coronary heart disease among Japanese men in Hawaii. J Behav Med 8:343, 1985.

Cohen JB, Syme SL, Jenkins CD, Kagan A, Zyzanski SJ: Cultural content of type A behavior and risk for CHD: A study of Japanese American males. J Behav Med 2:375, 1979.

Cook WW, Medley DM: Proposed hostility and pharisaic-virtue scales for the MMPI. J Applied Psychol 38:414, 1954.

Crawshaw JE: Community rehabilitation after acute myocardial infarction. Heart Lung 3:258, 1974.

Croog SH, Fitzgerald EF: Subjective stress and serious illness of spouse: Wives of heart patients. J Health Social Behav 19:166, 1978.

Croog SH, Levine S, Lurie, Z: The heart patient and the recovery process. Social Sci Med 2:111, 1968.

Cutrona CE: Causal attributions and perinatal depression. J Abnorm Psychol 92:161, 1983.

Dembroski TM: Reliability and validity of methods used to assess coronary-prone behavior. In Dembroski TM, Weiss SM, Shields JL, Haynes SG, Feinleib M (eds): Coronary-Prone Behavior, pp. 95–106. New York: Springer-Verlag, 1978.

Dembroski TM, MacDougall JM, Williams RB, Haney TL, Blumenthal JA: Components of type A, hostility, and anger-in: relationship to angiographic findings. Psychosom Med 47(3):219, 1985.

Dimsdale JE: A perspective on type A behavior and coronary disease. N Eng J Med 318:110, 1988.

Dobson KS, Shaw BF: The effects of self-correction on cognitive distortions in depressions. Cognitive Theory Res 5:391, 1981.

Dracup C, Guzy PM, Taylor SE, Barry J: Cardiopulmonary resuscitation (CPR) training: Consequences for family members of high-risk cardiac patients. Arch Intern Med 146:1757, 1986.

Dreyfus HL, Rabinow P: Michel Foucault. Chicago: University of Chicago Press, 1982.

Frankenhaeuser M, Lundberg U, Forsman L: Note on arousing type A persons by depriving them of work. J Psychosom Res 24:45, 1980.

French JRP, Caplan RD: Organizational stress and individual strain. In Marrow AJ (ed): The Failure of Success. New York: AMACOM, 1972.

Friedman GD, Dales LG, Ury HK: Mortality in middle-aged smokers and nonsmokers. New Engl J Med 300:215, 1979.

Friedman M, Rosenman RH: Association of a specific overt behavior pattern with blood and cardiovascular findings. JAMA 169:1286, 1959.

Friedman M, Rosenman R: *Type A Behavior and Your Heart.* New York: Knopf, 1974.

Friedman M, Thoresen CE, Gill JJ, Powell L, Ulmer D, Thompson L, Price VA, Rabin DD, Breall WS, Dixon T, Levy RA, Bourg E: Alteration of type A behavior and reduction in cardiac recurrence in post-myocardial infarction patients. Am Heart J 108:237, 1984.

Friedman M, Ulmer D: *Treating Type A Behavior and Your Heart.* New York: Fawcett Crest, 1984.

Glass DC: *Behavior Patterns, Stress and Coronary Disease.* Hillsdale, N.J.: Erlbaum, 1977.

Glass DC, Lake CR, Contrada RJ, Kehoe K, Erlanger LR: Stability of individual differences in physiological responses to stress. Health Psych 2:317, 1983.

Glock CY, Bellah RN (eds): *The New Religious Consciousness.* Berkeley: University of California Press, 1976.

Gouldner A: *The Coming Crisis of Western Sociology.* New York: Avon Books, 1971.

Gulledge AD: Psychological aftermaths of myocardial infarction. In Gentry WD, Williams RB (eds): *Psychological Aspects of Myocardial Infarction and Coronary Care,* pp. 113-129. St. Louis: C.V. Mosby, 1979.

Hackett T: Changing behavior following myocardial infarction. In Kellermann JJ (ed): *Advances in Cardiology,* pp. 100–108. New York: Karger, 1986.

Hackett TP, Perez-Gonzalez JF, Blumchen G, Almeida-Feo D, Hellerstein HK: Return to work after myocardial infarction and coronary bypass surgery. In Kellerman J (ed): *Advances in Cardiology,* pp. 170–177. New York: Karger, 1986.

Halhuber MJ, Modification of coronary-prone behavior and clinical application. In Kellermann J (ed.): *Advances in Cardiology,* pp. 109–115. New York: Karger, 1986.

Harrison RV: Job demands and worker health: Person-environment misfit. Doctoral dissertation, University of Michigan, 1976.

Harrison RV: Person-environment fit and job stress. In Cooper CL, Payne R (eds): *Stress at Work.* New York: John Wiley & Sons, 1978.

Hartfield M: Appraisal of anger situations and subsequent coping responses in hypertensive and normotensive adults: A comparison. Unpublished doctoral dissertation, University of California at San Francisco, School of Nursing, 1985.

Haynes SG, Feinleib M: Women, work and coronary heart disease: Prospective findings from the Framingham Heart Study. Am J Public Health, 70:133, 1980.

Haynes SG, Levine S, Scotch N, Feinleib M, Kannel WB: The relationship of psychosocial factors to coronary heart disease in the Framingham study: I. Method and risk factors. Am J Epidemiol 107:362, 1978.

Heidegger M: *Being and Time.* New York: Harper & Row, 1962.

Helman CG: Heart disease and the cultural construction of time: The type A behavior pattern as a Western culture-bound syndrome. Soc Sci Med 25:969, 1987.

Jenkins CD: A comparative review of the interview and questionnaire methods in the assessment of the coronary-prone behavior pattern. In Dembroski TM, Weiss SM, Shields JL, Haynes S, Feinleib M (eds): *Coronary-Prone Behavior,* pp. 71–88. New York: Springer-Verlag, 1978.

Kahn JP, Kornfield DS, Frank DA, Heller SS, Hoar PF: Type A behavior and blood pressure during coronary artery bypass surgery. Psychosom Med 42:407, 1980.

Krantz DS, Manuck SB: Acute psychophysiological reactivity and risk of cardiovascular disease: A review and methodologic critique. Psychol Bullet 96:435, 1984.

Krantz DS, Baum A, Singer JE: *Handbook of Psychology and Health,* vol 3. *Cardiovascular Disorders and Behavior.* Hillsdale, N.J.: Erlbaum, 1983.

Krantz DS, Sanmarco ME, Selvester RH, Matthews KA: Psychological correlates of progression of atherosclerosis in men. Psychosom Med 41:467, 1979.

Lovallo WR, Pishkin V: Type A behavior, self-involvement, autonomic activity, and the traits of neuroticism and extraversion. Psychosom Med 42:329, 1980.

Lynch JJ: *The Broken Heart: The Medical Consequences of Loneliness.* New York: Basic Books, 1977.

MacDougall JM, Dembroski TM, Musante L: The structured interview and questionnaire methods of assessing coronary-prone behavior in male and female college students. J Behav Med 2:71, 1979.

MacIntyre A: *After Virtue.* Notre Dame: Ind.: University of Notre Dame Press, 1981.

Marmot MG, Syme SL: Acculturation and coronary heart disease in Japanese-Americans. Am J Epidemiol 104(3):225, 1976.

Maslow A: A theory of human motivation. Psychol Rev 50:370, 1943.

Matthews KA: Psychological perspectives on the type A behavior pattern. Psychol Bull 91:293, 1982.

Matthews KA, Glass DC, Rosenman RH, Bortner RW: Competitive drive, pattern A, and coronary heart disease: A further analysis of some data from the Western Collaborative Group Study. J Chron Dis 30:489, 1977.

Mayou R, Roster A, Williamson B: The psychological and social effects of myocardial infarction on wives. Br Med J 1:699, 1978.

Merleau-Ponty, M: *The Phenomenology of Perception.* London: Routledge and Kegan Paul, 1962.

Merton RK: *Social Theory and Social Structure.* New York: The Free Press, 1968.

Miller SM, Lack ER, Asroff S: Preference for control and coronary-prone behavior pattern: "I'd rather do it myself." J Person Social Psychol 49(2):492, 1985.

Obrist PA: *Cardiovascular Psychophysiology: A Perspective.* New York: Plenum Press, 1981.

Osler W: *Lecture on Angina Pectoris and Allied States.* New York: Appleton, 1892.

Overmeier JB, Seligman MEP: Effects of inescapable shock upon subsequent escape and avoidance responding. J Compar Physiol Psychol, 63:28, 1967.

Radley AR: The embodiment of social relations in coronary heart disease. Social Sci Med 19:1227, 1984.

Ragland DR, Brand RJ: Type A behavior and mortality from coronary heart disease. N Eng J Med 318:65, 1988.

Review Panel on Coronary-Prone Behavior and Coronary Heart Disease. Coronary-prone behavior and coronary heart disease: A critical review. Circulation 63:1199, 1981.

Rosenman RH, Brand RJ, Sholtz RI, Friedman M: Multivariate prediction of coronary heart disease during 8.5 year followup in the Western Collaborative Group Study. Am J Cardiol 37:903, 1976.

Roskies E: *Stress Management for the Healthy Type A.* London: Guilford Press, 1987.

Ruberman W, Weinblatt E, Goldberg JD, Caudbury B: Psychosocial influence on mortality after myocardial infarction. New Engl J Med 311:552, 1984.

Sacks O: *A Leg to Stand On*. New York: Simon & Schuster, 1984.

Scheier M, Carber C: Self-focused attention and the experience of emotion: Attraction, repulsion, elation, and depression. J Pers Soc Psych 35:625, 1974.

Scherwitz, L, Berton K, Leventhal H: Type A behavior, self-involvement and cardiovascular response. Psychosom Med 40(8):593, 1978.

Scherwitz L, McKelvain R, Laman C, Patterson J, Dutton L, Ysim S, Lester J, Kraft I, Rochelle D, Leachman R: Type A behavior, self-involvement, and coronary atherosclerosis. Psychosom Med 45(1):47, 1983.

Schmieder R, Friedrich G, Neus H, Rudel H, Von Eiff AW: The influence of beta blockers on cardiovascular reactivity and type A behavior pattern in hypertensives. Psychosom Med 45:417, 1983.

Seligman MEP: *Helplessness*. San Francisco: W.H. Freeman, 1975.

Seligman MEP, Maier SF: Failure to escape traumatic shock. J Exper Psychol 74:1, 1967.

Shils E: *Tradition*. Chicago: University of Chicago Press, 1981.

Stallones RA: The rise and fall of ischemic heart disease. Sci Am 243(5):53, 1980.

Talbott E, et al: Biologic and psychosocial risk factors of sudden death from coronary disease in white women. Am J Cardiol 39:858, 1977.

Thoresen CA, Ohman A: The type A behavior pattern: a person-environment interaction perspective. In Magnusson D, Ohman A (eds): *Psychopathology: An Interactional Perspective*. New York: Academic Press, 1987.

Tipton SM: *Getting Saved from the Sixties*. Berkeley: University of California Press, 1982.

Weber M: *The Protestant Ethic and the Spirit of Capitalism*. New York: Charles Scribner's Sons, 1958.

Weidner G, Matthews KA: Reported physical symptoms elicited by unpredictable events and the type A coronary-prone behavior pattern. J Person Social Psychol 36:1213, 1978.

Wenger NK: *Coronary Care: Rehabilitation after Myocardial Infarction*. New York: American Heart Association, 1973.

Wenger NK, Almeida-Feo D, Rosenthal J: *Rehabilitation of the Cardiac Patient*. Proceedings of the Third World Congress of Cardiac Rehabilitation, Caracas, October 20–23, 1986. New York: Karger, 1985.

Wiklund I, Sanne H, Vedin A, Wilhelmsson C: Coping with myocardial infarction: A model with clinical applications, a literature review. Int Rehab Med 7(4):167, 1985.

Williams RB, Barefoot JC, Shekelle RB: The health consequences of hostility. In Chesney MA, Rosenman RH (eds): *Anger, Hostility and Behavioral Medicine*, pp. 173–185. New York: Hemisphere/McGraw Hill, 1985.

Williams RB, Haney TL, Lee KL, Kong Y, Blumenthal JA, Whalen RE: Type A behavior, hostitlity, and coronary atherosclerosis. Psychosom Med 42:529, 1980.

Williams RB, Lane JD, Kuhn CM, Melosh W, White AD, Schanberg SM: Type A behavior and elevated physiological and neuroendocrine responses to cognitive tasks. Science 218:483, 1982.

Yankelovich D: *New Rules in American life: Searching for Self-Fulfillment in a World Turned Upside Down*. New York: Random House, 1981.

CHAPTER EIGHT

Coping with Cancer

The patient began talking about how some of the relationships had changed in her life: "People don't call me anymore. I don't get calls to go out to lunch. I'm isolated." . . . So I became the person she could talk to when she felt really sick. She used me to validate that it was OK that she didn't feel well and that she felt blue some days and that she wasn't always up in this vibrant mood.   *Sharon Olsen RN, MS*

Cancer is singled out for discussion here for three major reasons: First, cancer is the second leading cause of death in the United States; one in four families will have a family member stricken with cancer. Second, the treatment and recovery trajectories of cancer can be particularly demanding for patients and caregivers. Third, cancer is culturally one of the most dreaded diseases. Although "increased success" has been highly advertised, actual appraisals of increases in survival times may have been inflated by earlier detection. Also, the decreases in mortality rates have been limited to certain types of cancers, such as acute myelocytic leukemia, Wilms' tumors, testicular cancers, and Hodgkin's disease. Progress has been small or negligible in melanoma and cancer of the pancreas, liver, cervix, adrenal cortex, and soft tissue (Brandt 1987, Sondik 1987). Even so, chemotherapy, radiation therapy, and immunotherapy or their combinations have created a need for a cultural redefinition of the disease as a chronic or potentially curable illness rather than an invariably fatal one.

Each kind of illness and disability creates different demands for nursing care. Providing nursing care for the oncology patient has the reputation of being extremely challenging and significant because the disease requries that nurses adopt ingenious strategies for providing comfort, nutrition, social support, rest, and activity in the midst of demanding and often debilitating treatment regimens. Expert oncology nurses set for themselves the goal of understanding the "insider's" illness experience. From the nursing perspective, disease and suffering must be approachable and not alienating if a nurse is to coach, comfort, and assist the patient in coping with an illness. As Fagin and Diers point out (1983):

> Nursing is a metaphor for intimacy. Nurses are involved in the most private aspects of people's lives, and they cannot hide behind technology or a veil of omniscience as other practitioners or technicians in hospitals may do. Nurses do for others publicly what healthy persons do for themselves behind closed doors. Nurses, as trusted peers, are there to hear secrets, especially the ones born of vulnerability. Nurses are treasured when these interchanges are successful, but most often people do not wish to remember their vulnerability or loss of control, and nurses are indelibly identified with those terribly personal times (p. 116).

Because nurses attempt to understand the illness experience from the patient's perspective, nurses report that they must personally come to terms with the disability and suffering of patients. Nurses work in the intimate regions, and patients typically rehearse the most frightening, tentative personal questions with nurses. It is not surprising that nurses report that they must come to terms with the illness for themselves before they can work effectively with patients. Of course "coming to terms with the illness" has varied meanings depending upon the nurse, but it always means that the nurse must develop particular coping skills and perspectives on the illness that she or he learns professionally, personally, and clinically from patients.

EXPERT COACHING, THE RESPONSIBILITY OF UNEVEN KNOWLEDGE

Knowing a particular illness trajectory well means that the nurse knows the range of possibilities for any one type of disease. The nurse's expert knowledge about the typical cancer trajectory may not match the patient's hopes or fears. The standard policy on patient education is to be as clear as possible with the patient about the nature of the disease, the treatment options, and the implications. However, information giving is usually tempered by what the patient asks and states. The health care worker has little control over how much the patient will hear and understand about the disease. Furthermore it is impossible to predict a *particular* patient's response to therapy and the range of side effects and complications.

Coaching the patient without violating the patient's self-understanding and sense of possibility requires informed and artful caring. Patients turn to nurses to discuss the implications and the meanings of the therapy and its side effects. Nurses must rely on knowing the patient and family as well as possible in order to interpret their concerns to one another and to the rest of the health care team.

During the treatment course, the nurse as expert coach can provide practical information to help the patient cope with the exigencies of the illness and treatment demands. However, this information must be given with a sense of timing and patient readiness, or else too much information, or information given before it is needed or understood, can unnecessarily frighten or overwhelm the patient. Unwarranted "advice giving" can damage the patient's sense of personal control and self-efficacy. The nurse's intimate knowledge of the illness and the disease, and the accessibility of nurses, makes nurses' dialogue with patients exceed typical medical or psychological counseling. The nurse-patient discourse typically covers a range of topics from management of symptoms, understanding of the disease and treatment, and how to accomplish personal goals in the midst of the illness and treatment, to issues of the meaning of the illness and self-understanding in relation to the disease, disfigurement, pain, and death. Consequently the need for specialized education in stress and coping is particularly germane for nurses working with cancer patients because the disease and treatment can be extremely demanding and because cancer is a stigmatized illness (Sontag 1979).

Clearly the person's stress level and coping options will vary considerably depending upon whether he or she understands the cancer to be curable or fatal. The potential for a cure, of course, depends upon the site, the type of cancer, and the stage of the cancer at detection. This chapter is divided into two major sections. The first deals with the possible role of personality and/or stress in the development of cancer and the cultural meanings of cancer. The second addresses stress and coping with cancer for the patient and for the caregivers.

Is There a Cancer Prone Personality?

Attributing certain personality characteristics to cancer patients has a long social history. In the second century, Galen noted that cancer occurred more commonly in "melancholic" women than those of "sanguine" temperament (Mettler and Mettler 1947). Gendron (1701) concluded that women who had serious depression and high anxiety were susceptible to cancer. Greer (1983) notes that the medical literature of the eighteenth and nineteenth centuries contained various references to emotional distress as a cause of cancer.

Susan Sontag (1979) names Wilhelm Reich, a disciple of Freud, as the primary source of the modern notion of "repression of passion" as a causal agent in cancer. She quotes Reich's definition of cancer as follows:

> . . . "a disease following emotional resignation—a bioenergetics shrinking, a giving up of hope." Reich illustrated his influential theory with Freud's cancer, which he thought began when Freud, naturally passionate and "very unhappily married," yielded to resignation. "He lived a very calm, quiet, decent family life, but there is little doubt that he was very much dissatisfied genitally. Both his resignation and his cancer were evidence of that. Freud had to give up, as a person. He had to give up personal pleasures, his personal delights, in his middle years. . . . If my view of cancer is correct, you just give up, you resign—and, then, you shrink." (as cited by Sontag, pp. 22–23).

Such personal attributions of "responsibility" for the development of cancer due to "resignation" are no doubt responsible for the popular health care admonitions that cancer patients must "fight for their life," or "take charge of their cancer." While it is true that fighting is usually preferable to giving up, the demand that the patient *fight* may come at a time when he or she has the least reserve and may increase the sense of helplessness and despair that often accompanies the fatigue, cachexia, and treatment side effects of therapy.

In order to understand the influence of cultural meanings on caregiving practices, it is instructive to contrast the typical approach of health care workers with burn victims to the almost-opposite stance with cancer patients, who may actually suffer similar levels of distress. Burn patients with only a fair prognosis are encouraged to "hang on" and not be discouraged because they *will* feel better. Such a promise is not always possible for the cancer patient, but the health care workers' consensus seems to be one of moral demand that they "fight" in a fairly narrowly prescribed way even at the point of the patient's lowest physical reserve. Such a strategy may actually deepen the patient's sense of hopelessness, and limit his or her own resourcefulness. This is a problem of trivializing distress (Lazarus 1985) and blaming the victim. Both of these issues will be discussed further under the section on "coping with cancer."

The role of stress and coping in the etiology of cancer is extremely difficult to research because cultural understandings of cancer may cause overinterpretation and may lead to the assigning of culturally undesirable traits to be the "cause" of the disease. The moral overtones of such research are evident, and the possibility of increasing the burden of the person with cancer is great.

Careful prospective studies are required to sort out the cultural myths from the actual patterns that may exist between stress and coping and cancer. Such prospective studies must take into consideration personality and stress issues as well as heritability, aging, carcinogenic exposures, and latency (growth time) of cancers. The latency period for cancer is the interval from beginning cell division to clinical detection and ranges from 2.1 years up to 11 years with 7 years the median. Cancer in very young children is therefore more likely to be inherited, and in older children a combination of genetic predisposition and early exposure to a carcinogen generally plays a larger role than personality and stress factors. In evaluating studies that examine links between personality and stress on the etiology of cancer, the likely influence of the amount and duration of carcinogen exposure and the role of decreased immune functioning with aging would place the personality or stress-and-coping hypotheses for development of cancer primarily in the middle-aged population prior to the decline of the immune system with aging (Fox 1978).

The psychosocial epidemiology of cancer is further complicated by the fact that the disease itself can affect emotions and behavior due to changes in aspects of the body such as fatigue, hair loss, anorexia, nausea, and pain. Hormonal changes also affect emotions and behavior. For example, cancer can affect the central nervous system, alter metabolic processes and electrolyte balance, or produce hormones, depending upon the site and type of cancer. As the disease progresses, paraneoplastic syndromes including cachexia, fever, clotting abnormalities, hypercalcemia, inappropriate secretion of antidiuretic hormone, along with a range of side effects and sequelae of treatment may affect mood, outlook, personality, and coping. Because the diagnosis *cancer* is often understood to be life-threatening and carries with it a sense of fear and dread, even the experience of having a diagnostic workup for cancer can create great distress and alterations in coping. The potential distress patients experience during a diagnostic workup casts grave doubts on the validity of studies assessing personality styles *during* this time of crisis.

Corticosteroids and epinephrine inhibit the immune system

(Borysenko and Borysenko 1982). Epinephrine levels increase during anxiety, novelty, anticipation, unpredictability, and general emotional arousal, whereas norepinephrine levels increase with physical stress, such as during exercise. The condition of uncertainty and depression can cause high cortisol secretion, although it is possible to hypersecrete cortisol without stress responses (Borysenko 1982).

The role of the immune system in the etiology and progression of cancer is far from clear. The immune surveillance theory that macrophages and lymphocytes police and interfere with the development of aberrant cells has spawned a host of new monoclonal antibody therapies (Dijulio 1988, Dijulio and Bedegian 1983, Oldham 1987, Basham et al. 1986) that add hope and yet new complications in the treatment of cancer. A subset of lymphocytes known as natural killer (NK) cells has been identified. NK cells can acquire cytotoxic properties spontaneously, without prior sensitization. This process is called spontaneous lymphocyte-mediated cytotoxicity (Pross and Baines 1976). Macrophages also have spontaneous antitumor activity (Haskill, Proctor, and Yamamura 1975). The picture is complex and still unfolding. Macrophages work on some tumors, while NK cells work on others (Chow, Greene, and Greenberg 1979). It has been demonstrated that stress decreases both NK cell activity and macrophage-mediated cytotoxicity (Borysenko 1982, Locke 1982).

Fox (1978) conducted an extensive review of the literature outlining the psychological characteristics that might theoretically be implicated in the development of cancer:

> (1) Those that change *behavior* so that a person increases or decreases his exposure to carcinogens such as those in cigarette smoke or those in organic vapors while at work, or excessive intermittent sun exposure and (2) those that change the *body* by means of humoral or cellular processes without the intervention of an external carcinogenic agent. Examples of (1) are personality characteristics associated with different probabilities of smoking and attitudes resulting from societal pressures leading to dangerous behavior, e.g. exposure to sun. An example of (2) is increased secretion of corticosteriods in dominant mice when they become submissive following removal to another cage and another group of mice (pp. 47–48).

It has been theorized that the production of abnormal amounts of adrenocortical hormones reduces immune capability, hence increasing cancer risk. Also, a broad range of defenses, such as strong social ties and good nutrition, may play a role in the prevention of cancer through strengthening the immune system as well as other bodily defenses (Fox 1978). This causal picture is complicated when one examines the differential effects of personality and stressful transactions leading to different hormonal responses in relation to site and type of cancer. This differential response must be kept in mind when one evaluates studies that search for "all cancer" as the outcome variable. For example, Kersey and Specter (1975) studied a group of subjects over twenty years of age who had immune deficiencies. They found that their group was at greater risk for lymphoreticular and stomach cancers but not at greater risk for lung, breast, or colon cancers than the normal population. Anthony (1970) found a similar pattern in children. Patients at risk due to immunosuppression after transplantation also are more susceptible to cancer of the lymphatic system, epithelial skin cancers, and brain tumors (Fox 1978) than age-matched controls. Patients with acquired immune deficiency syndrome (AIDS) are susceptible to epidemic Kaposi's sarcoma and malignant lymphomas of the central nervous system (Cohen 1987).

The key personality characteristics linked to cancer causation have *not* been adequately demonstrated. Major problems exist in study design, and almost no prospective studies have been done (Fox 1978, Greer 1983). In retrospective studies, it is easy for patients and researchers alike to reinterpret the past in light of the present distress. Also, it is impossible in retrospective studies to sort out the impact of the disease on personality. The following personality characteristics have been hypothesized (but not proved) to be linked with the development of cancer: poor emotional outlet, hopelessness, and tendency to self-sacrifice and self-blame (Kissen 1966, Schmale and Iker 1971); low in ratings of closeness to parents (Thomas and Duszynski 1974); low anxiety and suppression of anger (Greer and Morris 1975, Margarey et al. 1977). Optimism, a tendency to avoid conflicts, and emotional suppression have been associated with breast cancer (Wirsching et al. 1982).

The major theoretical perspectives for investigating links between personality and or stress to cancer have been psychodynamic theories (Bahnson 1980, 1981); life change or loss of important relationships (Greer and Morris 1975; Grissom et al. 1975; Grossarth-Maticek, Frentzel-Beyme, and Becker 1984; Schonfield 1972; Smith et al. 1984); lifestyle and coping patterns (Fox 1978, Kissen and Rao 1969). Each of these theoretical perspectives will be reviewed briefly and critiqued from a phenomenological perspective.

PSYCHODYNAMIC THEORIES

Claus Bahnson (1980, 1981) has developed the most extensive theory and program of research based on psychodynamic theory of the person. He postulates that the following early childhood patterns are associated with the development of cancer:

- Childhood trauma, loss of close figures, lack of a protected and loving childhood, and parental deprivation and coldness.
- An encompassing underlying main affect of hopelessness that colors all experiences—the certainty that everything must go wrong, coupled with simultaneous guilt feelings because of self-blame. (This affect may be considered to be the result of early "imprinting" or conditioning.)
- A repetition compulsion of self-destructive drives, attitudes and act, often manifested on anniversaries of other similar or related events.
- The development of a double life or double self within which realistic and adaptive ego operations unfold, separated from and independent of a parallel "shadow self" that feels isolated, unloved, hurt, and deserted (pp. 977–978).

These early childhood patterns are coupled with a "centrifugal family pattern" of early individuation, where mutual isolation and distancing are the rule. Emotional expression is discouraged, and the child must come to terms with her or his internal dynamics by a premature mastery that "most often depends upon denial and secondary repression of difficult wishes and feelings" (p. 979). As Fox (1978) notes, Bahnson speculates that the individual "chooses" the site of cancer based on his or her own internal conflicts. This is a good example of "pure intentionality." The mind is separate from the body and thinks in symbolic and conceptual terms even on an "unconscious" level. (See Chapter Three for a critique of this position.) In such a view, agency, motivated thinking, and action are somatic manifestations of disease. In this view, there is a meaningful cause of the disease—the somatization of internal conflicts. The person's own conflicts and coping become the cause of the disease. This places the ultimate responsibility on the individual and easily leads to a "blame-the-victim" stance.

Bahnson (1980) and Engelman and Craddick (1984) illustrate the psychodynamic view. For example, using the notion that the cancer serves to defend the ego, Engelman and Craddick hypothesize that cancer patients "create, at an unconscious level, a receptive physiological condition in which the cancer may prosper" (p. 69). They reason that cancer patients identify their cancer as ego syntonic, and the physician and cure as alien to their ego integrity. However, Engel-man and Craddick fail to confirm their hypothesis of an unconsciously motivated form of cancer causation in a study using projective testing of patients scheduled for surgical breast biopsy. There were no significant differences between patients with benign and malignant lesions in terms of "cancer acceptance" or in terms of cure being more ego syntonic.

Unfortunately, the large prospective cohort studies needed to document such a theory have not been carried out. Most of the evidence stems from clinical histories of cancer patients and controls (Bahnson 1980). This is particularly troublesome because cancer has such powerful personal and cultural meanings that the person may reinterpret much of his or her past life in light of the cancer experience. In other words, "being the kind of person who develops cancer" may become a new interpretive grid for retroactively understanding one's past life. Furthermore, from a social learning theory perspective, the health care researcher may unwittingly have a stake in proving that the person "creates" the cancer through internal conflicts in order to protect a sense of an orderly, "just" world where all events are explainable and controllable.

It is plausible that coping strategies and ways of understanding and being in the world developed in childhood could create a particular hormonal milieu that promotes particular diseases such as cancer or cardiovascular disease. A meaningful pattern of self-understanding and coping strategies might be linked to particular disease outcomes, but it seems superfluous to construct particular "motivated" conflicts that would target particular organs (Fox 1978). Such a motivated view assumes a therapeutic correction that would enable people to step outside their history and commitments and gain enlightened control over their conflicts and thus control over their bodies. This is a dualistic view of the mind and body, in which "mind over matter" is taken up as a means of controlling mind, body, and experience.

LIFE CHANGE AND LOSS OF SIGNIFICANT RELATIONSHIPS

The Schedule of Recent Experiences developed by Holmes and Rahe (1967) has been used as an "operational definition" of stress based on the premise that any change, positive or negative, requires adaptive energy and therefore creates stress. There are difficulties with using the life change definition of stress in cancer studies because it is based on recall. Since the latency period of cancer is relatively long (from two to eleven years), the hypothesis would have to be that a period of time with a large number of changes would decrease the immune capabilities and speed the growth of a preexisting cancer or interfere with effective natural surveillance of a cancer with a short latency period. It is difficult to associate the time period adjacent to the onset of disease for any particular population unless everyone went through a similar level of change at the same time.

Three studies of women with breast cancer have not shown any association of disease onset with stressful life events including the loss of important relationships in the recent or remote past (Greer and Morris 1975, Muslin et al. 1966, Schonfield 1972). Schmale and Iker's study (1966) departs from the usual measurement of life events only. They evaluated emotional responses to the life events as well as the events and found that women with cancer of the cervix differed little from healthy control subjects in terms of numbers of life experiences. However, women with cancer of the cervix were more likely to report feelings of hopelessness in response to these experiences than were control subjects.

Smith and colleagues (1984) examined the relationship between life change to the onset of cancer in twenty-two pairs of HLA-identical siblings. In each pair, one twin had hematologic malignancy and the other did not. Both were hospitalized at the time of the study for bone marrow transplantation. There were no significant differences between the pairs in life change units prior to the diagnosis of the malignancy. In the life change theory of causation, "stress" (change) triggers the proliferation of already existing cancer cells by decreasing immune function. Yet the latency period of cancer is an average of five to seven years. Any one period of high life change could not be implicated over such a long period unless chaos and change became a way of life and there was little adaptation to high levels of change.

LIFESTYLE AND COPING PATTERNS

Although Fox (1978) suggests separating physical lifestyle risks, such as smoking and exposure to sun, in reality, such lifestyle risks are bound up with coping patterns. For a person to develop cancer, Fox theorizes, a long exposure to a carcinogen is required if it has low or moderate mutagenic capability. When that exposure is accompanied by a fluctuating level of protection, and when the pattern of the individual is more nearly one of immunosuppression than of enhancement of immune capabilities, then such a lifestyle and coping pattern will increase the person's susceptibility to cancer. He postulates that people who are caught in "no-exit" situations are susceptible to sustained suppression of the immune system. Examples are people trapped in incompatible marriages where divorce is not considered an option, or immigrants who cannot go back to their country but find it impossible to adapt to the new country.

Research interest and emphasis have changed in the past ten years from the influence of personality and stress on the development of cancer to the impact of lifestyle on the incidence of cancer. For example, epidemiological studies estimate that one third of *all* cancers are directly related to smoking. High-fat, low-fiber diets are related to breast and probably colon cancer (Pitot 1986). Changing these lifestyle patterns requires a social as well as an individual response.

The research difficulties of sorting out the impact of personality and stress on the etiology of cancer may prevent definitive answers in this field. The question may be too complex and relational to be addressed by mechanical notions of causality. It is clear that whatever role personality and coping play in cancer causation, they are not the *only* cause.

We may be culturally predisposed to look for "individualistic" causes for societal and community problems instead of adopting responsible measures to change health policies about known risk factors such as food additives, toxic wastes, industrial hazards, and polluted air and water. Three cultural forces lead to the emphasis on "cure" rather than prevention:

1. In our individualistic society, disease causation has traditionally been held to be the individual's responsibility.

2. The strong profit motive in a consumer-oriented society limits environmental controls and controls on food production.

3. The Cartesian dissociation of body and self predisposes us to discount bodily issues and thus health issues—the body is considered as "other" rather than as central to the self.

In our consumer-oriented, individualistic society, it is politically safe but irresponsible to place full responsibility on the individual while avoiding policy changes in industry. Aflatoxin, a known carcinogen, is pervasive but not removed from foods because it would be extremely costly. However, food additives could be removed from commercially produced foods at little or no cost to the producers (Epstein 1978). But producers fear losing a competitive edge because they see the public as wanting their food colored and preserved with additives. Meanwhile, consumers have begun to read food labels and pay extra for food that has fewer additives, and this trend may eventually influence the food producers. In the long view, a switch from an emphasis on finding a "cure" for cancer to preventing cancer will require a shift in our cultural interpretations of self, disease, health, illness, and society.

The psychosocial factors related to length of survival of cancer patients are an equally controversial area of study. Cassileth et al. (1985), in a prospective study of 359 cancer patients with advanced malignant disease, found that psychosocial variables—e.g., social ties, marital and job satisfaction, use of psychotropic drugs, general life evaluation/satisfaction, subjective view of adult health, and degree of hopelessness/helplessness—did not individually or in combination influence the length of survival or time to relapse. These authors point out that cancer patients with advanced disease need not feel that they have failed if they cannot through their own efforts of personal and social change prolong their lives. These authors, however, miss the point that decreasing distress and improving the quality of life are of value in themselves. This prospective study did not include patients with disease detected in the early stages, nor did the researchers include a test of psychosocial interventions.

Cultural Meanings of Cancer

Parker (1981) points out that in Western society death and suffering have become taboo topics for the following four reasons: (a) loss of traditional religious beliefs; (b) medicalization and specialization in the care of the sick that separates the sick from common daily experience; (c) a consumer-oriented, materialistic focus in society that values the replacement of the old with the "brand new," thus de-emphasizing and avoiding loss; (d) an association of good health with "cleanliness" and a cultural obsession with youth and "clean and shining" bodies, which lead to an avoidance of death as a disintegration and decaying of the body.

Parker (1981) explains that traditional religious beliefs gave a central place to death and suffering. These lapsed beliefs, and the emerging secularized scientistic orientations promised cure and freedom from suffering. Death and suffering became a cultural embarrassment and taboo topics because society offered no meanings that made death and suffering explicable or approachable. Death and suffering become counterevidence to the illusion of progress and give the lie to the promise of imminent solutions for suffering and death through technology. Advances in medical science and technology created a division of labor, and the sick are now routinely separated from family and friends in their roles as caretakers. The sick are now placed in institutions, where they are cared for by professional workers. This separation of the sick from the well and the hiddenness of the means of recovery mean that people have little firsthand experience with illness and suffering. Many illnesses that formerly plagued us are now prevented, and the remaining ones are treated in institutions.

The trend to separate the well from the ill is being reversed with the increase in home care as a means of reducing medical costs. But people who are at the extreme stages of illness and suffering will likely continue to be cared for in institutional settings. During the past fifteen years, family participation in hospital patient care has increased. Lovejoy (1987) found that family members kept vigils with patients in order to protect, support, and care for their family member. In response to this trend, we need to increase the emphasis on caring for the family members in the hospital as well as the patient.

A technological self-understanding leads consumers to expect the replacement of old diseased parts with new parts. Parts are interchangeable; consequently, the recognition of change as loss and the experience of grief are covered over and avoided. In such a society, Parker (1981) argues, there are few opportunities to talk about or come to terms with genuine, unavoidable loss as a part of the human condition. Furthermore, Parker points out that the modern hygienic and cosmetic orientation to the body and the obsession with making the body good-looking, clean, and sweet-smelling limit our acceptance of the malodorous, decaying body. Parker concludes:

> In such a society the disease of cancer appears to have become the metaphor of the deepest fears held about the inevitable disintegration and decay of the body. Cancer is the disease which attacks the bodily organs about which greatest ambivalences are felt: those of sexuality, reproduction and excretion. The societal "battle" against cancer is then seen as the struggle to resist acceptance of the inevitability in life of death, decay and decomposition (p. 8).

In a study of widows' bereavement and stress and coping related to their spouses' final illness, Vachon et al. (1977) compared patients with cardiovascular disease and cancer. They conclude:

268

Factors of social desirability colored the experiences of patient and spouse. Cancer is still associated with evil, dirt, pain and death, whereas cardiovascular disease is seen as being more "manly" and the aftermath of working too hard. These unspoken social attitudes contributed to making the final illness and the bereavement period more difficult for the widow (p. 1153).

The truth of these observations is illustrated by an interview excerpt from Sharon Olsen's (1985) research:

> [A clinical nurse specialist in oncology is describing her first contact with a patient.] I remember her saying cancer is a dirty word. It's a dirty word and dirty people get cancer. She's a very prim and proper lady.

The patient's words illustrate the personal and social stigma attached to cancer in this society. Another clinical nurse specialist participant in Olsen's study describes what it was like for one of her patients socially as her cancer progressed:

> [The patient] began talking about how some of the relationships had changed in her life: "People don't call me anymore. I don't get calls to go out to lunch, I'm isolated." She was very angry at her minister. "This man should know how to minister to me and he doesn't. He's not meeting my needs. And many people aren't meeting my needs. My friends aren't calling. They don't ask me how I'm doing. It's like everybody avoids this issue that I'm sick and they all want me to feel wonderful and great and when I don't feel great there's nobody that I can talk to about that."
>
> So I became the person she could talk to when she felt really sick. She used me to validate that it was OK that she didn't feel well and that she felt blue some days and she wasn't always up in this vibrant mood.

Cancer patients face a double burden of having to make the illness not only bearable for themselves but also for their friends. For example, Gordon et al. (1977), in interviews with 136 patients diagnosed with breast cancer, lung cancer, or sarcoma, found that of the twenty problems most frequently cited by all interviewees, seven were of an interpersonal nature (e.g., "communication with friends about cancer difficult," "discussing future with family difficult," "people acting differently after cancer"). Friends and associates may require that the cancer patient be cheerful to lighten their own sense of fear and suffering (Wortman and Dunkel-Schetter 1979). In the above excerpt, the clinical nurse specialist illustrates the role of coach and confident insider who can listen and hear about the lived experience of cancer without insisting on polite cheerfulness or exacting a social cost to the patient's unburdening.

Susan Sontag (1979) analyzes the relationship between cultural meanings of cancer and current cultural self-understanding. She points out that cancer evokes a different sense of economic catastrophe than was true in the era when tuberculosis was the most-dreaded disease. In that era, the possibilities seemed limitless, and the major fear was about not having enough energy to spend. In the modern era, in which Sontag notes a destructive overproduction by the economy and excessive bureaucratic restraints on the individual, the language used to describe cancer reflects this shift in economic concerns:

> The language used to describe cancer evokes a different economic catastrophe: that of unregulated, abnormal, incoherent growth. The tumor has energy, not the patient; "it" is out of control. Cancer cells, according to the textbook account, are cells that have shed the mechanism which "restrains" growth.... (The growth of normal cells is "self-limiting" due to a mechanism called "contact inhibition.") Cancer cells do not simply multiply; they are "invasive." ("Malignant tumors invade even when they grow very slowly," as one textbook puts it.) Cancer cells "colonize" from the original tumor to far sites in the body, first setting up tiny outposts ("micrometastases").... Treatment also has a military flavor. Radiotherapy uses the metaphors of aerial warfare; patients are "bombarded" with toxic rays. And chemotherapy is chemical warfare (pp. 62–64).

It is little wonder that being confronted with a possible diagnosis of cancer creates terror and a sense of horror and even betrayal. These are freely bestowed cultural images of cancer. Sontag notes how often the word *cancer* is used metaphorically to represent deterioration and decay and how this metaphor burdens the cancer patient. She cites John Dean's well-publicized quote: "We have a cancer within—close to the Presidency—that's growing." Such metaphorical uses place a social burden and stigma on every cancer patient who may have a "cancer within." It may be that the militaristic metaphors, in a world that has not focused on preventing war, may unwittingly direct our efforts toward "winning" through a cure rather than preventing cancer.

These cultural interpretations become part of the illness experience and part of what the patient "copes with" when coping with cancer. Cancer is not considered a suitable topic for conversation, although this feeling may be changing somewhat as cancer patients discuss the illness more openly in the media. When the illness is discussed socially, it must be stripped of its militaristic metaphorical uses and "evil" connotations and be reinterpreted for the self and the other. Many patients do not have the social skill required for this reinterpretation, nor do they completely understand the culturally inherited shame they experience when they name their disease.

Sontag (1979) longs for a completely clear, scientific understanding of cancer, free of cultural metaphors and personal responsibility. She notes that the metaphorical thinking about tuberculosis disappeared when the tubercle bacillus (mycobacterium) was discovered. However, she unrealistically looks for a single causal agent for disease. She mistakenly sees the mycobacterium as the single cause and fails to acknowledge the social epidemiology of tuberculosis (Cassel, 1976; Schaefer, 1983). For example, social epidemiologists have demonstrated that people who are socially isolated are more susceptible to tuberculosis than those who are not. She longs for a simplistic biomedical model of disease that involves only agent and host. Such a simplistic view is untenable given the current understanding of the interrelationship among host, agent, and environment. She does parenthetically note in her discussion of cancer, without elaboration:

> Needless to say, the hypothesis that distress can affect immunological responsiveness (and, in some circumstances, lower immunity to disease) is hardly the same as — or constitutes evidence for — the view that emotions cause diseases, much less for the belief that specific emotions can produce specific diseases (pp. 52–53).

Here she seems to be making the theoretical distinction between a purely mechanistic (pure intentionality) view of the "motivated" relationship between emotion and disease evident in the psychodynamic paradigm, and the consequences of lifestyle and coping over time on the development of disease. Sontag takes issue with the former while leaving open the possibility that coping patterns and lifestyle may influence the immune system. She quarrels with the psychodynamic explanation that the cancer serves to keep the "ego intact" or else becomes a form of passive suicide.

The cultural metaphors and treatment of cancer fit in with the current technological understanding of the self as raw material to be shaped, developed, and created. Control is the major term in this mechanistic, technological self-understanding. It is not surprising that self-control and control of the disease become the major themes of the cancer patient and health care workers. But the fear of "loss of control" is never very far away in this understanding of the self as something to be managed and the "body" as being controlled by the "mind."

The diagnosis of cancer and the treatment for it causes patients to lose trust in their bodies and their sense of bodily integrity. The patient and health care worker alike may lose sight of the body's capacity for healing and recovery. This sense of trust in the body, a hope for recovery, and a renewed sense of bodily integrity are required if the patient is to recover from the illness of cancer as well as the disease. The Simonton method (Simonton and Matthews-Simonton 1981) of counseling patients seems to be aimed at restoring a sense of control, integrity, and possibility, although they openly acknowledge that their strategies seem highly beneficial to some and detrimental to others.

The discussion now turns to coping with cancer, but with the acknowledgment that no one copes with one totality called "cancer." Furthermore, the "cancer" that the person copes with is not just the particular disease but the cultural interpretations and burdens attached to it. Coping with cancer involves familial, economic, existential, social, and personal issues. We discuss coping under the headings of the role of the body, the role of the situation, the role of concerns, the role of temporality, help seeking and receiving, and coping with caregiving. Before this discussion, which is based on a phenomenological view of stress and coping, we present an exposition and critique of Avery D. Weisman's book *Coping with Cancer* (1979a), since that is a major alternative view to the one presented in this book and because Weisman's work is a major reference used by nurses.

Hoping Is Coping: A Normative Model of Coping

Weisman's book (1979) comes out of Project Omega, a research project designed to study the impact of coping on survival and quality of life of cancer patients. Weisman demonstrates impressive clinical skills in the book; however, the model of coping offered does not live up to the clinical knowledge presented. Inherent in his theory are problems of using a normative model. He proposes that there is a "good" way to cope with cancer and a "bad" way. This view of coping resembles the thinking of Norma Haan (1977), who defines three modes of coping:

> Coping involves purpose, choice, and flexible shift, adheres to intersubjective reality and logic, and allows and enhances proportionate affective expression; defensiveness is compelled, negating, rigid, distorting of intersubjective reality and logic, allows covert impulse expression,

and embodies the expectancy that anxiety can be relieved without directly addressing the problem; fragmentation is automated, ritualistic, privatistically formulated, affectively directed, and irrationally expressed in the sense that intersubjective reality is clearly violated (p. 34).

This is basically a psychodynamic view of the person as a rational problem solver who tests reality, and assumes total responsibility for feelings and actions. In this view, coping is a trait or talent that can be judged in a context-free fashion. Weisman frames it in moral terms:

> Defensiveness, or using defenses, means fending off an unspecified problem, and is ordinarily not considered very admirable. Coping is thought to be a good thing to do, provided that the strategy is socially sanctioned, i.e., not reckless, imprudent, revolutionary, or so on (p. 41).

This position overlooks the facts that typically one confronts more "unspecified" problems in life than well-defined ones and that defenses such as denial or avoidance may allow needed respite while one waits for the appropriate time or situation in which to take specific actions or alter one's perspectives (Lazarus and Folkman 1984). A context-free, trait approach to a transactional variable such as coping leads one to treat other transactional variables, such as hope, as trait variables as well. For example, Weisman (1979) defines hope as a trait unrelated to the person's circumstance:

> When hopeful people acquire cancer, they are tenacious and resourceful. Therefore, hope is not simply a wish to undo what cannot be changed, nor does it evaporate at bad news. Hopeful people, strangely enough, do not depend as much on goals as upon self-concept, even though self-concept is nourished by success in reaching goals. . . .
> Hope is a prerequisite for good coping. . . . Genuine hope does not need denial, because good copers seek and use resources of all kinds. Counterfeit hope only pretends to cope. Actually it covers passivity (p. 13).

By treating hope as a personal trait, one overlooks the relationship between the person, his or her world, and his or her situation. Indeed, treating hope as a personal trait overlooks the way the person is *in* the situation. Hope is a transactional variable, it is constituted both by the person and by the situation. To view hope as a context-free trait possessed by the person regardless of the situation sets the person up to be morally responsible for all feelings and to be blamed when hope is not available to the person. That such a trait position leads to a "blame-the-victim" stance is borne out later in Weisman's book, when he states

273

that "there are patients who are born losers, and expect the future to be no different than the past" (p. 23).

The major problem with defining some coping strategies as "good" and others as "bad" is that the person's concerns and context are not taken into consideration. This approach leads to an "outside-in" view and lends itself to the development of trivial lists of advice that offer little guidance and show little understanding of what that advice might mean to specific people in specific situations. For example, Weisman (1979) offers the following advice:

1. Avoid avoidance; do not deny.
2. Confront realities, and take appropriate action.
3. Focus on solutions, or redefine a problem into solvable form.
4. Always consider alternatives.
5. Maintain open, mutual communication with significant others.
6. Seek and use constructive help, including decent medical care.
7. Accept support when offered; be assertive, when necessary.
8. Keep up morale through self-reliance or resources that are available.
9. Self-concept is as important as symptom relief.
10. Hope is self-pride, not self-deception (pp. 42–43).

As lists of context-free advice go, this one is not too flawed; however, lists of advice are deceptively simple, tend to miss the real issues involved, trivialize the demands, and overlook the loss. Such lists of advice reflect the naive assumption that there can be "rules" for effective coping. It is assumed that the patient or caretaker will know and recognize when the "advice" might apply and what forms it should take, and that the person has the ability to follow the advice. The item "Accept support when offered; be assertive, when necessary" is a good example. The patient may not know how to accept support when offered or how to be assertive when necessary. (Indeed, the problem is often the lack of recognition for the need to be assertive.) Any rule or general directive can play havoc when applied in ways that do not take into consideration the patient's world, skills, history, concerns, and current circumstances.

The strength of Weisman's (1979) work comes from a recognition of the pervasive impact of a cancer diagnosis on the person's life. His insights on areas of predominant concern are incorporated below in the discussion of coping with cancer.

Coping with Cancer

THE ROLE OF PERSONAL HISTORY

Each person comes to an illness with a history relevant to that illness. Her or his prior experience with and knowledge of the disease may be scant or extensive. The person may invest the disease with particular personal terror or have few preconceptions about it. The person's response may be influenced by past experience with relatives or friends who have the disease. This personal history shapes the person's illness experience during all its phases, including the treatment-seeking and prediagnostic phases. Prior knowledge and experience may lead to vigilance or to denial and avoidance.

In addition to bringing his or her personal history with the disease, the person comes to any illness with a historical self-understanding in terms of vigor, resilience, vulnerability, effectiveness of medicine and nursing, dealing with institutional demands, and recovery experiences. As the disease trajectory unfolds, this is added to the patient's history. If early diagnostic and treatment efforts have gone smoothly, the patient may have a higher level of trust in health care workers during later treatment efforts. However, unnecessary delays or initial treatment difficulties may inspire in the patient a continuing sense of wariness and distrust. Such a patient may suffer a sense of being betrayed by the disease itself and by health care workers.

Understanding the patient's prior experience with the disease and historical self-understanding is central to addressing the first question of coping—"coping with what?" The patient's relevant history to the particular disease sets up a major portion of what counts as stressful and what may be considered as coping options.

THE ROLE OF THE SITUATION

The term *situation* is used to describe the person's particular context. The person's situation sets up some possibilities and precludes others. From the phenomenological perspective (Benner 1984b, 1985; Taylor 1979), the person has situated freedom, that is, the freedom to actualize and choose options from a particular situation and a particular history. In Chapters Two and Three we contrasted situated freedom with radical freedom, the view that one can simply choose to "feel" any way about any event.

A major portion of the person's situation is his or her own particular social network. A person's social network may be effective and resourceful or may be a source of demand. Strained marital relationships are not likely to be improved by the demands of a major illness. Even such a reasonable "predictive" statement in human science, however, can be turned over by the transformations in meaning that can occur in individuals and families experiencing a major illness. Past issues may seem trivial in the light of the illness, and new possibilities may emerge. To say that such a possibility exists is to acknowledge situated freedom. To acknowledge that such a possibility is diminished by a past of turmoil, conflict, and misunderstanding is to acknowledge the power past roles and self-interpretations have to continue to work themselves out in new circumstances.

The situation is also defined by history, adult developmental stage, and family stage. It has been demonstrated that older people typically respond to cancer with more equanimity than younger people do (Mages and Mendelsohn 1979). A life-threatening illness has different implications for the person with a young family than for the person with adult children. Likewise, career stage, work demands, and financial resources define the situation for the person. For example, for someone with heavy financial responsibilities, losing one's income may bring economic disaster that rivals the disease in creating distress and coping demands for the family.

In Chapter Three, we introduced the notion that the way the person is *involved* in the situation is a basis for understanding the person's stress and coping. If the person is alienated and distrusting of medical care, his or her response to health care workers and choice of treatment will no doubt be influenced by this stance. It is reasonable to respond to a life-threatening diagnosis with anger, anxiety, and fear. Each of these distressing feelings sets up the way the person is *in* the situation. For example, an angry person may not be able to allow people to get close; indeed, anger may be the least distressing emotion, keeping feelings of helplessness and sadness at bay. Anger or any other dominant feeling create certain possibilities for the person and preclude others.

In an extremely individualistic and atomistic view of emotion, people are seen as free to *choose* their emotions and therefore are ultimately responsible for their feelings. They can "control" their feelings. Although it is true that people can alter their feelings, this is not the same as controlling or "dictating" feelings. The notion that one can choose feelings at will is very much connected with modern views of radical freedom—freedom from suffering and from encumbrances (Borgmann 1984). The problem with this position is that the role of the situation—and the way the person is *in* it—are overlooked. The person is free to choose to change the situation, move to a different situation, or attend to a different situation, or deliberately focus on a different feeling state or different time in her or his life. But this kind of "indirect" control is not the same as creating one's feelings from the ground up.

Feelings have a validity on their own. They reflect one's relationship to a situation. Just because people may choose how they act on or express their feelings, it does not follow that they have complete control over the beginning and end of feelings. For example, many patients act cheerful and optimistic in order not to frighten their friends away (Wortman and Dunkel-Schetter 1979). But socially contrived cheerfulness is not the same as feeling cheerful.

If it were possible to choose feelings regardless of the situation, the person would no longer be related to the situation. Such a view places the person outside of his or her own history and meaningful context. In other words, such a complete freedom would mean that others or things outside the self could have no claim on the person's responses. Such a view of emotion is ultimately nihilistic.

Understanding the alternative position, situated freedom, is helpful when working with people who are extremely distressed (angry, anxious, fearful, sad) over a life-threatening or disfiguring disease. Patients need not be held responsible or blamed for their feelings. Feelings create the person's sense of possibility. Any movement, growth, or change must come from his or her own particular stance. People cannot move from a vacuum to a vacuum in terms of perspectives and feelings, nor can this move be dictated by another person. People can only begin from where they are, and their feelings indicate their stance, even when they cannot be explicit or articulate about them. Thus, understanding situated freedom increases access and possibility when caring for distressed patients. Because the person has not freely chosen his or her feelings, and because the only source of possibility for the patient is *from* the current stance, the intervention must be based on an accurate interpretation of the patient's current way of being in the situation. Change *to* a different way of being in the situation can only occur *from* the current situation.

The prediagnostic and diagnostic phases of cancer present different coping demands than the treatment selection phase, the treatment phase, the remission phase, or the terminal phase do. Each of these phases creates a different situation with distinct adaptive demands for the patient and family. Each of these phases constitute a large measure of the patient's *situation*.

PREDIAGNOSTIC PHASE. Clearly, coping and lifestyle play a major role in whether the person is screened for the detection of early signs of cancer or attends to early warning signals. The person may avoid seeking medical attention due to the subtlety or misinterpretation of the symptoms, out of fear, avoidance, or ignorance; or because of feeling overwhelmed with other life demands.

Patient education for early detection of cancer, to be effective, must realistically warn and inform without creating a level of alarm that would cause the person to withdraw and avoid taking action in response to the message. General public education must be coordinated with health care workers so that the public gets an appropriate response to their request for information on early cancer detection. It is extremely difficult for a patient to regain trust in medicine and nursing after a prolonged "missed diagnosis" when the patient had sought help early.

DIAGNOSTIC PHASE. The stressfulness of the diagnostic phase varies greatly depending on the patient's interpretation of the disease and its implications. During this phase, the patient must select a physician and follow through with the required diagnostic tests. This is an extremely demanding situation in terms of the amount of threatening information that must be evaluated and acted upon.

A great deal of interpersonal skill is required to get adequate information about how to choose treatment centers, gauge the expertise of physicians, get a second opinion, and evaluate one's options. It is here that effective counseling by expert nurses can be extremely valuable. Time spent in sorting out the options and best resources at this point can help the patient feel settled about the lines of action presented in the treatment phase. However, most patients are simply not able to mobilize an organized search for all treatment options.

The variability in patient coping is great. Some may be in crisis, and their anxiety level may be too high to attend to issues at hand. In such circumstances, the patient may appear disorganized and may have difficulty remembering appointments and instructions. Simple, direct, and concrete instructions and schedules may be necessary to help the patient arrange for tests during this period of crisis and disorganization.

Some patients are able to assume the best, if this has been their established style, and not "borrow trouble" until the results are in. Other patients may be extremely mobilized and vigilant during the diagnostic workup, gathering information, planning, and trying to meet the situation with their best problem-solving efforts. Other patients may effectively appoint a family member to secure the information they need in order to act.

It is, of course, not possible to catalogue all the possible responses. The point is to recognize that patients will meet this situation with their own particular coping history, meanings, and resources. They cannot simply "choose" a way to cope with the situation if that way does not fit their own history and resources. This is why it is of little use to identify preferred modes of coping. The patient will do what she or he can, and one can help the patient augment her or his own approach only by counseling that attends to that person's understanding and coping stance. For example, one man may cope by placing himself in the "hands" of people in the health care setting most familiar to him, regardless of what other options are available in the community. He may be given information about other, more specialized resources and options, but he may not be able to act on that information, preferring not to subject himself to new institutions and new health care workers in a time of crisis.

Therefore, information giving is not sufficient. Timing, assessing the patient's level of fear and trust, assessing the availability and resourcefulness of family members and friends, and being available to offer guidance when the patient seeks it and can use it are essential to effective coaching through the diagnostic phase.

TREATMENT PHASE. The patient may experience a lessening in anxiety during the treatment phase simply because the situation is now clearer, the goals are clearer, and the tasks and demands are clearer. The patient's world is structured by the demands of surgery, recovery, radiation, and or chemotherapy. The treatment situation is further defined by whether or not the patient has been experiencing disease symptoms that may or may not improve with the treatment. For cancer patients, the treatment phase may mark the beginning of feeling sick because of the side effects of the treatment. If so, it is not unusual for patients to have doubts about whether they have made the right choice in their therapy. Effective patient education and counseling must accompany the therapy in order for the therapy to be accepted with minimal distress. A patient who knows what to expect will not mistake the side effects for deterioration or advancement of the disease.

Since not all patients experience all side effects, health care workers may be tempted to develop a "wait-and-see" attitude, discussing only those side effects that actually occur and not worrying the patient with the full range of possibilities. This is an ethical breach of the patient's right to be informed about the nature and effects of treatment, but it is also a serious breach of faith when the patient misinterprets the side effect and experiences needless worry and fear. Peck and Boland (1977), in a study of fifty patients undergoing radiation therapy, found that 60% did not know what to expect in terms of side effects, but preferred more knowledge to not understanding their physical responses and misinterpreting them as signs of deterioration. More than one-third felt worse after treatment and judged their treatment to have been ineffective, not realizing that their new distress resulted from the side effects of the radiation. Sixty percent of these patients were actually free of signs of cancer at follow-up 18–36 months later. The fear and distrust of radiation, and the limited efforts to support patients during this therapy, reflect the view that the treatment works on "cells and tissues" and its efficaciousness is not influenced by the person's understanding or participation.

The problem cannot be approached as a simple issue of information giving. Assisting patients through difficult treatments requires expert coaching (Benner 1984a). The patient will be able to hear and understand the implications of the side effects at various times and may not grasp or remember the information given initially when the treatment is planned. Patients usually need additional teaching at the point of beginning therapy and clarification when the actual side effects begin to develop.

Many patients previously treated with chemotherapy experience anticipatory nausea and vomiting and pseudohallucination as a result of subsequent chemotherapy. From a phenomenological perspective, this is a good example of embodied intelligence. The body learns to respond to the situation in meaningful and predictable ways. This phenomenon can also be explained by the classical conditioned response paradigm. The patient learns to pair or associate the sight of the clinic, the nurse, or other "signs" of chemotherapy with the experience of nausea and vomiting. The body knows how to respond to that situation. Nesse, Carli, Curtis, and Kleinman (1983) report patients having a vivid sense of the chemotherapy odor that disappeared when they learned that others could not also smell the odors. Patients reported that the experience was different from a memory, that is, they did not experience it as distant and from a past time. It was a reliving of the prior experience that could be altered when they were confronted by the fact that no one else could smell the odor. This is a good example of an embodied, perceptual memory that has real contours and concrete referents. Nesse et al. (1983) conclude:

> Were the perceptions a result of medications still in the body? This is conceivable, but the phenomenon was most commonly experienced during the days immediately before a treatment, when drug levels in the body were the lowest. Also, some patients reported smelling the odor of the clinic, not of the drugs. Were these perceptions simply vivid memories? The subjects did not think so; they said that the stimulus seemed to be clearly outside of themselves. The fact that many subjects could not control the experience and were frightened by it also suggests that it is more than vivid remembering. The phenomenon is best described as a "pseudohallucination"; i.e., subjects experienced perceptions in the absence of external stimuli, yet they recognized that the experience was not an accurate reflection of reality. . . . Whether conceptualized as a "conditioned perception" or as a vivid intrusive memory, the phenomenon itself is more clear-cut than its explanation. The presence of vivid pseudohallucinations in most patients receiving extensive chemotherapy suggests that the phenomenon does not result from psychopathology but instead from some basic psychological capacity (pp. 484–485).

Clearly, the response is real and is learned from the chemotherapy situation. The body learns to respond with alarm and protective vomiting when considering the noxious experience of chemotherapy. The phenomenon is far from being explained scientifically, but it appears that the most plausible account will come from comparing this pseudohallucination with other bodily responses, such as phantom limbs or the automatic advance constriction of capillaries of experienced blood donors in response to entering a blood donation situation (Wolf 1981, see Chapter Two). It is an example of the skilled body's ability to respond to meaningful situations and of the body's ontological capacity to dwell in meanings (Merleau-Ponty 1962, Polanyi 1958).

As an embodied capacity, the phenomenon is similar to the capacity drawn upon in visualization. In visualization, patients are asked to "place themselves" in another place and time and feel all those feelings in their bodies. This is a planned and deliberate use of the body's capacity for reliving past situations. In the case of the pseudohallucinations, the capacity is uninvited and may be frightening to the patient. The pseudohallucination recedes as the patient reestablishes that he or she is, in fact, not in the noxious situation but in quite a different one. Visualization and attentiveness to the present circumstance may be useful strategies for getting rid of the pseudohallucination. Certainly, informing patients about the phenomenon and checking to see if they are experiencing pseudohallucinations can prevent unnecessary fears of hypochondriasis or mental illness as a result of this common side effect.

Treatment demands may be extensive, requiring that the patient forgo all other activities and concentrate on the treatment only. This is perhaps the most difficult trajectory because the patient is removed from his or her normal coping resources. For example, work and activity (Benner 1984b, Gal and Lazarus 1975) are major coping resources in our society. Work provides a sense of identity, structures the day, and offers an arena where people can demonstrate their capability. Work is also a major source of self-esteem and provides a sense of social value. This is why continuing work, even part-time, may be an effective coping resource during treatment. Work can relativize the treatment, can offer distraction, and place one in the normal context of social contact. This, of course, depends on the nature of the work and the degree of the patient's distress in response to the treatment. Health care workers need to attend to the positive benefits of maintaining work as a coping resource, as well as a financial resource even if work and treatment schedules have to be altered.

Coping with treatment can be effectively supported through a number of ways: counseling, social support groups, tension-reduction strategies such as guided relaxation, hypnosis, visualization, massage, leisure and recreation, therapeutic touch, and spiritual healing. (See Chapter Five for a further description.) These relaxation and hope-generating practices may be looked upon with suspicion or even ridicule by people who espouse a microbial model of disease and cure. However, nurses can counteract this by legitimizing these coping strategies for patients and helping them find resources that promote relaxation and mobilize hope. Dr. Kathleen Schneider-Braus (1986) gives an example of the effectiveness of hypnotism, yet the skepticism with which it is viewed. It was originally published in the *Journal of the American Medical Association:*

They billed me as a hypnotist. Granted, psychiatrists easily slip into the realm of shamans, priests and healers, but still it made me nervous to have the oncologists and residents promising I would deliver the magic of hypnotism. What did that mean to the young woman riddled with leukemia and needing her eighth bone marrow sampling? The last two procedures had been performed with the patient under general anesthesia because the previous five had made her famous for screaming, jumping from the bed and other hysterics. Now the anesthesiologist was squeamish because of her compromised lung function. Too apprehensive to "snow" her with medication, and knowing it hadn't worked well in the past anyway, the team of doctors felt backed into a corner. Time to call the hypnotist. The deck was stacked against me. The medical team received me with dubious respect, and the nursing staff had a more open skepticism in their manner. The woman herself appeared pale and very near the end of her rope, but I sensed a strain of stubborn courage through the tears and despair. She told me she felt she could get through the chemotherapy, the infections, even the high risk of death—-anything but the pain of the bone marrow sampling. I admired her, mostly for her imperfect strength and her blunt humanness.

The sampling was to be done, ASAP. If I believed the hypnosis wouldn't work after the half-hour induction, I was to call it off. The operating room was already scheduled for the next day. Beginning the induction and realizing the woman could not relax lying back because of her cough, and could not close her eyes because she was deaf and needed to read my lips, I nearly called to confirm the operating room reservation. But I couldn't think of a polite way to get out, so I began. I insisted she receive a tranquilizer and some morphine to increase my chances. I was, after all, trained in biological psychiatry, and my confidence needed a boost.

She was a surprisingly good subject—-able to warm and cool alternate hands. I motioned the team to begin. Using the 23rd Psalm as our cue, my hypnosis session felt more like a religious revival, holding her sweat-drenched hands, shouting to her about cool waters and green pastures, eyes locked, face to face six inches apart. Then it was over. She couldn't believe it. I felt exhausted and unable to bounce back to my medical persona. The oncologist gave a sly grin and said that he had a few other referrals for me. But as I walked out of the room my sense of miracle was shattered. The oncologist said, "So you call that hypnosis? Looked like relaxation to me." I admitted that I hadn't levitated anyone or pulled a rabbit from a hat, but that was hypnosis all right. We don't really know what it is, so how could I explain it? I read his procedure note: "Bone marrow was performed with 1 mg Ativan, 4 mg morphine, and relaxation technique." I thought a lot about what I did in that room. I doubt that it was more than or different from what old-time general practitioners used to do, or midwives, or Indian medicine men. The difference lay in the skepticism of the oncologist. Hypnosis relies on the human's ability to focus and relax; it contains little iatrogenic risk and is not costly. Yet it takes a back seat to medication in the Western world's approach to patients. The reluctance to accept hypnosis may be a question of efficiency or reliability, but perhaps it's more a question of faith (pp. 762–763).

Extreme individualism, where the individual is understood as solely responsible for feelings, meanings, and self, cuts the person off from others and diminishes our sense of responsibility for one another. But this position at bottom is "faithless." In the most extreme position, the person is left with no ability to draw on resources outside the self. This position works best when the person is not confronted with extreme suffering and with the limits of control. The technological promise of a handy abundance and an end to all suffering is "embarrassed" in the face of an incurable disease and in the circumstance of extreme suffering. Consequently, the patient may be blamed for not sufficiently "managing the self." This is the familiar "blame-the-victim" stance that only adds to the patient's sense of alienation and suffering.

With all the emphasis on techniques to decrease distress, the value of understanding and attending to the suffering and sense of loss in order to reduce the stigma and social isolation must not be covered over or avoided. Patients and family suffer not only from the disease but also from the great sense of social isolation and unanswerable questions about the cause and meaning of the disease. The only healing response to this illness side of the experience is for those caring to maintain their human ties and limit the sense of separation and alienation.

At the end of this chapter, such understanding and caring are illustrated by "Lara's Story," a mother's diary of the care and support she received during the treatment and dying of her teenage daughter, Lara.

REMISSION. Remission, too, is a distinct situation, with its own resources, demands, and constraints. Some leukemic patients report feeling better than they have ever felt. Some feel a sense of invulnerability and strength as a result of regaining their vigor. They now experience their vigor and health, and these stand in stark contrast to the fatigue and weakness they felt during their treatment. This very contrast may lend to the feeling of omnipotence.

Many patients experience remission as a period of uncertainty and limbo. Their cure is ambiguous. Consequently, any illness symptom, pain, weakness, fatigue, even headache may be a source of distress and worry. The illness continues, although the disease may be cured. Bard and Sutherland (1955) report on their study of people recovering from breast cancer:

> [Quoting study participants] 'You treat yourself like a soft-boiled egg. You might break your shell at any moment.' . . .
>
> A long time after discharge from the hospital and after the experience is no longer so fresh in memory, most women report that they cannot rid themselves of the constant feeling that they "will never be the same again." Often, intensive inquiry on this point reveals that, despite "good adjustment" or "acceptance" of the physical loss, a psychological wound remains, which these women are convinced will never heal (pp. 65 and 70).

Cancer survivors have not been studied sufficiently to know the impact of surviving cancer on subsequent health, morale, and stress and coping. It is clear that cure of the disease alone is not enough. Full recovery from illness means that the person is healed, reintegrated into the community, and able once again to take up life projects without excessive fear.

RECURRENCE. Recurrence ushers in a new situation for the patient. The "limbo" period is over, and now the patient must confront a new treatment regimen and new prognosis, but with a history and direct knowledge of possible side effects. Recurrence presents a different prognosis and of course has different implications depending on the site, stage, and type of cancer. In most cases, recurrence presents patients with the realization that they may be able only to lengthen their lives, but not to be "cured."

Recurrence presents the patient and family with decisions about how aggressive they want to be in the therapy and with issues about what quality of life will be satisfactory. There may be conflict within the family about what route to take. An oncology clinical nurse specialist, quoted in Sharon Olsen's research notes, provided an illustration of this conflict (see also Olsen 1985):

> [She describes a middle-aged woman with ovarian cancer who had a devoted husband and a ten-year-old daughter.] We tried her on one course of cisplatin therapy. That was in the days when we weren't putting people to sleep and it was miserable. She was vomiting and said: "What am I doing this for? I've had a wonderful life, a wonderful husband, a wonder-

ful kid, a wonderful career, I've enjoyed it. I've loved all of it. But if it can't be the same, I don't want any more. I just don't see why I should put myself through this. You say the chemotherapy might even fix it for a while, but it doesn't fix it permanently. It's going to come back. Then what am I going to have, another bowel obstruction? Why go through it again? For what?" Her husband wanted her to fight. [A difficult period of negotiation ensued in which the nurse clarified the husband's and wife's positions to each other. The wife refused further therapy. At the point of his wife's death, the husband reflected on the value conflict between him and his wife.] He said, "In all our married life together, the one thing we had problems with was risk taking. If there were 20-80 odds, I'd take the 20 and she'd take the 80. And that's what she's done in her illness. The odds were that it would come back. So she accepted that. To me, the odds said, you might get a cure, and I wanted her to take the chemo so badly. She could have been a concert pianist, but her fear that she might stumble over a piece sometime prevented her from doing that. She refused to do things where she might stumble. If we had an argument, it was over this. That's why this has been so hard."

This description portrays the conflict and turmoil that may shroud decisions when recurrence is a possibility. These decisions are not clear-cut medical ones, but human decisions made in the context of the person's own life situation and history.

The nurse may be caught up in the decision making during recurrence. The patient may look to the nurse for an "informal" opinion or a personal opinion about whether a demanding treatment is worth the suffering involved. The patient will read the nurse's response by what is said but also by the nurse's demeanor and tone of voice. This is perhaps the most difficult coaching situation because the situation is typically underdetermined. Outcomes are not very predictable. Length of survival and quality of life vary considerably even for patients with the same disease. The nurse can present the possibilities and help the patient interpret the possible outcomes in terms of the patient's concerns and perspective. In the case presented above, the nurse assessed that the husband was on one end of the continuum, wanting all the therapy possible. The wife was on the other end of the continuum, and the nurse could see both sides. She maintained open communication with the husband and wife and supported the wife's decision. Years later, the nurse wondered whether she would have been more positive and encouraging about therapy had the patient elected to have one more round of chemotherapy, and whether the woman could have had five to six more years of life as a result. The question has no final answers. It is an example of the life-and-death issues that arise in clinical dialogue. This nurse did not hide from herself her responsibility or her influence in coaching this husband and wife through this difficult decision. She does not minimize the seriousness or the difficulty of her helping role.

Recurrence has its own adaptive demands, and those demands occur in a different context (a different situation) than those of the initial diagnosis and treatment phase. Recurrence and treatment are defined as "living" with cancer, and the intent for therapy is either cure or prolonged management of the disease. The situation sets up the prospect of learning to live with disability and chronic illness. The focus is on living rather than dying.

DEATH AND DYING. Death and dying are difficult to write about not only because we are a death-denying society but also because our meanings are predominantly associated with future goals, progress, and becoming. Our language and meanings have less to say about being, arriving, and dying. Death has no technological fix; death is not a "problem" to be solved. For this reason, the normal instrumental, strategic language does not lend itself to discussions of death and dying. Consequently, it is not surprising that one of the predominant ways of "coping" with death is to identify progressive stages in the process and then turn the process of dying into a developmental achievement. Kubler-Ross's (1969) classic work on death and dying identified the stages of denial, anger, rejection, bargaining, and acceptance. Each stage was to follow the other. The major contribution of Kubler-Ross's work was to get the general public to talk about dying for the first time. Her work opened up a new dialogue about death and dying. She made people aware of the feelings and aspirations of the dying. Death became an acceptable topic, perhaps because we were given a "culturally" acceptable approach, a structure, a predictable set of stages. For the first time, death became the last career, the last achievement. However, a drawback of this work was that not everyone experienced these predictable stages. It was found empirically that the stages did not hold up (Kestenbaum and Costa 1977, Parker 1981). The problem with the achievement-oriented approach to dying was that, though Kubler-Ross (1969) did not intend it, the stages became a prescription for a "healthy" way to die. Kestenbaum (1979) points out that the quest for a "healthy death" in the current death awareness movement is paradoxical:

. . . The general public and our health care providers are now more prepared to integrate dying and death into their general view of life—but on the proviso that the terminal condition achieves standards of psychosocial health that are seldom encountered in ordinary daily life. Attention must be given to our assumptions and expectations as well as to the concrete reality of the terminal situation (p. 187).

Kestenbaum (1979) outlines the following factors that have led to the "healthy dying" movement:

1. A critique of the extensiveness and intrusiveness of biomedical technology that may assault human dignity and prolong dying and suffering.

2. A critique of the withdrawal and avoidance of the dying person by family and health care workers and of the "mutual pretense" (Glaser and Strauss 1965, 1968) that may surround the dying person.

3. A reaction against the "lingering" course of terminal illness. It is not surprising to find that our society prefers a quick transition between life and death.

4. A fear of being in a state between life and death, being kept alive but unconscious on life-maintaining machines. The patient and family may feel that the person is "trapped," suspended between life and death.

5. An increased apprehensiveness about the suffering that may be associated with dying. In the context of the modern era, even minor symptoms of discomfort are expected to be controlled. Consequently, our society has a low tolerance for pain and suffering.

6. Finally, the emergence of an image of a "good" or "acceptable" or "self-actualized" death. Kubler-Ross (1969) offers the positive image of achieving "acceptance," and Weisman (1979a, 1979b) offers the notion of an "appropriate death"—a death consistent with the person's lifestyle and one that the person would choose if he or she were able.

All of these factors may raise unrealizable expectations about the death experience.

At heart, the problem of the current death awareness movement is *not* the intent to restore the significance of the dying person as a person, as a member of a family and community. The problem lies in the inability of the technological era (in which the body is seen as a combination of replaceable parts and the dying person as a failed machine) to find a basis for significance in dying. Kestenbaum (1979) points out that in the premodern era:

> The way a person confronted death could be seen as of supreme importance, and a confrontation to be practiced in days of health as well as the final night of passage. This attitude stands in obvious contrast to the more contemporary orientation in which the dying person was seen as a useless or failed machine (p. 184).

Death in the modern era, even in the midst of the death awareness movement, lacks meanings and ways of understanding that provide comfort, ways of understanding and being at the time of death. The achievement-oriented approach to dying without a background of relevant meanings sets up what may be experienced as the ultimate frustration when the death experience neither meets these expectations nor brings about what has not been possible in ordinary living.

Clearly, the death awareness movement and the notions of "comfort care" and "appropriate death" all create possibilities for making death less isolating and the subject of death less of a taboo. However, in this context of high expectations, the nurse will be required to coach the modern patient on the realities often associated with death even while trying to maximize comfort and minimize mental confusion and suffering for the patient and family. The patient's social context and physiological condition set limits on what the patient and family can expect (Parker 1981). The context of a surgical ward, the home, or the hospice all offer different possibilities. Also, acceptance and tranquillity may be blocked by physical changes.

Many patients experience delirium in the last stages of the illness due to metabolic encephalopathy, which may be caused by electrolyte imbalance, sepsis, drugs, or vital organ failure (Massie, Holland, and Glass 1983). The patient may also suffer from brain metastases. Complications of analgesia, chemotherapy, or radiotherapy may also create neurologic changes that alter sensorium.

A patient's final delirium may pose special difficulties for the family, who may have a preferred death in mind for their loved one. The final stage will be recalled by family members and friends during bereavement. Families may need coaching to understand what their loved one is experiencing. For the patient with delirium, Massie et al. (1983) recommend short, frequent contacts with a supportive person who

reassures the patient quietly about the environment, correcting mis-
interpretations and orienting the patient to the immediate surroundings. This kind of family coaching is illustrated by a description given to
Sharon Olsen by an oncology nurse specialist (see also Olsen 1985):

> I was going by a patient's room. She was dying and was not to be
> resuscitated. She had several family members visiting. I didn't know the
> family members very well; I didn't know her very well. I went in the room
> because the patient was gasping for breath. I changed her position and
> suctioned her, talked to her. In the process of going toward the patient, I
> noticed that all the family members were backing toward the wall. There
> were six to eight people, and all of them had their backs just as close to
> the wall as possible and were as far away from the patient as they could
> be. They were watching her, big eyed, from the wall where they were
> standing. There was no closeness, no contact at all between the patient
> who was lying there, not quite as alert as they were used to seeing her. I
> realized that they were close family members and that they were not
> comfortable with the situation at all. I wanted to help them realize that
> she was still the person they loved and not a body lying here, because
> that's how they were behaving. As I was caring for her, I was talking to
> them and to her, trying to make some kind of contact. When I was
> through and she was breathing more comfortably after a change of posi-
> tion and suctioning, I held her hand as I talked with them and with her.
> She didn't say very much, but she was hearing what we were saying. You
> could see that in her expressions. They began to open up. I explained that
> she could probably hear what they were saying even if she did not
> respond. So I said, if you have anything to say to her just do it. You may
> come over here. You can sit close to the bed, hold her hand, and let her
> know that you are here. By the time I left the room, two of them came
> over. The daughter was sitting at the bedside, and I took down the side
> rail, explaining that they must replace it when they left, but that they
> could have it down so that they could be close to her (research notes).

This patient was not delirious but heavily sedated, and she seemed
changed and unapproachable to the family members. The nurse's intervention was simple, but it may have had profound consequences for
the family's memory of the last hours, which can have a major impact
on bereavement.

The hospice movement is an important counter to the terrors of a
strictly cure-oriented health care system. Comfort care focuses on
quality of life and providing comfort to the dying. The current hospice
movement has been most influenced by Dr. Cicely Saunders and the
opening of St. Christopher's Hospice in Sydenham, England (Corless

1985). The goal of comfort care or palliation is to provide relief from physical distress while paying attention to emotional distress, fatigue, tension, and dread. The patient and family as a whole are considered in improving the quality of life.

In summary, the patient's situation is largely but not completely defined by the phase of the patient's illness. Judith Parker (1981) notes that the mix of duration of the disease and context, home care, out-patient treatment, and hospitalization also define the patient's situation. She identified the following six patterns of treatment context, each of which may have a short or long duration:

1. Continuous hospital-based treatment. (Typically, this is of shorter duration and is the situation for a rapidly developing disease and/or a delayed diagnosis.)
2. Continuous hospital-attached treatment.
3. Continuous alternating hospital-based and hospital-attached treatment.
4. Episodic home-focused treatment.
5. Episodic home-based treatment.
6. Sequential treatment.

Each of these patterns of treatment create a different "institutional demand" on the patient and family. The patient may not have contact with health care workers who have a sense of the patient's outpatient, hospital-based, or home care. This is where the oncology clinical nurse specialist who sees patients in all three settings provides continuity and coordination of services. In addition, the nurse helps the patient and family select and effectively use the community resources available for care.

We have discussed in detail aspects of the situation the patient encounters as the patient's condition changes over time, but of course the patient's situation is not confined to his or her disease and treatment situation. The patient's situation is also defined by the family situation, the financial situation, the work situation, and whatever else the illness interrupts or impinges upon. For example, the patient who enters the illness experience with a well-functioning supportive network has a distinctly different situation and thus different coping resources than the patient who enters the illness in the context of disturbed family relationships or without close supportive relationships.

Work will be taken up further under the heading of personal concern. But here it must be pointed out that the diagnosis of cancer places a person in a circumstance of possible job discrimination. Feldman (1980), in a trilogy of studies covering white-collar and certain professional occupations, blue-collar occupations, and service occupations ranging from unskilled workers to highly skilled technicians, found that 54% of the respondents in white-collar positions identified one or more work problems due to their cancer history. In contrast, 84% of the blue-collar sample experienced work problems associated with their cancer. Nearly one-fourth of the white-collar respondents reported that they experienced discrimination and negative attitudes as a result of their disease. Blue-collar workers reported even more problems, including incidents of discrimination that included dismissal, demotions, reduced wages, or reduced employee benefits. Both groups reported job application rejections as a result of their diagnosis of cancer. Patients in all three of Feldman's studies reported a need and desire for more information from their physicians and more assistance in dealing with the emotional impact of cancer.

The patient's financial situation deserves special attention because cancer is a catastrophic illness that typically causes great financial burden. In addition to having to bear the initial cost of treatment, patients may feel trapped in their current jobs with their current insurance carrier because access to complete insurance coverage once the person has cancer is difficult (Cohen and Cordoba 1983). The California Planners survey studied the problem of insurance barriers for persons with a history of cancer and found the following:

- Cancellation of existing coverage under health insurance policies
- Reduction of benefits
- Increase in premiums
- Refusal of new applications
- Extended waiting periods for coverage
- Exclusions
- Loss of insurance due to loss of employment
- The experience of being "locked-in" to a current job for fear of losing insurance coverage

Both the insurance and work discrimination may serve to reinforce the patient's sense of isolation and stigma associated with having cancer.

292

The patient's situation influences what coping options and resources will be available as well as what distresses will be particularly acute. Having cancer is a private and public experience with real-world consequences. Coaching the patient and family through diagnosis, treatment, recovery, or dying requires an understanding of the patient's situation.

The Role of the Body

The experience of the body may be radically altered as a result of a diagnosis of cancer. The person may cease to perceive the body as a reliable dwelling place and set of capacities and come to see it as an alien source of disease and danger. Being at war with the disease may also be experienced as being at war with one's body. Furthermore, the person's embodied sense of self may change as a result of internal and external physical alterations in the body. The person's bearing may change. Instead of reflecting fluid motion and confidence, his or her bearing may reflect halting protectiveness and a sense of vulnerability.

Patients who have undergone radical mastectomy report reluctance to go out in crowds for fear of being "bumped" or injured. Their sense of physical integrity has been altered. For example, Bard and Sutherland (1955) report patient descriptions after a mastectomy:

> I don't want to go in the subway with the crowds. I am afraid of being pushed or bumped in the crowds. I feel sort of scared. It's the same way with shopping. I'm always afraid I'll be bumped.

> Everything I do around the house I'm afraid of. I'm always worried that it will open the cut. I don't want to bust anything or tear it. That's the way I feel.

Rehabilitation needs to include an assessment of the alterations experienced in embodiment and a renewed or recovered sense of bodily integrity. The experience of the body as a machine and object is a common outcome of the medical treatment of disease. However, this relationship to embodiment is alienating and distressing. Feeling "whole" and recovered must include feeling at home in the body once again. Alterations in the sense of embodiment as a result of cancer have not been studied systematically. Research in this area is much needed and has implications for the rehabilitation of the cancer patient.

293

The Role of Personal Concerns

Patients live in a world and have personal concerns. Things and people matter. That such an obvious statement needs to be made is reflective of the modern notion of the disengaged self, the self separate and autonomous, which was discussed in Chapters Two and Three. The participant, member self that is constituted by personal concerns and meanings is overlooked in the autonomous, highly individualistic versions of the self. When a major illness strikes, the person experiences his or her possibilities and limitations in the context of what concrete concerns constitute the person. It is the view of the body as lived meanings and concerns, even in its very comportment, and the view of the person as constituted by personal concerns that offer promise in the modern era of finding significance in death. Death is approached in light of personal concerns, and the body is experienced as the bearer of attitudes, meanings, and even intelligence.

The acknowledgment that people live in meaningful worlds allows the caregiver to provide care in the context of the patient's own world. For example, if the patient practices a religion, the resources and possibilities in that religion can be drawn on by the patient and supported by the caregiver. Such a stance is not prescriptive. It makes no sense to expect the agnostic to draw on religious faith. However, the agnostic's concerns and spheres of meaning provide meanings and possibility that may be elaborated and strengthened during a time of crisis.

People do not relinquish their concerns as a result of falling ill, indeed, their concerns lead them to take up their illness in a particular way. This is why it is so essential for the provider of care to solicit the patient's understanding of the illness along with an understanding of what the illness interrupts or threatens. The patient's particular concerns can give the patient the incentive to weather treatments and guide the nurse in helping integrate the treatments into the patient's concerns.

Patterns in Seeking and Receiving Help

Falling ill requires seeking help or at the least confronting the possibility that one will require help now or in the future. Seeking and receiving help are interpersonal issues in a culture where self-esteem is based on individualism, self-control, independence, and self-reliance. A distinction is made between seeking help and receiving help because some people find it extremely difficult to deliberately and explicitly ask for help but may have little difficulty receiving help when it is offered by appropriate others. Others may have the ability to ask for help but may not be sufficiently comfortable to appropriate or use help when it is offered.

Help seeking and receiving are the personal sides to theories about social support and social networks (Berkman and Syme 1979, Norbeck and Peterson-Tilden 1983, Schaefer 1985). Wrubel (1985) found that people could have elaborate social networks but literally be social isolates in terms of their ability to ask for and receive help from others.

One reason for the invisibility of nurses and nursing may be the culture's discomfort in acknowledging the need to be cared for by others. In their practice and theory, nurses attend to ways of providing nursing care that do not further damage the patients' sense of self-control or increase their sense of helplessness unnecessarily.

Temporality

A life-threatening diagnosis such as cancer confronts the individual with his or her finitude and temporality. As Merleau-Ponty (1962) notes:

> The subject, who cannot be a series of psychic events, nevertheless cannot be eternal either. . . . It is indeed true that I should be incapable of perceiving any point in time without a before and an after, and that, in order to be aware of the relationship between the three terms, I must not be absorbed into any one of them: that time, in short, needs a synthesis. But it is equally true that this synthesis must always be undertaken afresh, and that any supposition that it can anywhere be brought to completion involves the negation of time (pp. 410–415).

For the self-interpreting being who takes a stand on the kind of being he or she is, the news of a life-threatening illness causes the individual to reflect on his or her life with a new perspective, a new "synthesis" of his or her temporality. In our culture, even curable cancer confronts the individual with his or her mortality.

Hearing that one has a life-threatening disease alters one's perception of the future and may even cause one to reinterpret the past in terms of an altered present or limited future. This is especially true in the case of cancer. Cancer has such symbolic power that past injustices, disappointments, and losses may now be related to current sense of calamity and loss. Because a cancer diagnosis typically constitutes a crisis, past and future become more available. Patients may welcome an opportunity to deal with past disappointments as well as their current problems. Consequently, brief therapy and counseling may be particularly effective for the patient during the crisis.

Acute distress and pain can make the present moment seem interminable and can foreclose the past and the future (see Chapter Six, pp. 216–217). Alternatively, pain relief can create an opportunity for the patient to experience a pain-free period with great intensity and immediacy. Patients may learn to exploit the present, making the most of every symptom-free moment. In Merleau-Ponty's terms above, the patient develops a new synthesis of time.

The foreshortening of the future presents different difficulties at different phases and stages of the life cycle. People who have been working hard with a notion of a promised payoff in retirement may feel especially cheated when they receive a life-threatening diagnosis. Parents with young children grieve over the missed opportunity to see their children grow up. In each case, one's understanding of life is altered by the new perspective on his or her own temporality.

Stress and Coping for the Caregivers

The cancer patient's caregiver can experience extreme distress. Glaser and Strauss (1968) conclude that the trajectory toward death is more difficult for caregivers and survivors-to-be than for patients. The patient may be quite absorbed in the moment-by-moment situation and existence. Slowly he or she adapts to lower levels of functioning and reduced sense of well-being. The family member typically continues to experience the patient's current losses in terms of past capacities and may experience the loss with greater awareness than even the patient. The patient's perspective becomes constricted, and this is a great protective coping resource. The caretaker, too, narrows and constricts his or her sense of the situation. However, the caretaker always has a greater zone of awareness and must interact with more people and deal with a wider range of issues and problems than the patient. Therefore, he or she may have a greater and more painful awareness of the patient's plight.

Weisman (1981, p. 165) assesses the patient's and caregiver's plight in terms of:

1. The protocol—"What treatment is required at this time?"
2. The plight—"What problems does this patient face right now?"

3. The promise (caregiver question)—"What is being asked of me?"

Additional strain occurs when the caregiver's promise does not match the patient's plight or protocol. He concludes:

> It is wholly possible that some of the distress suffered by patients might be iatrogenic, namely, the result of emotional burdens felt by caregivers and secondarily placed on patients. A caregiver who feels exhausted and truculent can hardly be expected to carry out still other unrewarding duties with forbearance and understanding. Sooner or later, the patient will be blamed for being needy and sick, and as a result, will hesitate to ask for needed medication, nursing care, or even for information (p. 162).

Caregivers, whether professionals or family members, experience distress. Excessive fatigue, irritability, and impatience can be due to being overextended. Burnout—the general feeling of loss of connection and commitment—is a late effect of exhaustion (Wrubel, Benner, and Lazarus 1981). Burnout is a loss of interest and sense of extreme fatigue, along with loss of energy. The person in burnout has literally lost the ability to care. Avoidance and abhorrence are cited by Weisman (1981) as distress signals. The caretaker feels compelled to avoid the patient's situation. Avoidance and abhorrence should be an indication of caretaker distress and a signal for respite rather than a signal for guilt and continued demand. Caretakers cannot always be given extended respites, but even an afternoon off, a good movie, and a good night's sleep can restore perspective and bring back their ability to be *in* the situation again. In the example below, Lara's mother describes how meaningful brief respites were during her daughter's short and tragic illness. Even the mundane activity of knitting was familiar, normal, and soothing, a welcome distraction in the midst of painful alien experiences. The support and the care of Lara's caregivers sustained her in her grief; the staff in the distant medical center became her community.

A false, strained optimism and cheerfulness can also be a sign of caretaker distress. This form of "cheerfulness" has a fragile quality about it and is not the same as felt hopefulness (see p. 375.)

We end this chapter with exemplar presented by Robin Kramer, pediatric oncology clinical nurse specialist; Michelle Marin, a staff nurse during the time of Lara's illness; and Lara's mother. This exemplar instantiates the perspective presented in this chapter.

Remembering Lara

Robin Fireman Kramer, RN, MS
Clinical Nurse Specialist, Pediatric Oncology

On September 20, 1983, the pediatric oncology office alerted me that a teenager was on her way in with a preliminary diagnosis of leukemia. Even before I met Lara, I felt that I had begun to connect with her. I still remember the "pit of nausea" I felt in my stomach when I learned of her pending arrival. I knew that, because of her age, there was a good chance that she had acute nonlymphoblastic leukemia. It is a difficult type of leukemia to treat, and consequently, the prognosis is grim. We were facing an enormous challenge, both becuase of her complicated medical care and because of the psychological implications of being a teenager coping with a cancer diagnosis.

Unlike a toddler or a preschool child who does not understand the life-threatening implications of cancer, Lara undoubtedly would. I ached inside for someone in the prime of her youth—looking toward a future of independence, parties, college, a career, and the joys of intimate relationships.

Lara, as I intuitively expected, was a bright-eyed, blond fourteen-year-old girl who, despite her illness, managed to smile and show a spunky personality at our first meeting. She was trying to be brave, but the fear in her eyes was undeniable. I introduced myself as the pediatric oncology clinical nurse specialist and began to orient Lara and her family to the Medical Center of the University of California at San Francisco. I explained that my role was to inform them about diagnostic tests that would occur over the next few days, to educate them about the disease and treatment once the diagnosis was confirmed, to coordinate Lara's medical and nursing care, to act as a liaison to the medical staff, fielding concerns and grievances, to help in any way possible, and to just be a friend during this frightening experience.

I assured Lara and her family that although UCSF is a large medical center, Lara's care would be individualized. She would not be just "another patient" or "a case study" to us, but a very important person. She and her family would be the focus of our care. I also reassured the family that because UCSF is a large medical center, we have access to the latest knowledge and technology.

Over the next two days, while waiting for confirmation of the diagnosis, I did a lot of listening. I heard about the symptoms and events that had led to Lara's hospitalization. I listened to the expression of shock, fear, and guilt—how could this diagnosis of leukemia be possible? The nursing staff and I spent considerable time getting to know Lara and her family—their coping strengths, their weaknesses, who supports whom and how. We did not negate their concerns or try to offer false assurance.

We acknowledged their feelings as real and helped the family sort through them in a healthy and meaningful way.

It was clear to all involved that one of the most useful things we could do for this distraught family, who was in a strange and overwhelming place, was to assist them, little by little, in gaining control over their experiences. This involved helping them anticipate and be prepared for what was to come, for how it might feel or look physically and emotionally. It also involved helping them to continue in their usual roles as much as possible and engaging them as appropriate in the decisions affecting Lara's care. The sincerity conveyed to the family convinced them that someone would always be there for them during the low times.

As we began therapy, we quickly realized that Lara focused on her symptoms rather than on the possibility of dying. Although she knew that she had less than a 50% chance of survival, she concentrated on the here-and-now; the pain associated with frequent IV's, bone marrows, and lumbar punctures; the embarrassment of hair loss; the isolation from her friends; and the nausea and vomiting associated with the chemotherapy. So over the course of the following weeks, we followed her lead by responding to her immediate concerns:

1. We moved her to a room with a phone jack and encouraged her friends to call and visit.

2. We served her cocktails of antiemetics to help control nausea and vomiting.

3. We arranged for only the most experienced staff to carry out Lara's procedures.

4. When she required two subcutaneous injections every 12 hours, we devised a system to give them simultaneously. Lara maintained control by choosing and alternating who the "shot givers" were.

During the long weeks of trying to induce a remission, when Lara was still doing relatively well, I used a variety of approaches in working with her, depending on what kind of day she was having. Sometimes we would just joke around and listen to music; other times we would talk about more serious issues—not just her illness, but her personal life, as well as my own. I think Lara was able to open up to me because I shared a piece of myself, telling her about how I had met my husband, my college days, the movie I saw last weekend—the typical things any teenager would be curious about. There were days when I walked in the room and could tell by Lara's and her mother's faces and greetings that it was not a good day. I would sit down and listen—giving Lara unspoken permission to be angry or depressed—and allowed Lara to question me about the chemotherapy, the reason for her white blood count being so low, the possibility of remission or a bone marrow transplant. I was always open with her, accepted her feelings, and never made light of them. I did not assure her that "it would get better soon" or that "I knew how she must be feeling" because I truly did not know whether she would get better or how she actually felt.

After being off for a weekend, I was surprised to learn that a friend of Lara's family knew a young woman in her early twenties who had successfully undergone a bone marrow transplant (BMT) in Seattle. The friend had arranged to have this young woman come visit Lara and her mother. They were quite excited about meeting her, placing their hope in the possibility of a BMT. The young woman visited one afternoon, bringing pictures of her experience and touting the transplant as wonderful and as a relatively easy process. Clearly, this young woman's outlook had resulted from her fortuitously smooth and complication-free transplant experience. I knew, however, that there was a horrible underside of this story, i.e., the possibility of severe mouth sores, nausea and vomiting, graft-versus-host disease, diarrhea, and fever with shaking chills. In fact, there was a 20-30% chance of dying within the first month. I felt trapped in the dilemma of whether to present a more realistic picture of the BMT. But this would burst their bubble at a time when Lara and her family needed the boost provided by this young woman's contagious enthusiasm. We were not even sure that Lara had an acceptable BMT match as we were awaiting the HLA typing results.

Finally, I decided to just answer their questions generally and not pursue an in-depth explanation of the benefits or risks associated with a BMT. As it turned out, no one in Lara's family was a compatible bone marrow donor. Understandably, the family was terribly disappointed. This seemed like the perfect opportunity for me to share with them the unpleasant side of the BMT experience, which made them feel better about the fact that the transplant was not an option for them.

The next incident that stands out in my mind is Lara's birthday party. At first, Lara was barely lukewarm about the idea of a party in the hospital. The normally rebellious and moody side of any healthy teenager surfaced in this terribly sick young girl. Nothing was right and nobody understood. Lara was just plain miserable. All I could do with her was listen, acknowledge how awful it must be, and honestly say that she must feel like crying. Permission to cry was all she needed to let the tears flow. My eyes welled up, too, and I did not try to hide it. The next day, Lara's mood picked up, and she eagerly participated in planning that party, which was a huge success.

The days dragged on. Lara's white blood count remained low. The possibility of a discharge was still not in the near future. Remission was not yet a reality, and it was hard to sustain optimism. Something needed to be done for Lara's morale. I approached Dr. Katherine Matthay, Lara's physician, about the possibility of a hospital pass for a few hours. She was not sure that it was reasonable given Lara's condition, yet she admitted it was exactly what Lara needed to lift her spirits. I persisted, explaining how we could arrange her antibiotics so that she would not miss a dose, make sure she was all "tanked up" with transfusions of packed red blood cells and platelets, and cap off her IV with heparin.

I volunteered to take her out in my car on Saturday or Sunday and promised not to keep her out too long. Dr. Matthay gave in relatively easily. Although no one said it out loud, we all realized that this could be the only time Lara might leave the hospital alive. The excitement mounted as we planned for the great escape: Lara was to invite two friends to join us on the city tour.

The Sunday came, and the caper came off without a hitch. Just before we returned to the hospital, we stopped for ice cream in the Haight-Ashbury district. Lara would not go in because she was embarrassed about her IV board. We all tried to coax her, saying that, with so many weird people in this area, no one would even notice her. Lara held steadfast to her decision, which we respected by bringing her ice cream to the car. Looking back, I fully understand how self-conscious she must have been. After all, being different is one of the greatest curses that can befall any teenager. Why should Lara have felt any other way?

One day, after visiting with Lara in her room, I had an uneasy feeling. Her eyes looked dull, she still seemed tired despite a recent transfusion, and her skin color was pasty. She also had started spiking fevers. She had been neutropenic for so long that I feared the possibility of a fungal infection. Over the next few days, Lara's condition steadily worsened, despite WBC transfusions. She became dyspneic and needed oxygen. There was talk of moving her to the intensive care unit. Lara, her family, and the staff were worried. We all secretly feared that she might not be able to pull through this crisis, yet no one spoke of this fear. Joann, Lara's mother, was visibly distraught, although she still tried to maintain a positive outlook. I took her to the cafeteria for coffee and broached the fear that she clearly held within. I simply said, "I'm worried that Lara may not pull through this crisis: I'm sure you're worried, too." The tears quickly spilled forth as her worst fears were unleashed. Joann felt that her world was coming to an end. It seemed terribly unfair not only that her daughter had to die but also that she had to do so without ever returning home again. We talked about getting Barry (her husband) and Jody (Lara's sister) to come down. It was a time for the family to be together.

Lara needed to be intubated because her respiratory status continued to deteriorate. This was a terrible experience for her; she continuously gestured to us to remove the tube. The medical and nursing staff, along with Lara's family, acknowledged that Lara's death was imminent. Our greatest gift to Lara would be to give back her dignity by removing the respirator. She immediately started talking in a high, squeaky voice, and plans quickly developed to have a party "to toast Lara's awakening," as Joann aptly described it.

As I visited with Lara, she looked me directly in the eyes and said, "I'm so sick, am I going to die?" Although it was a matter of seconds before I answered, it seemed like hours as my mind groped for the right words. I did not avert my gaze and answered from my heart: "I'm frightened Lara, you are so sick that you could die. I know you must be terribly scared, too. Everyone you love is with you, and we won't leave." She nodded and quietly closed her eyes to rest. Shortly thereafter, the champagne arrived, and we toasted Lara—her extubation, her courage, and her spirit. She smiled and said, "I love you all very much." Two hours later, she died peacefully with her family nearby.

Lara's memorial was held ten days later. My presence was not just a supportive gesture for the family but a necessity for me. I needed to say good-bye to Lara and to pay tribute to her spirit. I needed to try to make sense out of her death and to exorcise the lingering memory of her ravaged body.

Something unique had happened during those eight weeks that Lara was hospitalized. The level of concern, the caring, the emotional and spiritual exchange cannot be pinned down in mere words. The experience was synergistic and far reaching. I was *just one* of many people who connected hard and fast with Lara and her family. And this family, in turn, enriched our lives beyond measure. If there is ever any sense to be made of losing a loved one, perhaps it lies in the inexplicable gifts one receives along the way.

Remembering Lara
Michelle Marin

All I could do is just look through the PICU window. Lara, lying still but with her eyes open, was intubated on a ventilator; IV's, arterial lines, and other tubing everywhere connected her to life. She had leukemia with sepsis and was rapidly failing. All, including fifteen-year-old Lara, agreed that if the sample of her mother's bone marrow HLA typing didn't match hers, Lara would be allowed the dignity to die.

For one week, Lara remained in the PICU. The nurses and physicians who had taken care of Lara on our medical unit for eight weeks rotated through Lara's room to be with her—she was rarely alone. All the staff went in—-except for me. I'd force myself to look through the window, but I just couldn't go in her room. I thought I had established a good rapport with Joann, Lara's mom. But during this week, I could not even talk to her. I was both overwhelmed with sadness and shame that I could not talk to Lara and her family. But I wanted them to know I grieved for their loss, too. So I left a copy of Rabbi Harold Kushner's book, *When Bad Things Happen to Good People,* anonymously in her room.

The day Lara was disconnected from her life-sustaining ventilator and IV's a celebration took place. Several nurses and family members toasted her "awakening" off the ventilator. Two hours later she died. A friend called me to tell me the news of Lara's death. I don't remember even crying.

This incident, although it occurred in November 1983,[1] remains vividly with me. I think it symbolizes for me something that I couldn't see at the time. As a pediatric nurse, dealing with acutely ill children at UCSF, I thought I could "deal" with dying. But looking back, every time I had the opportunity to be with a child nearing death and his or her family, I backed away. I was afraid to cry with the family, upset them, or make them angry. Maybe, too, it brought back remembrances of the past with which I could not cope. It's hard even now to write about Lara. I'm older and wiser and certainly less afraid of my emotions. And having had the chance to be with dying people, I can see what Lara's death meant to me.

Lara's Story
Joann Callister, Lara's mother

On November 15, 1983, our fifteen-year-old daughter died of complications of acute promyelocytic leukemia. Her death occurred exactly eight weeks after diagnosis. Except for a few hours she was allowed to leave, the entire period was spent in the University of California, San Francisco Moffitt/Long Hospitals. This is a fairly common experience these days, but I feel that, because we shared something extraordinary with many remarkable people, ours is a special story.

The huge financial burden of a catastrophic illness is outrageous and calamitous to any but the wealthiest families. But as we watched our child succumb to the dreadful disease, of equal important to the medical care were the sensitive acts of concern, kindness and support offered by the entire staff of care givers in Pediatric Oncology. These acts were treasures of immeasurable worth to a frightened teenager and her distraught family. I regret that space does not allow a more detailed list of all the unusual services provided us by the nonmedical staff, including secretaries, maintenance workers and social workers.

Day 1   The very red-eyed, tired-looking young resident doctor introduced himself to my brother, my husband, our daughter, Lara, and me. Our fears, doubts, and uncertainties must have been obvious to Dr. Dan

---

1. Michelle Marin wrote this account up for a class assignment on paradigm cases at a University of California School of Nursing graduate program in 1987. When she wrote this account she was working with AIDS patients.

Lowenstein, since he was quick to assure us that we would be treated with sensitivity, as people, not just as a case study. His promise revealed uncanny foresight. This gentle, quiet man rotated off our case the second day, but returned almost daily to check on Lara's condition, either personally or by reading her charts.

Nurse Robin   The compassion of Dr. Lowenstein was a tough act to follow, but Nurse Specialist Robin Kramer rose to the occasion. Her job, as she explained it, was to help us in any way possible: to answer questions, educate us, field grievances, to be liaison to the medical staff, and to just generally be our friend during our stay. Any degree of stability I was able to maintain over the next eight weeks was due largely to the unwavering support and encouragement of this dedicated young woman. Her daily concern was not only for the patient, but for each family member. She often called during weekends, once from Los Angeles, to see how things were going.

Our Doctor   Petite in stature, but obviously mighty in brains and character, Dr. Katherine Matthay carried us along our rocky path of treatment. The yo-yo existence, helplessness and frustrations were dealt with with sensitive candor and forthrightness. She agonized over every decision, consulting with us while examining our alternatives. On our first Sunday afternoon, Dr. Matthay and Robin Kramer both gave up precious hours of their day off to meet with nine members of our family to explain the disease, the treatment and the prognosis. And, in doing so, provided an opportunity for each of us to express our feelings. Her attention to Lara's older sister and the sibling's perception of the crisis immediately endeared her to the family.

Happy Birthday   A fifteenth birthday should be joyous and special. The staff knew that intuitively. Doctors and nurses went out of their way to share good wishes and cake with Lara and the family on her day. She was quite flattered that they would make such a gesture. The children's playroom was turned over to us exclusively for the party. Another concession to our particular need.

Brotherly Love   Young, soap-opera-handsome resident David Norton saw in Lara the little sister he left in Pittsburgh. His self-effacing humor and sincere caring provided a big-brother attitude. The repartee between doctor and patient made for a warm relationship. David often stopped to say "good night" before going home after a long shift.

Down Day   On one particularly bad day, Dr. Lowenstein and Robin talked at length with a depressed and very sick Lara. Each recognized and accepted her anger, fears and disappointments. All the while allowing her dignity and self-esteem, two short commodities in the hospital setting. Promises for a future hospital pass placated the patient and gave her hope for a respite.

Mind over Matter   Child Life Specialist Adrianne Burton tried so hard to convince a doubtful Lara of the advantages of thought control and imagery. She brought tapes, offered a visiting puppy and even bought two goldfish to appease the tortured psyche. Lara was finally converted, but was too sick to garner the discipline to be effective. Adrianne responded to many desperate calls for help.

Hair   Madison Avenue has conned all teenagers to worship their crowning glory. The prospect of going bald was the most appalling and humiliating side effect of treatment. Lara suffered more nightmares over that trauma than anything else. We found that braiding delayed the hair loss. Nurse Catherine Caserza came in during break time to weave French braids. Her very neat handiwork made Lara feel more secure. Thanks to this solution, Lara never did become bald. Unable to leave her work far behind, Catherine even sent a postcard greeting while on vacation in Mexico.

Rock and Roll   Nurse Janey Hiura offered to take Lara to a Men at Work concert. Conditions would not allow such an activity so Janey brought from the concert what she could: a souvenir T-shirt, ticket stubs, a police restriction tape and, best of all, a note-by-note report of the action. Janey's tranquil manner had a calming effect during many of Lara's difficult times.

White Blood Cells   Because white blood cells must be donated, processed and infused within hours, only local people can be used as donors. Our hometown was too far away and we were strangers in an unknown city. I wept with worry about this problem. Within minutes of knowing that we needed ten donors, three nurses offered to give up four hours of their day off to help us. We were dumbstruck by such a generous response.

A Male Nurse   Warned that the next shift nurse was a man almost created havoc. I convinced Lara to give him a chance by promising to take over any embarrassing situations. Bill Poole's dry wit and no-nonsense demeanor completely won her over in minutes. The two outspoken, up-front personalities found a great affinity and Bill became one of Lara's favorites—in spite of being male!

The Great Escape   With faultless planning, Lara was "capped off" the IVs and we were granted a four-hour pass from the hospital. Robin was our "keeper" and tour guide. Once again giving up a Sunday afternoon, she took Lara, two of her visiting friends and me on a grand tour of the places all teenagers are curious about—the Haight and Castro districts. It was a delightful diversion from the hospital routine and did Lara a world of good, mentally.

The Telephone   At the encouragement of the staff, we moved into another room because it had a phone jack. That became Lara's lifeline to the outside world and was the single greatest morale booster we found.

TV   Any strong relationship is based on some common denominator. Since many of the nurses shared Lara's interest in General Hospital, all who could swing it would take lunch at two o'clock in order to watch the soap with her. She enjoyed the discussions and speculations regarding the story line. No matter how terrible she was feeling, Lara rallied enough to share that time with the nurses.

The Typewriter   Because of IVs, swollen hands and weakness, writing was difficult or imposible. Nurse Michelle Marin brought in her personal electric typewriter so Lara could more easily do homework and write letters. She never was able to use it, but the offer was appreciated.

The Song and Dance Man   Dr. Alex Blackwood (in unorthodox attire) sang, danced and joked his way into our hearts. His quiet, corny humor could bring a smile where tears had been. At our first meeting, Lara and I were intrigued by a feathery apparition that seemed to be clinging to the doctor's neck. Only close scrutiny revealed it to be a stuffed animal attached to his stethoscope and not some exotic tribal paraphernalia from Africa. Alex was on duty the day the final crisis began. It befell him to help tell me what was expected to be Lara's death sentence. The anguish expressed by this man then and many times later showed a profound humanness and touched me deeply.

Music   Nurse Lisa Tudisco and Lara talked a lot about France and mutual musical preferences. One day Lisa brought in a David Bowie tape for the Walkman. She knew Lara listened to tapes during chemotherapy to help lessen the pain and nausea.

Literature   Dr. Lowenstein came by before going on vacation to Hawaii. He left a copy of *The Little Prince* for Lara. On the flyleaf was a beautiful inscription to her. She had planned to use the book as a source for a book report that was a school assignment.

Concert   A few of the mothers of patients were given free tickets to attend a concert near the hospital. We went with great anticipation and were not disappointed. It was a short time of beauty in a long time of despair. We all valued the opportunity to relax for an hour or so.

Chinese Food   One day, in casual conversation, Lara mentioned to nurse Michelle Spode that she was hungry for Chinese food. Michelle spent her entire lunch hour searching for THE restaurant. She returned with enough food for an entire family.

Double Shots   A new chemotherapy had to be administered by four shots a day. To minimize the pain to an already wracked body, two nurses gave two shots simultaneously. One nurse was doing this during her free time.

Knit and Purl   My urge to knit was fostered when nurse Lynne Roger brought in a dozen pattern books from which Lara was to choose a sweater for me to make. Next day, Lynne came to the hospital two hours before her shift in order to drive me to the yarn shop. I selected the yarn and started to pay for it. Lynne put the bag of ten skeins of yarn in my arms, saying, "Here! This is a present from the staff." It took me a while to choke down the lump in my throat. She explained that they all wanted to do something special for us.

ICU Lara's worsening condition required moving into ICU. The floor nurses were very disgruntled when not allowed to help move and set up Lara in her new quarters. During the last six days there was nearly continuously one or more off-duty nurses or doctors with us in ICU. They had become family and we gratefully accepted their presence.

A Book Someone left *Why Bad Things Happen to Good People* in the room. The act was an anonymous, loving gesture. Unfortunately, I was never able to thank the donor.

The Toast We decided to give back Lara her dignity by removing the respirator. Word quickly went out that she was alert and talking (in a funny, squeaky voice). A crowd was soon gathered around her bed. While we laughed and joked about her being speechless for three days, a bottle of chilled champagne mysteriously appeared. We celebrated her "awakening" with a toast cheered on by several nurses and family members. She smiled with obvious pleasure from the attention, said "I love you all very much," and went to sleep.

The End Two hours later, with nurses and family still nearby, she breathed her last, quietly and peacefully.

Goodbye It took a long time to pack up and leave the hospital. Staff and parents of patients kept a steady flow of farewells. Their hugs were a great comfort.

The Memorial Ten days later, the Saturday after Thanksgiving, five nurses and a social worker drove from as far as a hundred miles to attend Lara's memorial service. Robin Kramer spoke to the gathering of 400 friends and family, telling them how Lara had touched the hearts of the staff in Pediatric Oncology. This act of love, spoken in a tight voice choked with emotion, was the culmination of the promise made on our first day at Moffitt, "To show we do care about you as people, not just as a case study."[1]

COMMENTARY

Lara's death is tragic. There is no way to remove the sadness. The remarkable thing that occurred, as Robin Kramer, Michelle Marin, and Lara's mother Joann describe, is that University of California at San Francisco with all the encumbrances of bureaucracy, high technology, and multiple caregivers became a caring community for Lara and her

---

1. From: *UCSF Magazine,* Vol. 8, (October 1985), 40–45.

family. No one psychologized about the gravity of the situation, and everyone was careful to build as much hope as possible. The disease was overwhelming. Some diseases are. We are not given omnipotence. But in the face of this pain, Lara and her family reached out, and the caregivers responded.

Everyone seemed aware that there were no "techniques" that could solve the real problem, but technical expertise was marshalled to provide comfort and to assuage nausea, pain, boredom, fear, and isolation. The caring was creative. Someone understood that the brief, focused attention knitting provided could help Joann get through some hours. Lara's beauty and humanity were celebrated.

Michelle Marin's paper provided a missing piece to the picture. She had given what she could by providing a book that she thought would bring comfort. One can give only what they are able to give. Lara and her family in turn gave to Michelle by beginning a three-year dialogue about her feelings on death. This dialogue has enabled Michelle Marin to work with AIDS patients and to risk caring, even though her patients are young and gravely ill. By offering what she could at the time, she said yes to caring, and she grew.

Lara and her family were remarkable because they could all reach out and feel cared for in the midst of fear and threat. The ability to receive comfort when no preferred solution is available is a remarkable resource.

REFERENCES

Anthony JJ: Malignant lymphoma associated with hydantoin drugs. Archiv Neurol 22:450, 1970.

Bahnson CB: Stress and cancer: The state of the art, Part 1. Psychomatics. 21:975, 1980.

Bahnson CB: Stress and cancer: The state of the art, Part 2. Psychomatics. 22:207, 1981.

Bard M, Sutherland AM: Psychological impact of cancer and its treatment: Adaptation to radical mastectomy. Cancer 8:55, 1955.

Basham TY, Kaminski MS, Kitamura K, Levy R, Merigan TC: Synergistic antitumor effect of interferon and anti-idiotype monoclonal antibody in murine lymphoma. J Immun 137:3019, 1986.

Benner P: *From Novice to Expert: Excellence and Power in Clinical Nursing Practice.* Menlo Park, Calif.: Addison-Wesley, 1984a.

Benner P: The oncology clinical nursing specialist: An expert coach. Oncol Nurs Forum 12:40, 1985b.

Benner P: Quality of life: A phenomenological perspective on explanation, prediction, and understanding in nursing science. Adv Nurs Sci 8:1, 1985a.

Benner P: *Stress and Satisfaction on the Job: Work Meanings and Coping of Mid-Career Men.* New York: Praeger Scientific Press, 1984b.

Benner P, Roskies E, Lazarus RS: Stress and coping under extreme conditions. In

Dimsdale JE (ed): *Survivors, Victims, and Perpetrators: Essays on the Nazi Holocaust.* Washington, D.C.: Hemisphere, 1980.

Benson H: *The Relaxation Response.* New York: Avon, 1976.

Berkman L, Syme SL: Social networks, host resistance, and mortality: A nine-year follow-up study of Alameda County residents. Am J Epidemiol 109:186, 1979.

Borgmann A: *Technology and the Character of Contemporary Life.* Chicago: The University of Chicago Press, 1984.

Borysenko JZ: Behavioral-physiological factors in the development and management of cancer. Gen Hosp Psychiatr 4:69, 1982.

Borysenko M, Borysenko J: Stress, behavior and immunity: Animal models and mediating mechanisms. Gen Hosp Psychiatr 4:59, 1982.

Brandt EN: Cancer control objectives for the year 2000: The article reviewed. Oncology 1:34, 1987.

Cassel J: The contribution of the social environment to host resistance. Am J Epidemiol 104:107, 1976.

Cassileth BR, Lusk EJ, Miller DS, Brown LL, Miller C: Psychosocial correlates of survival in advanced malignant disease. New Engl J Med 312:1551, 1985.

Chow DA, Greene MI, Greenberg AH: Macrophage-dependent, NK-cell-independent "natural" surveillance of tumors in syngneic mice. Int J Cancer 23:788, 1979.

Cohen FL: The epidemiology and etiology of AIDS. In *The person with AIDS.* Durham JD, Cohen FL (eds.). New York: Springer, 1987.

Cohen J, Cordoba C: Psychologic, social and economic aspects of cancer. Surg Ann 15:160, 1983.

Cohen MS, Wellisch DK: Living in limbo: Psychosocial intervention in families with a cancer patient. Am J Psychother 32:561, 1978.

Corless IB: Implications of the new hospice legislation and the accompanying regulations. Nurs Clin North Am 20:281, 1985.

Coyle N, Foley K: Pain in patients with cancer: Profile of patients and common pain syndromes. Semin Oncol Nurs 1:93, 1985.

Craig TJ, Abeloff MD: Psychiatric symptomatology among hospitalized cancer patients. Am J Psychiatry 131:1323, 1974.

Dijulio J: Treatment of B-Cell and T-Cell lymphomas with monoclonal antibodies. Seminars Oncol Nurs 4:100, 1988.

Dijulio J, Bedegian J: Hybridoma monoclonal antibody treatment of T-cell lymphomas: Clinical experience and nursing management. Onc Nurs Forum 10:22, 1983.

Dreyfus HL: *Being-in-the-World: A commentary on Heidegger's Being and Time, Division I.* Cambridge, Mass.: MIT Press, in press.

Epstein SS: *The Politics of Cancer.* San Francisco: Sierra Club Books, 1978.

Engelman SR, Craddick R: The symbolic relationship of breast cancer patients to their cancer, cure, physician, and themselves. Psychother Psychosom 41:68, 1984.

Fagerhaugh S, Strauss A: *Politics of Pain Management: Staff-Patient Interaction.* Menlo Park, Calif.: Addison-Wesley, 1977.

Fagin C, Diers D: Nursing as metaphor: Occasional notes. New Engl J Med 309:116, 1983.

Feldman FL: Work and cancer health histories: Work expectations and experiences of youth (ages 13–23) with cancer histories. Oakland: American Cancer Society, California Division, Inc., 1980.

Fox BH: Premorbid psychological factors as related to cancer incidence. J Behav Med 1:45, 1978.

Gal R, Lazarus RS: The role of activity in anticipating and confronting stressful situations. J Human Stress 1:4, 1975.

Gendron D: *Enquiries into the nature, knowledge and cure of cancer.* London: 1701.

Glaser BG, Strauss AL: *Awareness of Dying,* Chicago: Aldine, 1965.

Glaser BG, Strauss AL: *Time for Dying.* Chicago: Aldine, 1968.

Gonda TA, Ruark JE: *Dying Dignified.* Menlo Park, Calif.: Addison-Wesley, 1984.

Gordon WA et al.: The psychological problems of cancer patients: A retrospective study. Paper presented at the annual meeting of the American Psychological Association, San Francisco, August 1977.

Greer S: Cancer and the mind. Br J Psychiatry 143:535, 1983.

Greer S, Morris T: Psychological attributes of women who develop breast cancer: A controlled study. J Psychosom Res 19:147, 1975.

Grissom, JJ, Weiner BJ, Weiner EA: Psychological correlates of cancer. J Clin Psychol 43:113, 1975.

Grossarth-Maticek R: Psychological predictors of cancer and internal diseases: An overview. Psychother Psychosom 33:122, 1980.

Grossarth-Maticek R, Frentzel-Beyme R, Becker N: Cancer risks associated with life events and conflict solution. Can Detect Prev 7:201, 1984.

Grossarth-Maticek R, Siegrist J, Vetter H: Interpersonal repression as a predictor of cancer. Social Sci Med 16:493, 1982.

Haan N: *Coping and Defending: Processes of Self-Environment Organization.* New York: Academic Press, 1977.

Haskill S, Proctor JW, Yamamura Y: Host responses within solid tumors: I. Monocytic effector cells within rat sarcomas. J Nat Cancer Inst 54:387, 1975.

Holmes TH, Rahe RH: The social readjustment rating scale. J Psychosom Res 11:213, 1967.

Kestenbaum R: "Healthy dying": A paradoxical quest continues. J Social Issues 35:185, 1979.

Kestenbaum R, Costa PT: Psychological perspectives on death. In Rosenzweig MR, Porter LW (eds): *Annual Review of Psychology,* pp. 225–250. Palo Alto, Calif.: Annual Reviews, Inc. 1977.

Kersey JH, Spector BD: Primary immunodeficiency and malignancy. Birth Defects 11:289, 1975.

Kissen D: The significance of personality in lung cancer in men. Ann NY Acad Sci 125:820, 1966.

Kissen D, Rao LGS: Steroid excretion patterns and personality in lung cancer. Ann NY Acad Sci 164:476, 1969.

Kubler-Ross E: *On Death and Dying.* New York: The Macmillan Company, 1969.

Lazarus RS: The trivialization of distress. In Rosen JC, Solomon LJ (eds): *Preventing Health Risk Behaviors and Promoting Coping with Illness,* vol 8. *Vermont Conference on the Primary Prevention of Psychopathology.* Hanover, N.H.: University Press of New England, 1985.

Lazarus RS, Folkman S: *Stress, Appraisal, and Coping.* New York: Springer, 1984.

Locke S: Stress, adaptation and immunity: Studies in humans. Gen Hosp Psychiatry 4:49, 1982.

Lovejoy N: Roles played by hospital visitors. Heart and Lung 16:573, 1987.

Mages NL, Mendelsohn GA: Effects of cancer on patients' lives: A personological approach. In Stone GC, Cohen F, and Adler NE (eds): *Health Psychology: A Handbook,* pp. 255–284. San Francisco: Jossey-Bass, 1979.

Margarey CJ, Todd PB, Blizard PJ: Psycho-social factors influencing delay and breast self-examination in women with symptoms of breast cancer. Soc Sci Med 11:229, 1977.

Massie MJ, Holland J, Glass E: Delirium in terminally ill cancer patients. Am J Psychiat 140:1048, 1983.

Merleau-Ponty M: *Phenomenology of Perception.* London: Routledge & Kegan Paul, 1962.

Mettler CC, Mettler FA: *History of Medicine.* Philadelphia: Blakiston, 1947.

Meyerowitz BE: Psychosocial correlates of breast cancer and its treatments. Psychol Bull 87:108, 1980.

Nesse RM, Carli T, Curtis GC, Kleinman PD: Pseudohallucinations in cancer chemotherapy patients. Am J Psychiatry 140:483, 1983.

Norbeck J: Coping with stress in critical care nursing: Research findings: Focus on Critical Care 12:36, 1985.

Oldham RK: Monoclonal antibodies: Does sufficient selectivity to cancer cells exist for therapeutic intervention, J Biol Resp Med 6:227, 1987.

Olsen S: Exploring the clinical practice of expert oncology nurses. Unpublished master's thesis, University of Wisconsin, Madison, 1985.

Parker J: Cancer passage: Continuity and discontinuity in terminal illness. Unpublished doctoral dissertation, Monash University, Australia, 1981.

Peck A, Boland J: Emotional reactions to radiation treatment. Cancer 40:180, 1977.

Pitot HC: *Fundamentals of Oncology.* New York: Marcel Dekker, 1986.

Pitot HC: The natural history of neoplastic development. Cancer 49:1206, 1982.

Polanyi M: *Personal Knowledge.* Chicago: University of Chicago Press, 1958.

Polivy J: Psychological effects of mastectomy on a woman's feminine self-concept. J Nerv Mental Dis 164:77, 1977.

Pross HF, Baines MG: Spontaneous human lymphocyte-mediated cytotoxicity against tumor target cells: I. The effect of malignant disease. Int J Cancer 18:593, 1976.

Schaefer C: The role of stress and coping in the occurrence of serious illness. Unpublished doctoral dissertation, University of California at Berkeley, 1983.

Schmale AH Jr, Iker HP: The affect of hopelessness and the development of cancer: Part 1: Identification of uterine cancer in women with atypical cytology. Psychosom Med 28:714, 1966.

Schmale AH Jr, Iker H: Hopelessness as a predictor of cervical cancer. Social Sci Med 5:95, 1971.

Schneider-Braus K: A piece of my mind: The hypnotist. JAMA 256:762, 1986.

Schonfield J: Psychological factors related to delayed return to an earlier life-style in successfully treated cancer patients. J Psychosom Res 16:44, 1972.

Schottenfeld D: *Cancer Epidemiology and Prevention.* Springfield, Ill.: Charles C Thomas, 1975.

Simonton OC, Matthews-Simonton S: Cancer and stress: Counselling the cancer patient. Med J Austral 1:679, 1981.

Smith CK, Harrison SD, Ashworth C, Montano D, Davis A, Fefer A: Life change and the onset of cancer in identical twins. J Psychosom Res 28:525, 1984.

Sondik EJ: Cancer control objectives for the year 2000. Oncology 1:25, 1987.

Sontag S: *Illness as Metaphor.* New York: Vintage Books, 1979.

Taylor C: *Hegel and Modern Society.* Cambridge: Cambridge University Press, 1979.

Thomas CB, Duszyniski BA, Shaffer JW: Family attitudes reported in youth as potential predictors of cancer. Psychom Med 41:287, 1979.

Vachon MLS, Freedman K, Formo A, et al: The final illness in cancer: The widow's perspective. Can Med Assoc J 117:1151, 1977.

Weisman AD: *Coping with cancer.* New York: McGraw-Hill, 1979a.

Weisman AD: A model for psychosocial phasing in cancer. Gen Hosp Psychiatry 1:187, 1979b.

Weisman AD: *On Dying and Denying: A Psychiatric Study of Terminality.* New York: Behavioral Publications, 1972.

Weisman AD: Understanding the cancer patient: The syndrome of caregiver's plight. Psychiatry 44:161, 1981.

Wirsching M, Stierlin H, Hoffman F, Weber G, Wirsching B: Psychological identification of breast cancer patients before biopsy. J Psychosom Res 26:1, 1982.

Wolf S: The role of the brain in bodily disease. In Weiner H, Hofer MA, Stunkard AJ (eds): *Brain, Behavior, and Disease,* pp. 5–7. New York: Raven Press, 1981.

Wortman CB, Dunkel-Schetter C: Interpersonal relationships and cancer: A theoretical analysis. J Social Issues 35:120, 1979.

Wrubel J: Personal meanings and coping processes. Unpublished doctoral dissertation, University of California at San Francisco, 1985.

Wrubel J, Benner P, Lazarus RS: Social competence from the perspective of stress and coping. In Wine JD, Smye MD (eds): *Social Competence,* pp. 61–99. New York: Guilford Press, 1981.

CHAPTER NINE

Coping with Neurological Illnesses

She talked to me about her life, about how active and independent she had always been and how much she had been looking forward to her retirement. "And I've always been so proud of my hands. It sounds silly, but I've always liked my hands." I just sat there and said, "They are nice hands." She told me how she loved to bake and work in the garden, and that she was frightened of losing all those things and becoming too much of a burden on her daughter. I felt that something very significant was happening. *Barbara Ridley, RN, CRRN*

Neurological illness creates coping demands quite unlike those created by the other illnesses described in this book. People with neurological illnesses sustain damage to their "selves" in a way that people with no other illness do. In the worst cases, people experience complete personality changes. They become strangers to their friends and families. In other tragic outcomes, people lose the ability to comprehend or to communicate. Even if the personality and linguistic abilities are spared, there can be motoric or sensory damage, damage of the sort that makes people feel that they are trapped in someone else's body. In contrast to medical illnesses such as diabetes and cancer, closed head injuries are associated with psychological problems that may intensify over time (Levin et al. 1987). Health care givers in this field must find a way to help patients and family endure tragedy and to facilitate whatever recovery is possible while keeping the door open to the unexpected possibilities.

Neurological illness encompasses a wide and diverse array of illnesses and results of injury. In this chapter we will limit the discussion to stroke and closed head injury. We focus on these neurological illnesses because they account for a significant proportion of neurological illness treated in the general population. Thus, a large (and in some

313

cases growing) percentage of ill or disabled people need to cope with this type of illness. Also, we believe that our view of what it is to be a person and our approach to stress and coping are particularly useful in understanding and helping people with neurological illnesses.

Brief Definition of Illnesses To Be Discussed

Stroke is a term commonly used for a cerebrovascular accident. It can cause death to parts of the brain through bleeding, clot, or other blockage. Stroke can be described in terms of the parts of the body affected (e.g., right brain hemiplegia) or in terms of its cause. The cause or etiology of stroke is classified as thrombosis, embolism, or hemorrhage.

Closed head injury is an impact injury, either from the head coming abruptly to a stop, as in a car accident (deceleration), or from the head moving abruptly, as after a blow (acceleration). This type of injury contrasts with penetrating head injury, as occurs with gunshot wounds, in that the skull is not broken and in that the resulting lesions are not usually focal. Brain damage from closed head injury originates from two kinds of lesions: contusions that cause hemorrhage, and diffuse injury to white matter from stretching or tearing of axons.

Epidemiology

STROKE

Stroke is the third leading cause of death in the United States, but two-thirds of people who suffer stroke survive. Stroke can be suffered by a person at any age, but older people are at much greater risk. The morbidity risk for adults up to the age of 40 is 0.1%, but for every subsequent five-year period, the risk factor doubles. Thus, the risk is 29% for a person of eighty-five and about 45% for a person of ninety (Espmark 1973).

According to the American Heart Association, risk factors for stroke are the same as those for heart disease because usually stroke is the result of the same cardiovascular disease that causes heart attacks. Women, particularly women over thirty-five who take birth control pills and smoke, are also at risk. Blacks, who have a higher prevalence of hypertension, are at greater risk than whites.

In the past ten years, because of success in the treatment and prevention of heart disease and hypertension, the incidence of stroke

314

has gone down. And, because of advances in medical technology, more stroke sufferers are surviving. In 1973, 214,333 people died from stroke or its complications. Nine years later, only 159,630 deaths were attributed to stroke (Kerson 1985). But success in preventing mortality has not been matched with similar progress in rehabilitation. As a result, stroke has become a major cause of disability among the elderly (Andrews and Stewart 1979).

CLOSED HEAD INJURY

Efforts have been made in the last decade to secure accurate epidemiological data on the incidence (i.e., number of new cases each year) and prevalence (i.e., number of existing cases, including new cases) of closed head injury. The findings of the National Head and Spinal Cord Injury Survey (HSCI), which began in 1974, have been reported by Kalsbeek et al. (1980). They report an estimated incidence of 200 per 100,000 population and a prevalence of 450 cases per 100,000 population. Levin, Benton, and Grossman (1982) observe that the incidence is undoubtedly underreported in the HSCI Survey because the data are based on hospital admissions and thus do not include those who died of severe head injury before receiving medical attention or those with mild injury who were treated in an emergency room and released. Likewise, the prevalence estimates are underestimated because the study encompasses only the years from 1970 to 1974 and thus does not include people injured before 1970 who were still alive but disabled.

If stroke is an older person's illness, closed head injury is an illness of youth. A look at the risk factors for closed head injury reveals a glimpse of our culture. The population at greatest risk for closed head injury is male and between the ages of fifteen and twenty-four (Annegers et al. 1980, Field 1976, Kraus 1980). About four times as many males as females are admitted to hospitals for severe head injury (the ratio goes down after age seventy) (Kraus 1980). Approximately half of these head injuries are sustained in automobile accidents (Annegers et al. 1980, Kalsbeek et al. 1980). And alcohol consumption has been implicated in 20% of the head injuries in males fifteen years or older (Field 1976). Although studies show that the incidence of head injury has increased over the last twenty years, the mortality rate has remained unchanged (Levin, Benton, and Grossman 1982). Thus, as with stroke in the older population, closed head injury is responsible for disability due to brain damage in a significant proportion of our younger population.

Outcome of Illness

SEVERE STROKE OR INJURY

According to *The National Survey of Stroke* (as reported in Kerson 1985), 31% of stroke victims in the United States die during their hospitalization. The mortality figures for people with severe closed head injury are comparable to those for stroke only in those geographic areas that can provide rapid evacuation to a center with a neurosurgical specialization and prompt evaluation with computed tomographic (CT) scanning (Becker et al. 1977, Marshall et al. 1979, Miller et al. 1981). Otherwise, mortality among those with severe injury seems to be approximately 50%.

As noted in the preceding section, the success in preserving life that new medical and nursing technology has made possible has not been followed up with equal strides in rehabilitation. Many people who are brain damaged through stroke or closed head injury remain severely disabled and dependent for the rest of their lives.

The Glasgow Outcome Scale (Jennett and Bond 1975) was developed to assess recovery at different time spans following either head injury or nontraumatic coma. It has been used in a number of settings in different countries and has proved useful as a research tool in evaluating and predicting outcome (Jennett 1984). In the context of this chapter, a brief look at the scale is useful as a basis for understanding to some degree the range of coping demands a brain-damaged person must face.

In the *vegetative state,* the person may be reflexively responsive but cannot make psychologically meaningful responses. "Patients who obey even simple commands, or who utter even a single word, are assigned to the next category" (Jennett 1984, p. 38). The next category, *severe disability,* encompasses a wide range of possible limitations and applies to patients one step above "vegetative" as well as to people who suffer no physical disability, but are so mentally handicapped that they require constant supervision. *Moderate disability* refers to that group of people who can live independently but who have some limitation upon their lives. Their physical and/or mental deficit prevents them from engaging in the same work or social life they had before injury. *Good recovery* means that the person can take up work and social life as before, even though some mental and/or physical deficits are present.

Note that "good recovery" does not mean that the person is fully himself or herself again. This fact reflects divergent perspectives in the field of treatment of brain damage. One perspective comes from the knowledge of how serious a disablement or risk of death the person faced. The other viewpoint reflects the notion that until the person can be fully reintegrated into his or her world, recovery has not been attained. As one group of authors put it:

> In general, neurosurgeons, who are primarily concerned with the survival of the patient and the prevention of devastating physical and mental impairment, tend to view persisting relatively minor disabilities as of little significance as compared to what might have been the fate of the victim of severe head trauma. On the other hand, rehabilitation specialists are likely to consider these minor disabilities as reflective of a poor outcome if, in fact, they interfere with the patient's interpersonal adjustment and vocational effectiveness (Levin, Benton, and Grossman 1982, p. 225).

Certainly the first view has merit. People who suffer from a variety of illnesses come to see themselves as much better off than they might have been. We understand this position and have described it in earlier chapters in terms of "situated possibility." However, for reasons to be discussed in a later section, it does seem that workers in the field have often been more pessimistic than necessary about the possibilities for recovery from neurological deficits following stroke or closed head injury.

MILD STROKE OR INJURY

Mild strokes or transient ischemic attacks (TIAs) can be precursors of more serious stroke, but they often go unnoticed. Retrospectively, after a major stroke or as the result of a complete neurological evaluation, the symptoms of mild stroke are identified. Often, though, symptoms such as forgetfulness, slowed cognition, clumsiness, distractibility, irritability, or dizziness are not remarked on or attributed to other causes, such as aging or high blood pressure. This is a problem for health care providers, since the early identification and recognition of the meaning of these symptoms (i.e., that the person has experienced a minor stroke or TIA) sometimes help prevent further, more damaging cerebrovascular accidents.

Quite paradoxically, the common effects and outcomes of mild closed head injury have been regarded, until recently, not as signaling neural damage but as reflecting a neurotic response. People with minor injuries who suffer only a brief loss or no loss of consciousness and who may not have even been hospitalized have for years been noted to complain of a variety of symptoms that include "headache, dizziness, fatigue, diminished concentration, memory deficit, irritability, anxiety, insomnia, hypochondriacal concern, hypersensitivity to noise, and photophobia" (Levin, Benton, and Grossman 1982). This group of symptoms is referred to as the postconcussional syndrome. One author (Miller 1961) terms the response an "accident neurosis" and theorizes that postconcussional syndrome is more prevalent among those awaiting legal redress for damages.

Currently it is acknowledged that even mild concussion can result in permanent brain damage. Jane et al. (1982) examined the effects of mechanical impact and nonimpact injuries on monkeys and found brain stem axonal degeneration from even very mild head injuries. Oppenheimer (1968) found microscopic lesions in the cerebral white matter of people who suffered minor concussion but died of other causes. He also found that subsequent minor concussions caused cumulative damage as evidenced by more severe behavioral symptoms with each successive injury.

It has been a recurring theme of this book that the assumption of a mind-body split contributes to an objectification of the body and person by health care givers. From a perspective of body reducible to physical mechanism, the patient is required to justify his or her suffering as based in "real" symptoms to qualify for medical and nursing interventions other than psychiatric ones requiring a change in the patient's "attitude." The postconcussional syndrome is a case in point.

At this time it is generally accepted that even minor injury can cause lasting symptoms, although why this is the case is still being studied. Epidemiological studies have shown that quite a few people with mild injury report experiencing impaired memory and concentration, fatigue, and irritability (Wrightson and Gronwall 1980). Because mild injury so often does not result in any highly apparent physical or mental deficit, neuropsychological investigations have been designed to pinpoint subtleties in mental functioning. Gronwall and Wrightson (1974) found that those patients returning to work who complained of symptoms more often showed slow decision making on the Paced Auditory Serial Addition Task (PASAT). The nature of the test involves divided attention, memory, mental transformations, and responding. The authors proposed that the symptoms were the result of the constant effort required to compensate for the slowed mental processing.

Following both the work by Gronwall and Wrightson described above and Lazarus' coping theory, van Zomeren, Brouwer, and Deelman (1984) offer a "coping hypothesis" to describe and account for postconcussional syndrome. They propose that since, unlike more severely injured people, these patients exhibit no visible signs of damage, both the people in their social (including work) context and the patients themselves expect that their functioning will be as before. Also, since no one usually explains that they will experience some slowing of mental processing for some time (six months to a year), people with mild concussion find that they must constantly exert more effort to perform at preinjury levels. This state of chronic effort results in the constellation of symptoms associated with the syndrome. Commenting on research that shows how often this group of posttraumatic "neurotic" complaints was found in mildly and moderately injured patients and not at all in severely injured ones, the authors note:

> One might speculate that the clue to understanding this discontinuity is once again found in the subjective perception of abilities and demands. Only when a gap is perceived, and when it is thought to be bridgeable, a patient will try to cope with the situation. If too much compensatory effort is invested for too long a period, neurotic-like symptoms may appear (van Zomeren, Brouwer, and Deelman 1984, pp. 98–99).

The situation of the person with postconcussion syndrome fully illustrates our approach to stress and coping. After mild trauma, the person takes up his or her life again with the expectation that things will go as usual. Although there is breakdown in the taken-for-granted functioning of the body, breakdown does not result in everything coming to a grinding halt. Reaction time is slowed, and it is difficult to attend to two things at once. Mental transformations take longer. The person "copes" with this discontinuity in bodily self-understanding by trying harder. As van Zomeren et al. note above, the gap seems bridgeable. But the whole point of the taken-for-granted body is that functioning be effortless. It is exhausting to attend to and try harder to perform functions that one normally executes without conscious attending.

Coping, as we have indicated throughout the book, is not an antidote to stress. Stress is the disruption of meanings, and coping is the attempt to maintain, restore, or manage the loss of disrupted meanings. In this case, the disrupted meanings are taken-for-granted bodily ways of being in the world, and the coping is the attempt to restore that bodily capacity through increased mental effort. The coping efforts are completely natural responses, but they involve further disruption as they become the person's new way of being in the world. The slowing down of mental functioning after mild head injury can be temporary, resolving itself anywhere from six months to a year after the trauma. But the new bodily attitude of effortful responding may become entrenched, even when it is no longer required.

Barth et al. (1983) propose a very straightforward answer to the problem: "Simply informing patients that minor head injury has the potential to interfere with normal functioning may significantly increase individual adaptation" (p. 532). One might ask why this completely obvious therapeutic intervention was not the common practice, why so many mildly brain-injured people have been labeled neurotic, and, quite possibly by extension to the stroke experience, why so many elderly people have probably been labeled (or have labeled themselves) senile or hypochondriacal. The answer, we believe, rests first of all in the dualistic notion of the person that some illness experiences are real and others are merely subjective, i.e., neurotic. This assumption not only sets up the postconcussion syndrome as neurotic but also prevents the health care giver from achieving a caring relationship with the patient. It creates in the health care giver an attitude of suspicion, a belief that suffering has to be justified by "real" symptoms. We have dealt with this problem more fully in Chapter Six.

There are other reasons that it took so long for this unfortunate result of mild concussion to be recognized for what it is. These reasons have to do with the predominant approaches to the study of the brain and theories about brain function. These are discussed below.

CONCLUSION

The striking feature of both severe stroke and closed head injury is that they are so seriously life-threatening and disabling. We will be dealing with the nature of that disability in a later section, but at this point it suffices to indicate that these are serious and not uncommon illnesses. And although they differentially affect the population, the elderly being at much greater risk for stroke and the young at greater risk for closed head injuries, they share much in common in the kinds of disabilities they cause and the unpredictability of the course of recovery. Recovery and rehabilitation are the focus of another later section.

The striking feature of mild closed head injury is that it also has serious effects that can impair return to normal functioning. In a later section, we turn to a discussion of the brain's amazing "plasticity." The reader should keep in mind all the while that, from the individual sufferer's point of view, there is no such thing as "minor brain damage."

Theories of Brain Function and Recovery: Localization versus Holism

LOCALIZATION OF BRAIN FUNCTION

When theories come to be viewed not as theories but as coincidental with "truth," they cease to be used as theories and become paradigms, that is, lenses through which scientific researchers observe the world and determine what counts as a fact, what counts as an affirmation, and what counts as an anomaly (Kuhn 1977). Finger and Stein (1982) propose that the localization of brain function has become a paradigm in contemporary neuroscience, a paradigm that has had a major impact on how recovery from brain damage is regarded and pursued. They argue for a "paradigm shift" to a more holistic view.

Researchers supporting the theory of the localization of brain function use the brain lesion method to expand their knowledge of the role of the brain in various functions. By localizing the site of the lesion and observing the associated physiological or behavioral deficit, they make inferences about function. Experimental work with animals allows the production of very specific lesions. In humans, the damage done by stroke or closed head injury is usually much more generalized. But advances in scanning technology have allowed neuroscientists much greater access to the exact areas damaged and have provided information that previously would have been obtainable only by postmortem examination.

The theory of the localization of brain function proposes that specific parts of or points in the brain are responsible for specific functions, not only nonconscious physiological regulative processes but also complex cognitive behaviors. Pursuit of this theory has influenced conceptions of recovery from brain damage in several ways. Since neuronal damage is considered to be permanent and irreversible, and since function is supposedly localized, damage to the structure means loss of function. Recovery of function is sometimes attributed to the subsiding of neural shock (i.e., the neural tissues were not destroyed in the first place). Other observations of recovery are attributed to the person's having learned new ways to perform old functions (which is not the same as undamaged parts of the brain taking over functions). And sometimes recovery is attributed to the insensitivity of tests to measure deficits in the first place.

Because of this insistence on the identity between structure and function, possibilities for recovery have been played down, almost to the point that they are disregarded. The learning of new ways to perform old functions is not in itself so much of interest; it is just a way to account for anomalies in recovery after neural damage, anomalies that would, if unaccounted for, disprove the theory that neural damage is irreversible. Finger and Stein (1982) spell out the implications of this position for the study of recovery:

> Clearly, one effect of this theoretical predisposition against the concept of recovery of function has been to diminish the attraction of doing research on recovery. The paradox is that the importance of understanding the effects of brain damage and the ability of an individual to resume seemingly normal or near-normal functioning [have] never been denied. Thus, on the one hand, recovery of function is sometimes treated as a threat or an embarrassment to established doctrines. Yet, on the other hand, there are certainly very practical reasons for increasing our understanding of recovery phenomena, regardless of our theoretical biases (p. 8).

When a theory approaches the stature of a paradigm, researchers in the field necessarily pursue certain avenues and ignore others as not productive. Early findings of the failure of neural regeneration in mammals have long been a correlative of the theory of localization. Further research in the area of regeneration did not seem productive, and research in the identification of functional locations appeared most useful. Now, of course, we are experiencing a veritable explosion of research in neural regeneration, from studies of what forms of regeneration can occur on their own to experiments in ways to facilitate regeneration. These are discussed below.

Another way in which the theory of localization of function has worked paradigmatically is in the interpretation of available data. Investigations in the neural functioning of infants and children have shown that neural specialization does not occur until the end of infancy. Prior to that time there exists great adaptability in the assuming of function when structures are damaged. Under the theory, however, these data are interpreted to mean that there is not localization of function before a certain point but that once a structure becomes the fixed locus of a function, adaptability in taking over function post-trauma is lost.

BRAIN FUNCTION AS HOLISTIC

The holistic approach to neural organization views the brain as complex and dynamic, as an organ of considerable plasticity both physiologically and in terms of its behavioral effects. The holistic approach does not reject the notion of the localization of function, it simply reexamines the meaning of function. Alexander Luria (1966) has captured the central issue here in his definition of the two meanings of function.

> On the one hand, the term *function* denotes a particular property of a tissue. In this sense we are justified in speaking of the function of bile secretion characteristic of liver cells. . . . It is easy to see that such a function is firmly associated with particular morphological structures and cannot be conceived independently of them. However, the word *function* may also . . . denote a *complex adaptive activity of a whole system*, and sometimes of a whole organism, establishing certain relationships with the external environment, and producing some form of adaptive effect. . . . In this sense we frequently speak of the function of spoken communication, the function of memory, and even of certain intellectual functions.
>
> Whereas function in the first sense of the term is always a narrow, clearly defined activity of a particular tissue or particular organ, function in its second meaning is the complex result of the work of an entire *functional system*, the links of which may be interchanged and which, employing different intermediate stages, preserves the constancy only of its final effect (Luria 1966, pp. 17–18).

And so the issue is not so much a question of localization as it is a question of what is being localized. The simple functions of certain cell groups differ radically from the activities of dynamic functional systems. This distinction is extremely pertinent because in neuroscience even seemingly simple functions have been found to involve the participation of a whole system of different cells. Luria, citing the work of I.N. Filimonov, describes the patellar reflex as involving "both the posterior and anterior horns of the spinal cord, and cells of the pyramidal and extrapyramidal systems" (1966, p. 20). So even the function of this apparently simple reflex does not involve neurons at one point but at different places and levels in the central nervous system.

If this is the case for a simple reflex, then imagine what must be involved in any nonreflexive, purposive form of motor activity. It is in the consideration of motor performance that the notion of "function" gains further clarity. The functional system that directs and effects motor activity is not the same kind of system that controls the patellar reflex. The patellar reflex, while not locatable at one specific point, has been identified with a group of neurons. A motor activity is more complex, not simply because it requires more neurons at different places to be accomplished. A motor activity is also more complex because it has two aspects, what it aims to do and how it does what it aims to do. In humans and in animals the same end can be accomplished by a number of different methods. Karl Lashley (1960) dramatically revealed this quality in a series of lesion experiments on rats. The rats had been trained to run through a maze. After surgical creation of lesions of the spinal cord or the cerebellum, the rats still went through the maze but by means of a different set of motor impulses. For example, one rat somersaulted the entire distance. The functional system that needs to be identified and researched here is the one that organizes and regulates not the motor function, but which motor pattern is used.

Yet another approach to the meaning of function is revealed when we consider what are usually termed "the higher functions." When human psychological processes are considered, the role of the world outside that of the individual organism becomes readily apparent. The social context is essential to the creation and existence of human beings.

Merleau-Ponty (1962) has developed the most elaborate refutation of a mechanistic physiology that expects stable pathways and precise localization of functions.

> As in the case of the reflex arc theory, physiology of perception begins by recognizing an anatomical path leading from a receiver through a definite transmitter to a recording station, equally specialized. The objective world being given, it is assumed that it passes on to the sense-organs messages which must be registered, then deciphered in such a way as to reproduce in us the original text. Hence we have in principle a point-by-point correspondence and constant connection between the stimulus and the elementary perception. But this "constancy hypothesis" conflicts with the data of consciousness, and the very psychologists who accept it recognize its purely theoretical character. For example, the intensity of a sound under certain circumstances lowers its pitch; the addition of auxiliary lines makes two figures unequal which are objectively equal; a coloured area appears to be the same colour over the whole of its surface, whereas the chromatic thresholds of the different parts of the retina ought to make it red in one place, orange somewhere else, and in certain cases colourless. . . . Normal functioning must be understood as a process of integration in which the text of the external world is not so much copied, as composed (pp. 7–9).

The "compositional" nature of perception is overlooked in the meta-phor of physical receptors for "specific stimuli" and "specific motor abilities." As Merleau-Ponty (1962) points out, an injury extending to nervous tissue does not destroy one after another, ready-made sensory contents but instead makes the active differentation of stimuli in-creasingly unreliable. For example, in the case of color perception, at the beginning of the injury, the saturation of all colors are affected, but their basic shade remains the same. Even in late stages, when colors appear as monochromatic grays, color perception may be restored briefly by favorable conditions, such as contrast and long exposure. Similarly, in the case of noncortical injury affecting the sense of touch, the specific sensation can be restored if a stimulus is extensive and strong enough. Merleau-Ponty's strong refutation of the localization hypothesis made in the late 1950s and early 1960s is even more persuasive when one considers current empirical findings:

> Central lesions seem to leave qualities intact; on the other hand they modify the spatial organization of data and the perception of objects. This is what had led to the belief in specialized gnostic centres for the localiza-tion and interpretation of qualities. In fact, modern research shows that central lesions have the effect in most cases of raising the chronaxies [the minimum time an electric current must flow to cause a muscle to con-tract], which are increased to two or three times their normal strength in the patient. The excitation produces its effects more slowly, these survive longer, and the tactile perception of roughness, for example, is jeopar-dized insofar as it presupposes a succession of circumscribed impressions or precise consciousness of different positions of the hand. *The vague localization of the stimulus is not explained by the destruction of a localizing centre, but by the reduction to a uniform level of sensations, which are no longer capable of organizing themselves into a stable grouping in which each of them receives a univocal value and is translated into consciousness only by a limited change* (p. 74) [empha-sis added].

Mechanistic views of central nervous system functioning fail to recognize the integration and interrelatedness of the system. The localization paradigm (looking for specific structural locations for specific functions) misses the ways embodiment and being in the world organize and structure perceptions, understanding, and motor abilities. For example, from a localization perspective it is not at all clear why pointing and grasping, which may involve the same motor activity, are organized differently so that one can lose the ability to point to an object on command but may not lose the practical ability to grasp the same object in the context of normal activity. As Merleau-Ponty (1962) points out:

> A patient, asked to point to some part of his body, his nose for example, can only manage to do so if he is allowed to take hold of it. If the patient is set the task of interrupting the movement before its completion, or if he is allowed to touch his nose only with a wooden rule, the action becomes impossible. It must therefore be concluded that "grasping" or "touching," even for the body is different from "pointing." From the outset the grasping movement is magically at its completion; it can begin only by anticipating its end, since to disallow taking hold is sufficient to inhibit the action (pp. 103–104).

The localization paradigm looks for the structure that generates the ability without consideration of the person's world and bodily intentionality (see Chapter Three). A structural account that looks for specific functions without considering the phenomenal world necessarily overlooks the way the world creates and solicits human capacities and the possible multiple pathways and accesses to any one motor activity.

Without a minimum social context (which we take to include positive contact with a caretaker, spoken language and communicatory interaction, and some visual and motoric stimulation), a person's cognitive development will be retarded. In truly deprived circumstances, as Rene Spitz' (1965) classic study has shown, life itself is threatened. The very content of one's experiences alters the way physiological structures function.

As Luria (1966) puts it:

> Innate factors and direct individual experience shape the behavior of an animal, but with human beings there is a third aspect, namely, the assimilation of the experience of mankind in general, which is incorporated in objective activity, in language, in the products of work, and in the forms of social life of human beings. This social experience not only forms the methods of human work and operations with objects in the external environment, but it also creates complex and plastic methods of controlling the individual's own behavior and the wide range of generalized images and ideas composing human consciousness (pp. 21–22).

IMPLICATIONS, CONTRASTS, AND CONCLUSIONS

Thus, in a holistic view, function is understood in terms of what kind of function. In complex, adaptive activity, an integration of systems is involved. The same activity can be described anatomically, physiologically, neurologically, behaviorally, or phenomenologically. Pursuit of the understanding of human activity on these multiple levels could enhance our knowledge of how the brain functions and particularly could give clues of possibilities for recovery. Insistence on finding the single location in the brain from which complex, adaptive activity originates appears, in this light, to be a wrongheaded kind of reductionism.

If the theory of the localizaton of brain function is to be valid, function has to be fixed. But since both the development and the execution of complex, adaptive activity depend on a context, function cannot be thought of as static or fixed. The same ends may be achieved through various means in a neurologically intact organism, a fact explored in a later section on the meaning and role of plasticity in recovery.

At heart, the two theories of brain function differ in their view of the person. Localization theory has become a deficit model, with all the mechanistic implications inherent in the term *model*. The important focus is on the accurate assessment of what the neurologically damaged person cannot do, because that, along with the location of the brain lesion, provides information that supposedly leads to the localization of function. Because of this focus, much attention has been paid to "explaining" recovery in terms of compensatory mechanisms or of lack of sensitivity in deficit assessment techniques. In other words, the interest is in distinguishing between *true* recovery of function, that is, the recovery of the use of the same neural pathways as before injury, and *compensatory* recovery, which is either the nonconscious use of other pathways or areas of the brain or the conscious learning of different ways to achieve the same ends. This distinction between kinds of recovery allows the researchers to hone in on an accurate assessment of deficits, which may not be in any way behaviorally evident.

Organismic theory, by contrast, is an asset approach. The neural system is viewed as having parts that work together. It is a dynamic system. In other words, it is in flux, changes over time, and is flexible in response. In this view, the neural system has anatomical parts that function as a whole. And that whole is a part of the person, who in turn functions as a whole in a social world. When neural damage occurs, the focus of interest is not on what is lost, but on what remains: what remains in terms of undamaged, functional parts of the whole and what remains in terms of capacities for adaptation. Capacities for adaptation now are known to include under some conditions neural regeneration, automatic takeover of function by other parts of the brain, and the learning of new, more conscious ways to perform formerly automatic functions. The damaged brain is part of a person, and that person is still involved in a social world and has concerns and intents.

Recovery

THE INDIVIDUALITY OF THE CENTRAL NERVOUS SYSTEM

As the previous section has demonstrated, attitudes toward recovery on the part of neuroscientists have been influenced in important ways by the theory of localization of brain function. When the goal is mapping out the functional sites of the cerebral cortex, normative data are very important. The focus necessarily must be on the significant proportion of a sample who show the same association between lesion and deficit. The anomalous case, for example, the patient with a seemingly identical lesion but no deficit, needs to be explained, certainly, but it is not the focus of interest.

However, those neuroscientists who work with human patients all recognize the tremendous individuality of each case. Finger and Stein (1982) comment: "Although group norms may set guidelines and be appropriate for summarizing data in an experimental setting, there is no such thing as an "average brain injury" (p. 332).

The same theme is taken up by Geschwind (1985), who describes the differential levels of recovery from aphasia between right-handed and left-handed people. He found that left-handed people are much more likely to make a good recovery. Even right-handed people who have a close blood relative who is left-handed have a greater chance of good recovery from aphasia. Geschwind comments: "One cannot stress strongly enough the importance of individual differences in the nervous system" (pp. 3–4). These individual differences are certainly due to genetic factors, as is handedness, but also to differences in developmental level and personal, social, and historical experiences (e.g., educational level and prior illnesses).

The individuality of the human nervous system is a factor to be reckoned with in all studies of recovery. Lezak and Gray (1984) discuss high variance in group data as a perennial problem in head injury research because such research depends on group means that hide individual variance. Brooks et al. (1984) suggest that cases should be grouped in terms of the recovery patterns they follow. This procedure would certainly help to reveal which recovery trajectories are typical and which are not typical but still possible. This could provide useful guidelines for clinicians.

The normative approach makes it impossible to examine stability and variance *within* the individual over time. Recently a number of researchers have been calling for both ipsative (intra-individual variation) and normative research (Allport 1962, Broverman 1962, Lazarus and Folkman 1984, Marceil 1977). In ipsative research, the individual is studied across time and contexts to observe stability and variance as well as to discover actual patterns of recovery or functioning. Once these patterns have been discovered within the individual, comparisons can be made between individuals. These comparisons can be of whole patterns (such as a pattern of returning functioning) or of more typical norms, such as standard deviations and means.

The emphasis on individual differences is clearly a useful corrective in a field that in some areas of research is characterized by an overconcern with normative findings. For the expert nurse, the suggestion of Brooks et al. (1984) for grouping patterns to account for both the norm and the variant is the heart of expert clinical practice (see Chapter 10, p. 393–394). Expert nurses are concerned about both the usual expression and outcome of an illness as well as the individual experience of that illness. Perhaps an apt metaphor is that the caregiver walks a line with normative symptoms and outcomes on one side and individual illness experience on the other.

As Benner (1984) has demonstrated, to attain expertise, the giver of health care must reach a point at which she or he recognizes patterns and commonalities. For the beginner, each patient represents a new and individual illness experience. With further experience with many patients, the health care giver can begin to recognize patterns. This advanced clinical skill of pattern recognition is crucial for the identification of symptoms or symptom patterns that represent either a positive or a negative change in status. The expert nurse learns to recognize individual patterns of symptoms or even subclinical signs because they are like ones she or he has seen before, even though they may be very individually expressed. And so, in this way, the expert nurse must be concerned with a grasp of the commonalities in illness trajectories without relying on statistical summaries. In a clinical setting, the caregiver can take into account more variations and more similarities because the commonalities that the clinician observes do not rely entirely on summary data or the standard normative accounts.

The expert nurse is concerned with the individual because the nurse is involved in treating the whole person. Although a rise in intracranial pressure signals a negative change in status and the fading of posttraumatic amnesia signals a positive change in status, the experience of the illness is still individual. And the possibilities for recovery from even seemingly identical lesions can vary greatly from person to person. Expert nurses guide care of the patient not only by monitoring changes in status, but also by interpreting the illness to the individual and uncovering individual possibilities.

THEORIES OF RECOVERY OF FUNCTION

As has been discussed in an earlier section, attitudes toward recovery have been shaped in part by the theory of the localization of function. Some theories that account for recovery reflect this interest in the localization theory; other theories emphasize the plasticity of the brain. Controversy abounds concerning all of these theories, and none of them is universally considered to be proven. They are presented very briefly here as background and context against which to discuss the central fact for which these theories strive to account: After insult to the central nervous system, recovery of function does occur in some cases and to some degree.

DIASCHISIS. *Diaschisis* is a term proposed by Constantin von Monakow (1853–1930) (see Finger and Stein 1982, Marshall 1984) to describe the transitory impairment of neural activity in the immediate area of neuronal injury. Diaschisis can account for the recovery of function because the areas that recover are seen as not irreversibly damaged but only suppressed.

The theory of diaschisis has not achieved a wide following in the West. It has been to some extent misunderstood as a theory, and the term has been borrowed to refer to other possible causes of neural shock (e.g., decreased cerebral blood flow) than that postulated by von Monakow. For this reason, experimental testing of the theory has had quite uneven and contradictory results.

In the Soviet Union, Alexander Luria (1963) has taken up the idea of diaschisis as one important approach to treatment. Von Monakow's idea was that diaschisis was a temporary state that would resolve itself naturally over time, but in some instances the impairment of function *can* be permanent. Accordingly, Luria has developed pharmacological interventions to restore the neural excitability and reports great success with the technique.

On the whole, diaschisis is regarded as a descriptive rather than an explanatory account of recovery. The question is still open as to its validity as far as Western researchers are concerned. It seems likely that if histochemical experimentation can uncover the underlying process of suppression of excitability, there will be a rise in interest in the use of the kind of pharmacological interventions described by Luria to restore lost function.

REDUNDANCY. According to the theory of redundancy, recovery can be accounted for by the activity of undamaged neurons that participated in the behavior before the trauma. Marshall (1984) observes that redundancy can be accounted for either because functions have a hierarchical organization in the nervous system or because neurons necessary for a particular function are spread throughout a brain structure.

A notable degree of redundancy has been found within the sensory and motor systems (Frommer 1978). Beck and Chambers (1970) provide an example of this kind of research. They demonstrated that sparing of even a few fibers of the pyramidal tract in monkeys will allow some degree of recovery.

Of course, what is left out of this theory is the process by which the surviving neurons are enabled to assume a greater role in functioning. The more recent work on the morphological changes that are possible in the central nervous system may fill in the gaps here. This new research on neural plasticity is discussed in a later section.

VICARIOUS FUNCTIONING. Like the notion of redundancy, the theory of vicarious functioning proposes that undamaged neurons take over the functions of damaged neurons. Whereas the theory of redundancy holds that spared neurons that are related to the damaged neurons or that perform the same function take over entire function after insult, the theory of vicarious functioning proposes that entirely different structures of the central nervous system take over the lost function.

Like the theory of redundancy, this theory can be tested only on animals subjected to controlled lesions and behavioral testing. An example of this kind of experiment is found in the work of Spear and Braun (1969; see also Spear 1979). Ablation of the visual cortex in cats results initially in impairment, but with training the cats can learn to discriminate patterns.

Also, like redundancy, vicarious functioning may eventually be shown to be the result of morphological changes in the central nervous system. If this is the case, the theory will have to be modified to reflect an even more dynamic and flexible notion of the brain. The idea of one structure just taking over the function of another without changing its anatomical form still suggests mechanism. It is somewhat like the image of plugging into another circuit. But if modifications take place at the cellular level, as current research now seems to indicate, the brain has to be seen as far more "organismic" and in flux than most theories account for.

All of the theories of recovery just discussed have the same limitations. First, they are all difficult to prove empirically. Experimental work has proved inconclusive, either because the experiments were not replicated or because there were always other possible explanations of the observed phenomena. Second, the functional anatomy of the central nervous system is not monolithic. Different areas respond differently to damage and afford different possibilities for recovery. Because experimental work must necessarily focus on a particular area, often a very highly defined area, it has proved difficult to replicate experimental results in other anatomical areas.

BEHAVIORAL COMPENSATION. It has long been observed that humans (and animals) frequently develop alternative strategies (sometimes called tricks) to compensate for lost functions. This holds true even for people with very severe physical handicaps, including those that result from damage to the central nervous system. As mentioned earlier, localizationists have shown great interest in accounting for the "tricks" used by people with brain lesions to "create the impression" of recovery of damaged neural functioning. The reason for their interest is that accounting for recovery in terms of these substituted strategies presented no challenge to the theory of localization of function. However, the precise identification of the occurrence and nature of behavioral compensation is of even greater importance to the study and enablement of recovery.

An interesting example of a behavioral compensation is described by Geschwind (1974). A patient who suffered damage to the corpus callosum, a major communicatory pathway between the cerebral hemispheres, devised a way for his left hand to respond to a verbal command that only the left hemisphere could understand.

Consider a patient with a callosal lesion who apparently carried out verbal commands correctly with both the right and left hands. . . . The patient would first carry out the command with his right hand and would only then carry out the movement with the left arm. . . . The patient, or rather the left hemisphere of the patient, had learned that by signalling nonverbally it could get the right hand to imitate the movement. Clearly, no language comprehension by the right hemisphere was necessary for this performance, but one could be easily fooled (p. 501).

The theories of redundancy and vicarious functioning may seem to overlap with the theory of behavioral compensation. For example, it can be difficult to ascertain from behavior alone whether the individual is using spared neurons in a new way or has developed a new strategy using available sensory and motor capabilities. The value of this theory is that it leads to the observation and description of the means by which goals are achieved. Only these very precise accounts can enable health care givers to become aware of the possibilities open to their patients with central nervous system damage and to devise ways to teach them alternative strategies.

It is currently impossible to proceed from observed behavior in humans to a study of the brain circuitry involved in the behavior. Until the invention of some nonintrusive technology that allows the locating and tracking of firing neurons, some of the questions inherent in the theory of behavioral compensation will remain unanswered. However, although the physiological basis for compensation is not known, the fact that such compensatory strategies are possible is known. And this has become in itself the basis for the systematic study of rehabilitation.

NEUROPHYSIOLOGICAL PLASTICITY AND POSSIBILITIES FOR RECOVERY

There has long been interest in the possibility of regeneration and repair of damaged neural tissue. Early experiments failed to find such regeneration, and the success of localization theory in uncovering functional areas of the brain directed interest away from concerns with regeneration. Now the pendulum has swung in the other direction, and the most dramatic and new findings in neuroscience concern neurophysiological plasticity. This section offers a very brief and general summary of what has thus far been determined about neural regeneration.

There are two basic areas of current investigation. One involves structural changes that might permit restoration of lost function. The other area is neurochemical adaptations at synaptic sites. Structural changes involve morphological adaptations such as regeneration of axons, collateral axon sprouting, and neurogenesis or neurotransplants. The first is the regrowth of damaged neural tissue. The second (sometimes known called "sprouting") involves the growth of new synaptic endings from nearby undamaged neurons. The third refers to the natural creation and growth of new neurons or to the repair of an existent lesion through nerve cell transplant. Neurochemical adaptations involve variation in the rate of chemical transmission after trauma. All of these have been experimentally demonstrated and replicated in adult vertebrates.

Neuroscientists are now struggling with this problem: On the one hand, it has been demonstrated that it is possible for the central nervous system of the adult to repair or rebuild damaged circuits. On the other hand, most injuries that can be sectioned and microscopically examined are seen not to have been repaired. This is undoubtedly due to the effects of neural injury, which include both additional neural death and sealing off of the lesion. Death of neural cells not originally injured probably causes greater secondary loss of surrounding neurons (Cotman and Nieto-Sampedro 1985). A major challenge now facing neuroscientists is to identify the causes of this secondary loss and to provide methods for its prevention. (See Cotman and Nieto-Sampedro 1985 for a discussion of the role of metabolic imbalance of neurotrophic factors in secondary nerve cell death.)

The sealing off of the area of the lesion by what is called the glial "scar" is another impediment to the processes of regeneration because axons sprouting from nearby neurons cannot penetrate the barrier. Furthermore, the sprouting of axons may not be in itself an unmitigated good. Sprouting has been implicated in the development of epilepsy, a not uncommon but late outcome of brain damage (Bowen, Demirjian, Karpiak, and Katzman 1973). Also, collatoral sprouts may compete with regenerating axons for synapses, thus preventing the reestablishment of disrupted connections (Devor and Schneider 1975).

Thus, it is now widely accepted that neurophysiological adaptation aimed at restoring lost function is a general response to neural injury. Morphological changes like sprouting may in fact be an ordinary occurrence even in the absence of a lesion (see Sotelo and Palay 1971). This plasticity of the central nervous system has wide experimental support. And the quality of flux should not be applied just to surviving healthy tissue. As Geschwind (1985) comments:

It is a salient principle that one can probably never speak of a *fixed* neurological lesion. Damage in every location is followed by a sequence of changes, both local and distant, some instantaneous and others proceeding over the years (p. 2).

The lesion itself is shaped (sometimes positively, sometimes negatively) by the central nervous system, and it also interactively influences processes in the surviving tissue (again sometimes positively, as in the promotion of regenerative growth, and sometimes negatively, as in the loss of regained functions years later and the shrinkage of brain observed postmortem).

The techniques available for viewing brain tissue, that is, sectioning brains of dead animals, necessitate stopping time. The plastic quality of change and adaptation is not readily appreciable with such methods. There is a tendency to think of the living brain as always just like that specimen permanently frozen on the slide. This tendency has undoubtedly encouraged mechanical images of the central nervous system. But the amazing recoveries of severely damaged people, recoveries occurring far later than the usual time required for the passing of "neural shock," have intrigued numerous neuroscientists for a century or more. The links between neurophysiological plasticity and unexpected recoveries have still not been uncovered, but the miraculous recoveries of a few have inspired researchers to try to make the miracle commonplace.

Much of the current research in this area involves animal experimentation. The applicability of this research to a study of recovery of function in humans is not always readily apparent. This research nevertheless sets a tone. Although we still do not know what causes recovery, there are now possibilities that were not considered before. Even without pharmacological or surgical interventions based on this current work, we can design behavioral rehabilitation and recovery regimens based on the general principle of a dynamic central nervous system that has both resources and deficits. And these resources and deficits are not defined solely by lesion location but also by contextual interactions, both in the past and in the present.

Recovery and the Individual

Neurological illness that results from stroke or closed head injury points up the distinction made between disease and illness in Chapter One. Until the recent work on neurophysiological plasticity, which uncovers the interactive process between the regenerative forces in the remaining healthy tissue and the degenerative forces in the area of the lesion, the person who had sustained a closed head injury or a stroke and survived any secondary complications was not thought to be in a diseased state. The disease, as in the case of stroke, was considered to be the causative factor of the stroke. Once the stroke had occurred and the person was released from the hospital, the disease to be treated was hypertension or whatever was thought to have precipitated the stroke.

Now we know that both regenerative and degenerative processes can continue for a long time in the central nervous system. But neuroscience is just beginning to deal with possible ways of intervening in this process. And the strongly prevailing view of people with neurological damage is not that they have a disease but that they are disabled. As a result, heroic measures are undertaken in the hospital to save the lives of people with central nervous system damage, but rehabilitative efforts to ensure the highest possible level of recovery over months and even years are often lacking. In the 1970s, professor Bryan Jennett began a major and influential study of closed head injury. His work led to the international use of a standardized scale of simple assessments for making prognoses in patients with closed head injury. He comments incisively, "The tremendous efforts expended on intensive treatment in the early weeks after injury are often largely wasted by the failure to provide the means whereby the full potential for recovery can be achieved during the later stages" (Jennett 1975, p. 267).

The survivor of a stroke or closed head injury may not be considered to have a disease, but he or she certainly experiences an illness. The person has experienced a major interruption of life, and the possibilities of taking up former activities are greatly reduced.

This section deals with the issue of the individual and recovery. We have presented some of the problems of normative studies of recovery from neurological damage. Here we take up the theme again by presenting some contradictory findings about normative recovery and discussing what has been seen to be possible for individuals. Then we take up the issue of rehabilitation and recovery, presenting various approaches and showing how the notion of embodiment is useful both for developing rehabilitative approaches and interpreting their success. Finally, we discuss stress and coping of individuals with neurological damage.

NORMATIVE RECOVERY VERSUS INDIVIDUAL RECOVERY

The rule of thumb for recovery from stroke or closed head injury is "the more severe the injury, the greater the disability." Rules of thumb are extremely useful in guiding an exploration of what process might make the rule generally hold true. But rules of thumb are generalizations, and their usefulness ends when they become truisms or entrenched ways of thinking that prevent a person from being open to anomalous possibility.

For example, age is often cited as a factor in recovery from brain damage, but the research findings are not clear-cut. In a two-year study of cognitive recovery from closed head injury, Bond and Brooks (1976) found that a greater proportion of older patients died of head injuries and a greater proportion were left with severe disability compared to younger patients with similar injuries. *Older* here does not mean *elderly,* however, since the predominant age group was fifteen to thirty years. It might be useful to know if the findings about recovery and age would still hold if pretrauma physical condition were a controlled variable. A major risk factor for closed head injury is consumption of alcohol, and in the group of people who suffer closed head injury, there are more alcoholics among older than younger patients, for whom consumption of alcohol immediately prior to injury, not alcoholism per se, is a risk factor.

In contrast to Bond and Brooks, Andrews, Brocklehurst, Richards, and Laycock (1982) did not find associations between age and degree of recovery in their one-year follow-up study of severely disabled stroke patients. In this case, the groups compared were those under and those over sixty-five years of age. The authors cite six studies in which an association between age and recovery level was found and four studies in which, like theirs, no relationship was found. Again, it would be useful to know if prestroke physical condition (or educational level) is a stronger predictor than age.

Later we discuss what pre-illness aspects of the person might affect level of recovery. But at this point we simply wish to indicate that the association between age and recovery is not clear-cut. There is a chance that our general cultural understandings about older versus younger, which have become more visible as anthropologists and sociologists have interpreted them (see Chapter Four for examples), may be just as influential for potential recovery as simple chronological

337

age. Certainly no one would argue that we typically react with a sense of the tragedy of a wasted life when we hear of a young person who has suffered severe cognitive disability as a result of brain damage. By contrast, we often react with a sense that these things happen to old people when we hear of an elderly person who has suffered similar disability.

Our caveats about using normative data for assessing recovery from brain damage are worth repeating here. Normative data by their nature disguise variance. And yet most studies of brain recovery are normative. The unusual and anomalous become "out-liers," which concern researchers because they affect the significance level of the statistical measure. But apparently there is always considerable variance in studies of recovery from brain damage, and not surprisingly so. As we pointed out, not only are brains highly individual, but so are lesions. In laboratory studies, we can create a series of identical lesions in experimental animals, but closed head injury and stroke are not so neat. Also, the lesion changes in interaction with the brain, resulting in another individual aspect.

We have normative data about recovery of cognitive functions after closed head injury. The Bond and Brooks (1976) two-year follow-up study showed that "the greater part of recovery of function arising directly from the brain's activity in adults occurs within a short time of injury and that changes after six months, although present, are only slight" (p. 131). Further, the study revealed that the people who attained the lowest levels of recovery reached their best state sooner, and those were the people with the most severe injuries.

The Bond and Brooks study is a very careful one. For example, it follows the patients over a two-year period rather than the more common six-month or one-year follow-up period. It attends to the issue of different patterns of recovery for different cognitive functions as measured by different assessment tools. The study's conclusions indirectly suppose the hypothesis that there are critical times for relearning, and the authors propose that the sooner rehabilitation begins the better.

An interesting contrast to the Bond and Brooks study of recovery from closed head injury is the study by Andrews et al. (1982) of recovery from stroke. A one-year follow-up study of fifty-three people severely disabled two weeks after stroke found that roughly half improved so as to be classified as either mildly or moderately disabled and the rest remained severely disabled. Since the people who remained severely disabled in this study were the ones who received the most rehabilitative therapy, the author concludes:

> The value of prolonged therapy is debatable. Whilst it is appreciated that it is difficult to discontinue treatment for a patient who has not recovered, it must be questioned whether rehabilitation resources could not have been better used. This is particularly the case for the very long period of therapy provided for many of those who did not improve. It is of note for instance that 38% of those patients who did not improve were still receiving therapy one year following the onset of the stroke (p. 229).

From our perspective, it is of note that discussions of cost-benefit analysis must of necessity use normative data and argue for the allocation of resources for the good of the many. And in using such normative data, outcomes must be statistically measurable. Even in the thoughtful study by Bond and Brooks, the outcome measure (other than statistically significant change on cognitive measures) was the Glasgow Outcome Scale, which assigns to one category totally bed-ridden people who can obey only simple commands and people with no physical disability who are too mentally impaired to live unsupervised (see the beginning of this chapter for a fuller description of the scale). The groupings on the Glasgow Outcome Scale are clearly very large and include quite diverse levels of functioning. Thus, it is not surprising that Bond and Brooks observe that only a very few people moved up from one category to another after the first six months after injury. But even though they were in a very small minority, one might wonder, who are those people? What happened to them that was different, or in what ways were they different from the others, that they could make such a major change?

Nonnormative data, otherwise known as case studies, reveal a different picture. Geschwind (1985) cites the case of a severely aphasic patient he first saw six years after brain trauma. Twelve years later, the man made a substantial recovery. Craine and Gudeman (1981) cite several case studies in their rehabilitation manual. One case concerns a thirty-three-year-old former chef who suffered acute head injury in a car accident. He came to the rehabilitation center five weeks after the accident with problems in ambulation, minimal verbal communicatory function, loss of memory in all areas, and difficulties with fine motor movements in his hands. His goal and the goal of his training was to return to work as a chef. After two years of therapy, he works part-time as a cook and cashier.

Another case study describes a forty-five-year-old professional woman who, following a stroke, was left with right spastic hemiplegia and aphasia to such a degree that she had no functional speech. After three years of therapy she works as an independent saleswoman. Neither this woman nor the man discussed above could be said to be "normal." They have not returned to their preinjury states. The man would still be considered "handicapped." The woman is not cured of her aphasia but has found ways around it, and she has some lack of feeling and motor control in her right hand.

How can these cases be assessed in terms of outcome? The case studies make no mention of cognitive tests, so we do not know where these people would fall on the Bond and Brooks measures. But by their own measures, their recovery was significant. A man who has serious memory problems and difficulties with fine motor control of his hands improves enough to work as a cook. A woman who is unable to answer the telephone because she cannot speak improves enough to work as a saleswoman and make telephone sales calls. But if outcome is to be assessed in terms of how long it takes (and thus how much it costs in dollars), then a different criterion may have to be used. The man required two years of therapy, and the woman three, to reach the levels described, and they still continue rehabilitative therapy. Geschwind's (1985) recovered aphasic, about whose rehabilitative therapy (or lack thereof) nothing was said, took eighteen years to recover lost function.

The ideal outcome is a full recovery of function and return to life as it was lived before neural damage occurred. This ideal outcome has strongly influenced studies of recovery because the person's actual recovery is always judged against this ideal. In reality, a good recovery is like that of the man and woman cited above, namely, sufficient return of functional ability to allow independence and the ability to work, at least part-time. By shifting the assessment of recovery from an ideal-based model, to an individual model based on situated possibility, we can formulate other goals for recovery.

In a study of the phenomenology of recovery in a stroke rehabilitation center, Gold (1983) found that the goals of recovery at the center were a change of the meaning of the illness for the individual and an ability to present an image of health and normality regardless of disability. Of the change of meaning, Gold observes, "In the stroke center, rehabilitation is accomplished by teaching the participant to redefine stroke from a life-shattering medical ailment to a conquerable inconvenience" (p. 243).

340

Gold goes on to examine the aspects necessary to project an image of wellness and how these aspects are taught informally in the course of the daily activities of the rehabilitation center. Many of these aspects were taken-for-granted ways of being in the world before stroke that now need to be relearned. The rehabilitation center creates a miniculture in which these meanings are present as part of the culture, and this facilitates their being learned by the stroke patients.

Gold illustrates several examples of ways of being in the world taught by the center. He puts these under the heading "time orientation." As intepreted by Gold, time orientation refers to an awareness of when activities are scheduled, a sense of timing (that is, when to be attentive and when to participate), and the American cultural meaning that, over time, working produces results.

Other examples of ways of being in the world are found in what emotions are expressed and how they are interpreted. The workers in the rehabilitation center encourage a cheery outlook and discourage expressions of anger and depression. However, it is recognized that stroke survivors are often emotionally volatile and also may have reason to feel unhappy. Gold describes how the workers in the center deal with patients' crying:

> First, crying is often defined as a physiological rather than emotional by-product of stroke in medical literature. Second, according to the center's staff, stroke victims, like all people, become frustrated, depressed and angry. Crying is a means of expressing this. Third, by taking a group therapy approach, crying can be defined as a legitimate form of valued communication. The crying person is then comforted by the staff, so demonstrating the supportive and understanding environment which exists (p. 252).

This study exemplifies recovery goals and outcomes quite different from the ones applied in normative studies of recovery. It is possible to conceive of a rehabilitation that aims to deal with the meanings of the illness for the person, because, at some level, recovery has to mean a reintegration of a sense of well-being. Even if a person is irreparably damaged, even if a person is at risk for another stroke, he or she can still understand the self in terms of well-being and wholeness, not in ideal terms, but in a situated sense. For example, the person can see the self as a fighter, or the person can see the self as having made significant gains, or as fortunate because it could have been so much worse.

Rehabilitation also has to deal with the reconstitution of the meanings of everyday life because people have to be enabled to live in an interpretable world and relearn if necessary how to be interpretable in that world. The stroke survivors at the rehabilitation center in Gold's study may or may not recover a statistically significant degree of cognitive and motor functioning, but they probably will recover some meanings that make existence possible. Although they may learn meanings that promote useful behavior for social living, such as being on time for scheduled appointments, dressing attractively, and appearing cheerful, they will more particularly learn that it matters to others that they are alive and that they are participants and members, not outsiders.

For us, the bottom line of recovery from brain damage is the reintegration into the world of care and concern, where people and things matter to the person and the person matters to others. We have all read and heard accounts of people who have emerged from lengthy coma or people who have made amazing recoveries after brain damage, like Patricia Neal and Agnes de Mille. Only in the context of the unpublicized number of people who do not survive or achieve recovery can these anecdotal accounts truly be appreciated. But these miraculous recoveries all have one thing in common, people who loved and cared, who through their love and care engaged others to care also.

PATHWAYS TO REHABILITATION

The successes of certain rehabilitation programs for people with brain damage, sometimes called neurotraining programs, make sense in the light of a phenomenological view of the person. In this section we highlight the central aspects of successful neurotraining approaches.

CAPACITY-SPECIFIC NEUROTRAINING. We have discussed the neurophysiological plasticity of the central nervous system as it is currently being discovered by neuroscientists. Rehabilitation programs tap into plasticity as it is exemplified on another level, that is, the flexible ability of the human nervous system to accomplish the same ends by different means. This capability was described earlier as "behavioral compensation" (see p. 332). Behavioral compensation was of interest to neuroscientists committed to localizing brain function because the ability to identify a behavior as "compensatory" meant that the area of the lesion was responsible for that behavior before the trauma. But the careful and accurate accounting of such compensatory behavior is invaluable to the clinician involved in rehabilitation because it illuminates the possibilities for neurotraining.

Luria (1966) identifies two kinds of behavioral compensation. One is automatic; the other, conscious. An example of an automatic compensation is the reorganization of the visual field that occurs after partial loss. He observes that some patients did not even know they had lost part of the visual field in both eyes but thought they had lost part of the vision in one eye.

> Special investigations showed that this peculiar interpretation of the defect was due to the fact that the patients were not really left with only a partial, or "half" visual field: the defect of the visual field led immediately to its functional reorganization, as a result of which the macula, now located not at the centre but at the periphery of the constricted visual field, lost its dominance, and an area became isolated in the centre of the new, constricted visual field which possessed all the signs of increased sensitivity. In other words, a new centre of the visual field or a new "functional macula" developed, around which the whole remaining visual field became organized. This reorganization appeared to take place automatically, unconsciously and by direct adaptation of the remaining visual field to the object scrutinized by the eye. As a result . . . the patient developed a new, constricted visual field which, however, possessed all the qualities of the normal field and gave the patient relatively normal visual adaptation (pp. 56–57).

The other form of behavioral compensation is conscious and deliberate. We have all heard of or witnessed the amazing ability of people with deformed or amputated limbs to call into use different parts of the body to perform the functions of the missing limbs. So in the human central nervous system other functional parts can be trained to take over the role of the damaged area.

> Clinical practice supplies examples of cases in which a patient had lost the ability to calculate aloud, but was still able to recite the multiplication tables with the aid of a visual image of the number to be multiplied or in which a patient compensated for an inablity to perceive shapes directly by means of eye movements with which he traced the outline of the object (Luria 1963, p. 72).

These clinical examples make sense in the light of a holistic notion of the person. And they provide an idea of how the rehabilitation clinician can draw on the plasticity of the human body, of which the central nervous system is an integrated part. In order for rehabilitation to lead to recovery, the patient must be assessed very carefully to locate not only the type and the source of the loss in terms of actual function but also the remaining capacities and strengths. Thus, understanding the specific deficit, for us, includes an assessment of similar functional abilities that arise in practical activity. For example, a patient with aphasia who cannot say "la, la" might still be able to lick gravy from the upper lip. In other words, the patient has retained the capacity to make the tongue movements necessary for saying "la, la." The same tongue movement that is lost in the practical activity of speaking can still be evoked in the practical activity of licking the lips. Because these capacities may not be available in deliberative action, acute care nurses and rehabilitation clinicians must be careful observers. For example, a stroke patient who was unable to raise his hand deliberately did raise his hand in a habitual social gesture to cover a yawn (Doolittle 1987).

Assessing deficits and capacities requires studying the person in context. Oliver Sacks (1985) describes the contrast between identifying the deficit through context-free testing and understanding capacities in normal contexts in his description of Rebecca, a nineteen-year-old girl who averaged 60 on IQ tests, though doing notably better on the verbal parts of the test:

> When I first saw her—clumsy, uncouth, all-of-a-fumble—I saw her merely, or wholly, as a casualty, a broken creature, whose neurological impairments I could pick out and dissect with precision: a multitude of apraxias and agnosias, a mass of sensorimotor impairments and breakdowns, limitations of intellectual schemata and concepts similar (by Piaget's critera) to those of a child of eight. A poor thing, I said to myself, with perhaps a "splinter skill," a freak gift, of speech; a mere mosaic of higher cortical functions, Piagetian schemata—most impaired.
>
> The next time I saw her, it was all very different. . . . I wandered outside—it was a lovely spring day— . . . I saw Rebecca sitting on a bench, gazing at the April foliage quietly, with obvious delight. Her posture had none of the clumsiness which had so impressed me before. . . .
>
> And then there came out, in Jacksonian spurts, odd, sudden, poetic ejaculations: "spring," "birth," "growing," "stirring," "coming to life," "seasons," "everything in its time." I found myself thinking of Ecclesiastes: "To everything there is a season, and a time to every purpose under the heaven. A time to be born, a time to plant, and a time. . . ." She had come apart, horribly, in formal testing, but now she was mysteriously "together" and composed. . . .
>
> Our tests, our approaches, I thought, as I watched her on the bench—enjoying not just a simple but a sacred view of nature—our approach, our "evaluations," are ridiculously inadequate. They only show us deficits, they do not show us powers; they only show us puzzles and schemata, when we need to see music, narrative, play, a being conducting itself spontaneously in its own natural way.

Rebecca, I felt, was complete and intact as "narrative" being, in conditions which allowed her to organise herself in a narrative way; and this was something very important to know, for it allowed one to see her, and her potential, in a quite different fashion from that imposed by the schematic mode (pp. 171–173).

Nurses have long emphasized the importance of identifying strengths and capacities, and nurses often have the advantage of seeing patients engage in practical activities. Nurses who visit patients in their homes have additional access to the patients' interests and concerns. Such nurses can plan rehabilitation that matches the person's interests and concerns to the resources available in the home and community.

People working in traditional rehabilitation programs have tended to become somewhat pessimistic about working with brain-damaged patients. This is true primarily because controlled evaluation studies have demonstrated that rehabilitation programs do not promote greater recovery than would be expected spontaneously, without the assistance of rehabilitation. We believe the reason traditional rehabilitation of the brain-damaged patient has not been more successful stems from the failure to specify in detail the deficits and capacities of patients and subsequently to structure rehabilitative activities to be deficit and capacity specific (Craine and Gudeman 1981, p. 18), building on similar capacities solicited by different contexts.

An example of a capacity-specific rehabilitation process is neuro-training for agraphia (the inability to write spontaneously). Sometimes attempts have been made to treat this kind of aphasia by having the patient copy words. But the deficit is not in the visual-motor system, which is called upon in the process of copying, but in the internal saying of the word that precedes the writing of it. Training in the articulation and sounding out of words is the appropriate method of rehabilitation (Luria 1963). Capacity-specific rehabilitation aims to discover and strengthen aspects of the habitual body that offer alternative capacities similar to those lost, e. g., covering the mouth for a yawn (Doolittle 1987), swatting a mosquito, or swimming. Once discovered, these capacities can be elaborated and extended. In the case of loss of smooth normal action, deliberative action may be practiced often enough to reinstate a new habitual body (Sacks 1985). Building on alternative capacities and strengths is discussed more fully below under the headings "The Context and Rehabilitation" and "Embodiment."

THE CONTEXT AND REHABILITATION. We see examples of how the person is constituted by his or her world in experiments examining the differential effects of environment on neural development and in studies of ways to rehabilitate lost neural function. The experiments, mostly performed on rats, are believed by neuroscientists to generalize to human experience, since it has been known for years that a deprived early environment can lead to failure to thrive in babies. The experiments all involve raising rats under different conditions, one "enriched," the other impoverished. Researchers have found that rats raised in the enriched conditions show increased dendritic branching (Greenough 1975), larger synaptic boutons (West and Greenough 1972), significant differences in size and weight of the cortex (e.g., Bennett, Rosenzweig, and Diamond 1969), and, of course, quite significant differences in maze learning (e.g., Rosenzweig 1971). Rosenzweig and his group of investigators assert that the observed differences are the result of active interactions with the environment and not just the result of greater activity per se. They also maintain that the observed anatomical, physiological, and behavioral changes not only are a result of early exposure to an enriched environment but also are possible in older rats.

Rehabilitative work with brain-damaged patients also reveals the importance of interaction with context for recovery. It is possible to elicit different levels of response from patients if the same task is made either internal or external. For example, Luria (1963) cites research on range of movement in people with injured elbows. Researchers found that patients achieved sequentially greater range of movement when asked to perform each of this series of tasks: Raise your hand as high as you can, raise your hand to a certain number on a screen, grasp an object suspended at a height. Although the experiment was designed for people with elbow injuries and not brain damage, it nevertheless illustrates an important principle. Each task requires a different level of neuromuscular coordination. On their own, patients are able to reach just one level. In interaction with a context, two other possible levels of coordination are made available.

Another way of seeing how this works is to look at experiments and neurotraining that involve adding a meaningful organization to the context of the task requirement. For example, in experiments with children two-and-one-half to three years old, Luria found that when the children were asked to press a button when they heard a certain sound, they could not coordinate the pressing movement with the sound nor

346

could they inhibit other motor movements not related to the sound stimulus. But when they were given a word instead of a sound as the stimulus for pressing the button, their movements became coordinated.

Likewise, when Luria was neurotraining a brain-damaged patient who could not "perceive more than two meaningless shapes and reproduce them in outline" (1963, p. 68), he gave the patient shapes that looked roughly like the silhouette of the letters of a word. The patient could then easily perform the task. Thus, the role of context is crucial to rehabilitation.

EMBODIMENT. If context is important in eliciting different levels of organized response in the person, embodiment is crucial to the ability to respond to context. The situated capacity to respond to situations in a precognitive, habitual way is a level of neurobody organization that can be used to help people regain lost function. Those habitual bodily actions that are retained in brain-damaged people can be elicited by the neurotherapist and then consciously used as the basis for helping the patient regain other lost functions. For example, Luria (1963) describes the starting point for reteaching speech in patients with "afferent motor aphasia":

> Usually . . . the imitative or symbolic movements of the articulatory apparatus disintegrate, whereas the elementary "instinctive" and "purposive" movements of the tongue and lips remain intact. Thus the patient who cannot touch his upper lip with the tip of his tongue or perform the movement of spitting in response to an instruction, can do so easily in a real situation, when licking his lips or spitting out unpleasant food; he can just as easily smoke a cigarette or pipe, chew his food, and blow out a lighted match. These residual movements of the lips, tongue and larynx, which form part of the patient's reaction to a given situation, can be made the starting point for restoration of the disordered speech function (p. 138).

Identifying the "residual movements" and capacities takes deliberate planning since most testing focuses on diagnosing the deficits.

A rehabilitative approach based on the principle of embodiment has been developed by physical therapist Berta Bobath and Dr. Karel Bobath (Bobath 1978, Gee and Passarella 1985). The therapy is based on the notion that hemiplegics should be taught to use their affected side in as normal a way as possible in order to stimulate neural repair and restore function. The therapy focuses on posture, tone, and movement. Patients are taught how to maintain normal posture sitting and standing. Restoration of muscle tone and prevention of spasticity are aided by weight-bearing activities, such as sleeping on the affected side. Normal movement patterns that were once automatic are now re-learned consciously. Patients are instructed in both principles and techniques that allow bilateral rather than unilateral movement.

This therapeutic approach contrasts with the more traditional one in which patients are taught to use their unaffected side to perform tasks. Rehabilitative therapy based on the Bobath principles has two advantages over the traditional therapy. First, it develops movements that are more like those typically used in normal activity (e.g., in rising from a chair, or in putting on clothes). Thus, movements are less effortful. Second, by evoking the preconscious body through conscious maintenance of normal posture, weight bearing, and movement, it counters spasticity and disuse of the affected side.

Studies of the usefulness of the Bobath principles in rehabilitation have found that patients show an improvement in their ability to perform activities of daily living (Lewis 1986), and that they show significantly greater degrees of functional improvement than patients treated with the traditional method (Passarela and Lewis 1987). Although the therapy is rehabilitative, therapists following the Bobath principles recommend that it be started during the acute care stage of the illness (Gee and Passarella 1985).

COPING WITH STROKE AND CLOSED HEAD INJURY

The question that must always be asked in studying coping is "coping with what?" We have taken pains in every chapter to show that it is a mistaken assumption to think one knows in advance what is difficult for a person or what is the source of suffering. One can have the basis for understanding what is stressful for a person, but then one needs to encounter the individual as an individual to interpret his or her own meanings. This chapter has proceeded through a series of perspectives, the epidemiologist's, the neuroscientist's, the outcome researcher's, the rehabilitation clinician's. Each successive perspective has gradually shifted the focus of concern from a grossly normative one to a more fine-grained and individualized one, the goal being to provide the reader with the basis for understanding the many aspects that contribute to both the stress of and the coping with closed head injury or stroke. Now we turn to the individual, and we present aspects of the experience of suffering brain damage from the perspective of the person. We first present selections from two first-hand accounts of the stroke experience, then we look at aspects of the illness experience research has illuminated: the kinds of coping demands encountered and the coping resources available to the individual, the context in terms of demand and of resources, and common meanings of the illness.

STROKE FROM THE PATIENT'S POINT OF VIEW. The following are selections from a personal account of the experience of stroke by Professor P. Smithells, Emeritus Professor of the University of Otago, New Zealand, Director of the School of Physical Education.

In July, 1975, shortly after retiring, I found it difficult to hold a chisel, could not tie my shoe laces and became a little confused about left and right, and in fact found my body very disobedient when doing practical tasks. In August 1975 I fell off a ladder breaking six adjacent ribs on my left side, a singularly painful experience. I realized that long-established neuro-muscular patterns were not working or were at least impaired.

I went then to an ophthalmologist who was testing my optical fields routinely and he immediately rang the neurologists at the hospital who agreed to see me the following day. After a few tests it seemed possible that I had had a parietal lobe stroke, which explained to me the lack of feedback from the muscles and joints on my left leg and arm. . . . I continued to walk whenever I could but there was speech impairment and ptosis of the left eye and weakness of the cheek and mouth. All function of my left hand disappeared but I could still walk with a dragging action for I had not kinaesthetic sense, the bio-feedback mechanisms having been knocked out.

I continued to write, but my handwriting, always difficult, became even more undisciplined, losing both horizontal and vertical accuracy, even though carried out by my unimpaired dominant hand. The worst blow was the loss of will-power. I had often pondered on where the seat of the will could be neurophysiologically speaking, and now conclude that it must in the intact upper motoneurone. It is a blow to the ego not being able to move a limb when you want to. It also is a very strange experience and as such disorientating. This led to a lot of sartorial confusion buttoning shirts and cardigans wrongly and putting on ties inaccurately. One has the feeling of shabbiness. Eating is a messy performance at first, but then one learns to use a combined fork and knife with the one hand and not to eat soups that require full control of mouth and throat. Cutaneous sensations being diminished, one is unaware about what is on the face on the affected side where the menu is there for all to see. One's total postural reflexes alter and in walking one's pendant useless arm is apt to become very cold and oedematous, producing a

349

general spinal twist, of a scoliotic kind. . . . One general reaction was a perpetual state of drowsiness and ennui, so that if I took my usual post-prandial sleep, it was apt to go on far too long. I used a timer with an alarm to control this tendency. . . .

One of the curious effects of the stroke . . . was a loss of timbre in my voice which has always been deep and resonant. . . . I used to read poetry in public and broadcast and my voice became to me an instrument which I could no longer play properly. I do not know who coined the word "stroke," but it is such a one-fell-swoop experience that I think stroke is a singularly appropriate term for the sudden cutting-off of competence. I had always been in previous illnesses a quick healer, so living with the slow recovery of a stroke has been a salutary lesson in accepting the inevitability of age and inevitable decrepitude of old-age.

Remarkably the one mechanism that has never wavered has been my appetite for food, and for learning, and for delving into the past. I am blest with almost total recall in terms of memory. . . . I have no difficulty with names and faces . . . visits from old graduate students passing through bring instant recall and much pleasure through being able to reminisce about the past. I hope I have not become a bore, the most unforgiveable of senile traits. I have had a very happy and exceedingly busy life with interesting people and challenges all the way (Smithells 1978, pp. 396–397).

The personal account of a stroke provides what is central to an understanding of the stress of coping with stroke, namely the meaning of the illness for the person. Physical disability understood in personal meaning terms is "the sudden cutting off of competence." In specific encounters of everyday life, physical disability leads to a "feeling of shabbiness." And in its specific effect on his voice, disability made it "an instrument which I could no longer play properly."

The nonspecific effects of stroke are felt as a "loss of will-power," and a "perpetual state of drowsiness and ennui." The loss of will is felt to be the "worst blow." It provides such a stark sense of discontinuity that he, somewhat facetiously, decides that willpower must occupy a localized site in the brain, which was damaged by his stroke.

He copes with his stroke in one way by maintaining as much as possible the continuity of his life. Although one leg is impaired, he still walks whenever he can. He also still writes (witness the account he has provided). His handwriting is affected, but then his handwriting was never very good. He can still write, that is the important thing. He adapts new habits where necessary to maintain the important aspect of meaning. For example, he changes his eating habits in order to avoid mess. He imposes external control to replace lost inner control, e.g., using a timer to wake himself up from a nap.

When the discontinuity is too great, he reinterprets his illness experience as typical of aging. In psychopathological parlance, this could be termed "denial." But in a phenomenological view, this shows up as a reweaving of the web of meaning in his life. It is a way of understanding the self as connected to the world of everyday life experience rather than as separated out as deviant, as ill. He can accept the extreme discontinuity the illness has created in his life, the persistence of disability, the failure to "heal quickly" if he understands them as part of the normative changes of aging. This coping strategy would be ineffective only if drugs, surgery, or therapy could restore the lost functions, and he were prevented from taking advantage of them because of his understanding of his illness as normative aging. Likewise, he uses humor, at least in the telling of his story. This provides the sense that he is not denying but is enabled to have a perspective on his illness that makes it more bearable.

He also copes with his illness by recognizing and relishing the important things in his life that remain. He still enjoys eating and learning. His memory is unimpaired, and reminiscing about the past is a source of great pleasure. Realizing that one still retains the aspects of one's life that matter is a main, and often ignored, way of coping. It is not simply a form of "cognitive coping" (Mechanic 1962), that is, something one says to oneself to feel better, such as, "it could be worse." It is a way of acknowledging the network of concerns that ties him to his world, the concerns that make life both possible and meaningful.

Another person's account of her stroke experience emphasizes both different and similar issues. The following are selections from Dr. Cindi Goldberg's account of her recovery from stroke. Like Professor Smithells, Dr. Goldberg is a professional (a clinical psychologist). Unlike Professor Smithells, she is young (thirty-six years old), and her stroke affected the left hemisphere of her brain, whereas Professor Smithells's affected the right. (Note: Different sequelae do follow depending on the location of the brain damage, but any damage to any area can affect the whole body. For example, Professor Smithells had difficulty writing with his dominant right hand, even though the paresis was on the left side of his body.)

Once it was clear that I was going to survive, the hard part began: recovery. My mind was shattered. It was like a million veils prevented me from experiencing life clearly and directly. For four days I couldn't speak—not one word. On the fourth day I said my first word. It was "no." After that, the ability to say simple words returned, but when I tried to say the complicated things I was capable of thinking, no one understood me. About one week after the stroke I felt panicky, very depressed, hopeless, desperate and afraid of everything.

I could count inside my head, but not verbally. I lost song lyrics and tunes. I retained English as a thinking mode, but couldn't express myself. I thought the stroke had drastically reduced my intelligence level. My self-esteem was abysmal.

I felt dull. It was hard to organize my thoughts and I could only think of one thing at a time. I didn't want to see anyone. It was too tiring to see friends because I had to concentrate too hard. And I wasn't easy to get along with. I had lost my sense of humor and my generosity. I complained most of the time.

Some friends avoided me. Others ignored what I was going through and proceeded to make arrangements to do activities that I was not ready to cope with. A few friends stayed with me, even when I felt really black and dismal. These friends I am really grateful for because they hastened my recovery. But on the whole, I became very isolated, lonely, and dependent upon my husband and the people taking care of me. I felt guilty—as if I had done something wrong.

While most of my feelings were despairing ones, a tiny corner of my mind said, "you have to get better." So I dutifully underwent therapy, not convinced it would do any good. My speech pathologist asked me to read and I told her I couldn't. She insisted I try and gave me a novel, *Portraits*. Reluctantly, I tried to read it. I was surprised that I understood it. After that, my reading skills progressed quickly. . . . Most importantly, my therapists treated me as an intelligent person who deserved respect. I needed that tremendously because I felt stupid and worthless. . . .

About two years after the stroke, I felt that my intelligence and emotions were coming back to normal. Now I feel 90–95% normal. . . .

There was even a positive side to the slow-down the stroke caused in my life. I have more capacity to listen now and that makes me more intuitive. In spite of losing so much, this is a special gift that I can take back to my counseling practice.

The feelings of frustration and isolation are largely gone. In spite of my speech problems, when I communicate a thought now, it eventually gets through. I don't know how, but it does. It amazes me. As a matter of fact, on rare occasions, I think of myself as normal (Goldberg 1986, pp. 1–2).

Dr. Goldberg's illness experience contrasts with Professor Smithells' in that the stroke affected different abilities. Professor Smithells retained all language abilities and memory. Dr. Goldberg lost expressive language, the ability to understand complex written language, and some ability to organize and remember. These abilities are centrally meaningful in her personal life and work life. Her loss of the ability to remain connected to her world, to the things that mattered to her, in the way that mattered to her created feelings of loss, despair, isolation, and lowered self-esteem.

The very resources that made it possible for Professor Smithells to adapt to and accept his illness were taken from Dr. Goldberg. But she retains that one part Professor Smithells so felt that he lacked—willpower. In spite of her despair and her fatigue, she listens to an inner voice and goes to rehabilitative therapy. After two years, she feels almost herself again. But because she no longer possesses the taken-for-granted capacity to speak, but has had to relearn how to speak using other functional systems, it "amazes" her when she actually communicates a thought.

Dr. Goldberg's experience with her friends points up important points about social support. First, having social support is not the same as being able to use it. She could not be buoyed up by visits from friends when their visits proved too exhausting for her. Second, not all social support is supportive. The friends who arranged activities without regard for her ability to participate made her situation more stressful for her. Third, being able to be present with a cared-for other in a direct, nondemanding way, without doing anything else, is in itself experienced as supportive. None of these aspects of social support can be captured by a social network questionnaire (Wrubel 1985), and yet each one is crucial to understanding how social support works.

The role of the rehabilitation therapists was clearly central. By treating her as an intelligent person deserving of respect, by giving her manageable tasks, and by initially insisting that she could do it, they provided more than the training necessary for the recovery of function. They provided her with a sense of self-worth when her self-esteem was at a low ebb. And they aided and abetted her own inner voice that willed her to work to get better. In short, they were caring, and their caring enabled recovery.

Professor Smithells was grateful for the meaningful capacities that were left him; Dr. Goldberg sees the positive side of her stroke in having gained a capacity to listen. These are lived examples of how within each person's situated life, each person's being in the world, there exist possibilities for new meanings and new connections.

COPING DEMAND AND COPING RESOURCES. The personal accounts included above provide a vivid sense of some of the coping demands stroke survivors encounter and some of the coping resources the person brings to the situation. Although the personal accounts were by stroke survivors, survivors of closed head injury could have told their stories just as well. Professor Bryan Jennett (1984) provides a succinct summary of the challenge that faces people with brain damage:

> That some patients can come to terms with overwhelming physical disability has been demonstrated many times, but there is a fallacy in extrapolating this to survival after severe brain damage—when the reserves of emotional drive, the stability of personality and the intellectual resources that are all so essential to coping with disability are themselves affected (p. 42).

Professor Jennett points out one aspect of brain damage that makes it so difficult to deal with. The same injury that deprives the person of normal functioning also deprives him or her of the resources the person would draw upon to deal with the loss. The sapping of resources is different in different people and according to injury. In Dr. Goldberg's case, the damage to the left hemisphere and resulting pattern of aphasia was a devastating loss. As a clinical therapist, Dr. Goldberg used oral communication as her primary way of encountering problems. This capacity was now denied her. She had to cope with her brain damage without the very skill she would invoke first. Damage to the left hemisphere that results in aphasia is often accompanied by depression, sometimes quite severe. Emotional outbursts of tears and/or rage are not uncommon and have been termed "catastrophic reactions" (Binder 1983). Thus, there is a linkage of coping demands that requires the person to emerge from despair to take up the arduous tasks of rehabilitation.

In Professor Smithells's case, the damage to the right hemisphere involved mainly motor function. His powers of expression and memory were preserved. But he noted a loss of willpower. This is not surprising, since all normal behavior and activity require the integrated function of both hemispheres. In the last section of Professor Smithells's account (not included in the selections above), written a year after the description of his stroke, he briefly describes having suffered a second stroke, being completely paralyzed on the left side, and having great difficulty sustaining consecutive thoughts unless cued by his wife.

Another and not uncommon effect of stroke is usually called a denial of illness or anosognosia, in which the person has no sense that anything is wrong. This can be manifested in "hemi-inattention" in which the person ignores the paralyzed half of the body and everything else on that side. These patients have been known to draw one-sided people, or comb only one side of the head, or shave only one side of the face.

Furthermore, damage to the frontal lobes is often associated with a kind of personality change in which the person loses motivation for recovery, becomes insensitive to appropriate social cues, behaves inappropriately, or becomes very "superficial." These kinds of changes create primarily a coping demand for the caregivers, both the health care providers and the family. The person is seemingly unaware that anything is amiss.

It is believed that a major personal resource for the person with brain damage is his or her life experience before damage. People with more education seem to fare better than people with comparable damage but less education. Recent work in neurophysiological plasticity suggests that the more learning or "overlearning" that has taken place, the greater the possibility for recovery of function (Finger and Stein 1982).

As the person moves out of the acute stage of recovery and into rehabilitation, health care providers are usually quite interested in assessing the patient's ability to manage independently, outside of either the acute care setting or a long-term convalescent home. A measure of primary sociobiological function—the Activities of Daily Living (ADL) (Katz and Akpom 1976)—is often used to assess level of function. The degree to which one is able to manage the requirements of everyday life can obviously determine whether one can live independently or not. But everyday coping as measured on the ADL is not the same as it is understood by the person.

Other physical factors not measured on the ADL (e.g., fatigability, impaired cognition, and fine motor function) can significantly affect how one gets on in the world, and even more importantly, how one feels about how one is getting on. In a study of quality of life in stroke survivors, Ahlsio et al. (1984) found that "perceived quality of life did not improve in follow-up, athough ADL function did" (p. 890). They concluded that there had been too much effort placed in physical rehabilitation and not enough placed in psychological support. This may be true. But it may also be true that not enough attention has been paid to what the patient is coping with. For example, the person may be able to dress himself or herself, but with difficulty and not always neatly. The person may be able to feed himself or herself, but not without spilling some or being unaware that he or she needs to wipe food from the numb part of the face. The "feeling of shabbiness" that Professor Smithells describes may be much more to the point for the person.

Further, performing the daily tasks of self-care must be much more arduous, physically and mentally, for a brain-damaged person than for one who is not. It is in itself stressful to have to think about reflectively what is normally smooth and taken for granted. Even in someone who has had a very successful recovery, the rehabilitated function is no longer taken for granted. Dr. Goldberg describes herself as "amazed" when she is able to communicate a thought to someone else. This constant awareness of what used to be taken for granted, along with the need to attend consciously and expend effort, would seem likely to affect anyone's assessment of the quality of his or her life.

Finally, gaining a rating of ADL-independent does not reflect ability to carry out such "nonessential" activities as visiting friends, fishing, going to a movie, or engaging in sexual intercourse. Sjogren and Fugl-Meyer (1982) found that frequency of sexual intercourse decreased for about three-fourths of the people in their study. This decrease correlated mainly with ADL-dependence and lack of sensation. But for decreased leisure, the association was with degree of motor disability and lack of sensation. In a later study, Sjogren (1982) found a relation between a sense of stigma and decrease in leisure activity. Whatever the reason for decreasing or ceasing usual leisure activities, the loss of such a source of pleasure must surely affect one's sense of the quality of life or the sense of what makes life meaningful. Over the long haul of a lifetime, without respite, without "breathers," without the little things that boost one's spirit, without those brief times of being pleasantly distracted, not all the will or effort or possession of coping resources will suffice.

THE SHIFTING CONTEXT OF COPING DEMAND. It is not always easy to answer the question "coping with what?" Personal meanings and concerns determine to a large extent what in any situation will be experienced as stressful. However, in the situation of coping with brain damage, as in any situation that endures over time, both the context and the personal meanings shift. What is at stake for the person and the nature of the coping demands are different at different points in time. This observation may seem completely obvious, but it is surprising how often it is ignored in studies that compare coping in the same individual at different times.

Initially, in the acute care setting, the specific context can be foreign and confusing for patient and family alike. Bourdon (1986) describes the intensive care context from the patient's point of view.

> The patients in the NICU are critically ill; some are near death. There are sounds of people moaning in pain. A slight "woosh" of the respirator and another alarm sounds. A family member cries. Another is anxious and paces the floor. A spouse, in anger, shouts at the nurse. She realizes he is feeling helpless and alone. Another family keeps a constant vigil, playing soothing tapes of Mozart and ocean sounds to their loved one, who is brain dead. This is the NICU. Both patient and family feel overwhelmed by these sights and sounds. One experiences a lack of privacy. All of these displays of emotion—sadness, anger, grief—are such personal matters. Yet, the patients' rooms must be open and visible to the staff at all times (p. 631).

Bourdon goes on to point out the ways in which the context created to save lives becomes in itself something with which to cope. The patient, already confused, is placed in a setting that would confuse a fully oriented person. Careful nursing management and interventions where necessary can minimize the worst of the problem.

The patient does adjust. The context becomes familiar, but the strangeness of a paralyzed body or an aphasic brain persists. As the physical signs improve and posttraumatic amnesia abates, the patient may become increasingly aware of the damage done. (Sometimes, as indicated earlier, there is a gross lack of awareness of any problem.) But even if the patient is aware of deficits, he or she may not grasp the implications of the damage. This is often described as "denial." We have discussed our perspective on denial several times in this book. At this point, we will briefly note that from a phenomenological perspective, *denial* is a term that covers a very large group of actions and meanings. If the goal is understanding, it is far more useful to examine both what the meanings are in the particular situation for that particular person and the adaptive nature of those meanings.

Health care providers who have seen many people with neurological damage know that recovery almost never means return of pretrauma functioning. Nonetheless, the exact outcome and degree of recovery are impossible to predict. So it seems less pathological than adaptive to live with the expectation and hope that one will get better as long as there is ambiguity and uncertainty about the outcome.

When the patient stabilizes, he or she is moved from the acute care setting to a rehabilitation unit. This setting is much less confusing, and life there is more normal than in the acute care setting. The full awareness of the loss often strikes patients when they enter the rehabilitation setting. Successful rehabilitation requires full, willing participation on the part of the patient. But such participation is very difficult for a person who is still dealing with the meaning of what has been lost. A caring intervention, such as the one described in the following exemplar, can make all the difference in finding the new meanings that will help a person engage in the process of rehabilitation.

PARADIGM

A Woman Who Had Always Been Proud of Her Hands
Barbara Ridley, RN, CRNN
Herrick Hospital, Berkeley, California

I work on a stroke rehab unit on the day shift. One morning I was, as usual, assigned three patients, one of whom was Mrs. B. She had been admitted the day before from the acute hospital. She was in her early sixties and had had a cerebrovascular accident with resulting left hemiplegia about ten days previously. When I reviewed her care plan and chart at the beginning of the shift, she appeared to me a very "light" patient. Compared to the problems of many of the patients on our unit, her problems seemed minor to me. She had no aphasia, no major problems with dysphagia, and was continent of bowel and bladder. When I went into the room to assess her, I found her to be alert and oriented. She was of small build, and I knew I would have no difficulty transferring her in and out of bed.

The beginning of the shift is always very hectic, as everyone has to be prepared for therapy on schedule. I was busy with my other patients and did not have much time to spend with Mrs. B. She was reluctant to go to the community dining room for breakfast, but that is not unusual on the first morning. I did not think much of it until I went into her room at about 10:00 A.M., when things had quieted down, and found her sitting in her wheelchair looking very despondent, her head buried in her hand. I sat down to talk to her, and she immediately started crying, telling me how useless she felt without the use of her left hand, how ugly she felt since her stroke, and how frightening the onset of the hemiplegia had been. My initial response was to want to say something to cheer her up, to say that she was not as badly affected as many people, that she might have return of function, or that through therapy she would learn the use of one-handed techniques. But something stopped me, and instead I just took the time to sit and *listen.*

She talked to me about her life, about how active and independent she had always been and how much she had been looking forward to her retirement. "And I've always been so proud of my hands. It sounds silly, but I've always liked my hands." I just sat there and said "They are nice hands." She told me that she loved to bake and work in the garden, and that she was frightened of losing all those things and becoming too much of a burden on her daughter. I felt that something very significant was happening. Perhaps it was because I had recently experienced a major loss in my own personal life that I felt that I could really *understand* her grief. I felt that it had been wrong to categorize her as a "light" patient. I realized that what might appear to be fairly minor deficits to me could seem totally devastating to her, and that the loss of a particular function has a different meaning for each individual.

I could tell that it meant a lot to her that I could listen to her in that way. After about half an hour I showed her how she could exercise and massage her left hand to reduce the edema, and she seemed to like that idea. She remained fairly subdued for the rest of the day, but she had an air of calmness about her.

I was off for three days, and when I returned to work I was not assigned to her. I found her in the community dining room, and her eyes lit up when she saw me. She beckoned me over to show me how she now had very slight movement in her left fingers, and how she had mastered the art of opening the milk carton with one hand. She now looked like a patient who was fully involved in her rehab program, and I knew that I had made a difference in helping her do that.

Discharge from the hospital involves another major contextual shift. Blazyk and Canavan (1986) call this shift in context a "crisis" when the patient has suffered a catastrophic illness or injury. They emphasize psychological factors, such as the difficulties families face in accepting that the health care givers in the hospital have not effected a cure, the need to realign role responsibilities in the family, and the unresolved emotional reactions to the illness or injury. Suggestions for intervention focus on making the family less dependent on the hospital and enabling them to work through their emotions. It is also suggested that the family be helped to reframe their understanding of the discharge in positive terms.

Coaching and guiding patients and families into new meanings that offer greater possibility are very important roles for the health care provider. However, it is not clear that discharge is a universal crisis. Research could clarify the meaning of discharge for the patient and the family, but anecdotal evidence indicates that there are several ways of understanding the meaning of discharge. For some families, it clearly means that the patient has survived the illness, and going home is highly meaningful regardless of level of disability.

More to the point from a coping perspective is the changed context of being at home instead of in the hospital. The coping demand of this context is experienced more over time as the enduring difficulties of home care persist. Families undoubtedly have to deal with a variety of emotions, but they also have to deal with limited support services for home care.

Research on the usefulness of giving spouses information about stroke and encouraging their involvement in patient care during the hospitalization and coping outcomes over six months postdischarge highlights the importance of considering the role of both shifting context and personal meaning in coping. Field, Cordle, and Bowman (1983) report that the intervention did seem to have an effect on practical management, but psychological coping was not measurably affected. For example, although anxiety increased upon discharge and then decreased, it did not go away altogether. Couples gave a positive presentation of their situation, but only a few regarded the future positively. Most were "taking things a day at a time" or were uncertain about the future.

Having a positive effect on practical management is a worthwhile outcome, since so much effort must be directed in that direction in these cases. It seems unrealistic, though, to aim to reduce anxiety unless the anxiety is groundless. The couples' approach to the future reflects more of their sense of the situation. There is a risk of another stroke or, when both spouses are elderly, of illness in the caretaker spouse.

Field's et al. findings show how people cope in order to maintain continuity of meaning in their lives and, when there is disruption, how they find ways of making new connections through new concerns:

> Many of these [coping] problems persisted throughout our study period, although typically couples deemphasized their significance. A recurrent theme in the interviews was their stress on independence and a great reluctance to call on others for help, even where this was clearly needed. . . . Some of the difficulties then, which couples experienced, were exacerbated by their strong emphasis on being independent, which pre-

vented them from getting all the help which was available. Their strategy was to "normalize" their problems and to emphasize the more positive aspects. . . . For example, several couples reported that the stroke "had brought them closer together," that they were "now more understanding" and some said that they were "better people" (p. 99).

The importance of the personal meaning of independence leads the couples to do tasks themselves, even when they had people available they could call on for help. They are coping with maintaining their independence. This is hard to understand as coping when one's understanding of coping is as a cure-all. Coping does not (necessarily) make life easier. It is possible to normalize one's problems when one's meanings and connections that create one's world are still intact. And it is possible, even in this most devastating of illnesses, to find new meaning. That is always possible.

REFERENCES

Ahlsio B, Britton M, Murray V, Theorell T: Disablement and quality of life after stroke. Stroke 15:886, 1984.

Allport GW: The general and the unique in psychological science. J Pers 30:405, 1962.

Andrews K, Brocklehurst JC, Richards B, and Laycock PJ: The recovery of the severely disabled stroke patient. Rheumatol Rehab 21:225, 1982.

Andrews K, Stewart J: Stroke recovery: He can but does he? Rheumatol Rehab 18:43, 1979.

Annegers JF, Grabow JD, Kurland LT, Laws ER: The incidence, causes, and secular trends of head trauma in Olmsted County, Minnesota. Neurology 30:912, 1980.

Barth JT, Macciocchi SN, Giordani B, Rimel R, Jane JA, Boll TJ: Neuropsychological sequelae of minor head injury. Neurosurgery 13:529, 1983.

Beck CH, Chambers WW: Speed, accuracy and strength of forelimb movement after unilateral pyramidotomy in rhesus monkeys. J Compar Physiol Psychol 70:1, 1970.

Becker DP, Miller JD, Ward JD, Greenberg RP, Young HF, Sakalas R: The outcome from severe head injury with early diagnosis and intensive management. J Neurosurg 47:491, 1977.

Benner P: From Novice to Expert: Excellence and Power in Clinical Nursing Practice. Menlo Park, Calif.: Addison-Wesley, 1984.

Bennett EL, Rosenzweig MR, Diamond MC: Rat brain: Effect of environmental enrichment on wet and dry weights. Science 163:825, 1969.

Binder LM: Emotional problems after stroke. Stroke 18:17, 1983.

Blazyk F, Canavan MM: Managing the discharge crisis following catastrophic illness or injury. Social Work Health Care 11:19, 1986.

Bobath B: Adult Hemiplegia: Evaluation and Treatment, 2d ed. London: William Heineman, 1978.

Bond MR, Brooks DN: Understanding the process of recovery as a basis for the investigation of rehabilitation for the brain injured. Scand J Rehab Med 8:127, 1976.

Bourdon SE: Psychological impact of neurotrauma in the acute care setting. Nurs Clin North Am 21:629, 1986.

Bowen FP, Demirjian C, Karpiak SE, and Katzman R: Sprouting of noradrenergic nerve terminals subsequent to freeze lesions of rabbit cerebral cortex. Paper presented at the Society for Neuroscience, Third Annual Meeting, San Diego, California, November, 1973.

Brooks DN, Deelman BG, van Zomeren AH, van Dongen H, van Harskamp F, and Aughton ME: Problems in measuring cognitive recovery after acute brain injury. J Clin Neuropsychol 6:71, 1984.

Broverman DM: Normative and ipsative measurement in psychology. Psych Rev 4:295, 1962.

Cotman CW, Nieto-Sampedro M: Progress in facilitating the recovery of function after central nervous system trauma. In Nottebohm F (ed): *Hope for a New Neurology,* pp. 83–104. New York: The New York Academy of Sciences, 1985.

Craine JF, Gudeman HE: *The Rehabilitation of Brain Functions: Principles, Procedures, and Techniques of Neurotraining.* Springfield, Ill: Charles C. Thomas, 1981.

Devor M, Schneider GE: Neuroanatomical plasticity: The principle of conservation of total axonal arborization. In Vital Durant F, Jeannerod J (eds): *Aspects of Neural Plasticity,* pp. 191–202. Lyon, France: Colloque INSERM, 1975.

Doolittle ND: Relevance of the Habitual Body for Neuroscience. Doctoral paper. University of California at San Francisco, 1987.

Espmark S: Stroke before 50: A follow-up study of voactional and psychological adjustment. Scand J Rehab Med [Suppl 2] 1973.

Field JH: *Epidemiology of Head Injury in England and Wales; with Particular Application to Rehabilitation.* Leicester: Printed for H.M. Stationery Office by Willsons, 1974.

Field D, Cordle CJ, Bowman GS: Coping with stroke at home. Internatl Rehab Med 5:96,. 1983.

Finger S, Stein DG: *Brain Damage and Recovery: Research and Clinical Perspectives.* New York: Academic Press, 1982.

Frommer GP: Subtotal lesions: Implications for coding and recovery of function. In Finger S. (ed): *Recovery from Brain Damage,* pp. 217–280. New York: Plenum, 1978.

Gee ZL, Passarella PM: *Nursing Care of the Stroke Patient: A Therapeutic Approach Based on Bobath Principles.* Pittsburgh: AREN-Publications, 1985.

Geschwind N: Late changes in the nervous system: An overview. In Stein DG, Rosen JJ, and Butters N (eds): *Plasticity and Recovery of Function in the Central Nervous System,* pp. 467–508. New York: Academic Press, 1974.

Geschwind N: Mechanisms of change after brain lesions. In Nottebohm F (ed) *Hope for a New Neurology,* pp. 1–11. New York: The New York Academy of Sciences, 1985.

Gold SJ: Getting well: Impression management as stroke rehabilitation. Qualitative Sociol 6:238, 1983.

Goldberg C: Coming back from stroke. Heart Briefs 36(2):1, 1986.

Greenough WT: Experiential modification of the developing brain. Am Sci, 63:37, 1975.

Gronwall D, Wrightson P: Delayed recovery of intellectual function after minor head injury. Lancet 2:604, 1974.

Jane JA, Rimel RW, Pobereskin LH, Tyson GW, Stewart O, Genarelli TA: Head injury:

Basic and clinical aspects. In Grossman RC, Gildenberg PL (eds): *Outcome and Pathology and Head Injury.* pp. 229–237. New York: Raven Press, 1982.

Jennett B: The measurement of outcome. In Brooks N (ed): *Closed Head Injury.* pp. 37–43. Oxford: Oxford University Press, 1984.

Jennett B: Who cares for head injuries? Br Med J 3:267, 1975.

Jennett B, Bond M: Assessment of outcome after severe brain damage. Lancet *i*:480, 1975.

Jennett B, Teasdale G, Galbraith S, Pickard J, Grant H, Braakman R, Avezaat C, Maas A, Minderhoud J, Vecht CJ, Heiden J, Small R, Caton W, Kurze T: Severe head injuries in three countries. J Neurol Neurosurg Psychiatr, 40:291, 1977.

Kalsbeek WD, McLaurin RL, Harris BSH III, Miller JD: The national head and spinal cord injury survey: Major findings. J Neurosurg [Suppl] 53:19, 1980.

Katz S, Akpom CA: A measure of primary sociobiological functions. Int J Health Serv 6:493, 1976.

Kerson TS, with Kerson LA: *Understanding Chronic Illness: The Medical and Psychosocial Dimensions of Nine Diseases.* New York: The Free Press, 1985.

Kraus JF: Injury to the head and spinal cord: The epidemiological relevance of the medical literature published from 1960 to 1978. J Neurosurg [Suppl] 53:3, 1980.

Kuhn TS: *The Structure of Scientific Revolutions,* 2d ed. Chicago: University of Chicago Press, 1977.

Lashley KS: *The Neuropsychology of Lashley: Selected Papers.* New York: McGraw-Hill, 1960.

Lazarus RS, Folkman S: Coping and adaptation. In Gentry WD (ed): *The Handbook of Behavioral Medicine.* New York: Guilford Press, 1984.

Levin HS, Benton AL, Grossman RG: *Neurobehavioral Consequences of Closed Head Injury.* New York: Oxford University Press, 1982.

Levin HS, High WM, Goethe KE, Sisson RA, Overall JE, Rhoades HM, Eisenberg HM, Kalisky Z, Gary HE: The neurobehavioural rating scale: Assessment of the behavioral sequelae of head injury by the clinician. J Neurol Neurosurg Psychiatr 50:183, 1987.

Lewis NA: Functional gains of CVA patients: A nursing approach. Rehabil Nurs 11:25, 1986.

Lezak MD, Gray DK: Sampling problems and nonparametric solutions in clinical neuropsychological research. J Clin Neuropsychol, 6:101, 1984.

Luria AR: *Human Brain and Psychological Processes.* Haigh B (trans). New York: Harper & Row, 1966. Originally published 1963.

Luria AR: *Restoration of Function after Brain Injury.* Zangwill OL (trans). New York: Macmillan, 1963. Originally published 1948.

Marceil JC: Implicit dimensions of idiography and nomotheses: A reformulation. Amer Psych 32:1046, 1977.

Marshall JF: Brain function: Neural adaptations and recovery from injury. Am Rev Psychol 35:277, 1984.

Marshall LF, Smith RW, Shapiro HM: The outcome with aggressive treatment in severe head injuries. Part I: The significance of intracranial pressure monitoring. J Neurosurg 50:20, 1979.

Mechanic D: *Students under Stress: A Study in the Social Psychology of Adaptation.* New York: The Free Press, 1962. (Reprinted in 1978 by the University of Wisconsin Press.)

Merleau-Ponty M: *The Phenomenology of Perception.* New Jersey: The Humanities Press, 1962.

Miller H: Accident neurosis. Br Med J 1:919, 1961.

Miller JD, Butterworth JF, Gudeman SK, Faulkner JE, Choi SC, Selhorst JB, Harbison JW, Lutz HA, Young HF, Becker DP: Further experience in the management of severe head injury. J Neurosurg 54:289, 1981.

Oppenheimer DR: Microscopic lesions in the brain following head injury. J Neurol Neurosurg Psychiatry 31:299, 1968.

Passarella PM, Lewis N: Nursing application of Bobath principles in stroke care. J Neurosci Nurs 19:106, 1987.

Rosenzweig MR: Effects of environment on development of brain and behavior. In Tobach E, Aronson LR, Shaw E (eds): *The Biopsychology of Development.* New York: Academic Press, 1971.

Sacks O: *The Man who Mistook his Wife for a Hat and Other Clinical Tales.* New York: Simon & Schuster, 1985.

Sjogren K: Leisure after stroke. Int Rehab Med 4:80, 1982.

Sjogren K, Fugl-Meyer AR: Adjustment to life after stroke with special reference to sexual intercourse and leisure. J Psychosom Res 26:409, 1982.

Smithells P: A personal account by a sufferer from a stroke. New Zeal Med J 87:396, 1978.

Sotelo C, Palay SL: Altered axons and axon terminals in the lateral vestibular nucleus of the rat. Possible example of neuronal remodeling. *Lab Invest* 25:633, 1971.

Spear PD: Behavioral and neurophysiological consequences of visual cortex damage: Mechanisms of recovery. In Sprague JM and Epstein AN (eds): *Progress in Psychobiology and Physiological Psychology,* vol 8. pp. 45–83. New York: Academic Press,1979.

Spear PD, Braun JJ: Pattern discrimination following removal of visual neocortex in the cat. Exper Neurol, 25:331, 1969.

Spitz R: *The First Year of Life; A Psychoanalytic Study of Normal and Deviant Development of Object Relations.* New York: International Universities Press, 1965.

van Zomeren AH, Brouwer WH, Deelman BG: Attentional deficits: The riddles of selectivity, speed, and alertness. In Brooks N (ed): *Closed Head Injury: Psychological, Social, and Family Consequences,* pp. 74–107. Oxford: Oxford University Press, 1984.

West RW, Greenough WT: Effect of environmental complexity on cortical synapses of rats: Preliminary results. Behav Biol 7:279, 1972.

Wrightson P Gronwall D: Time off work and symptoms after minor head injury. Injury 12:445, 1980.

Wrubel J: Personal meanings and coping processes. Unpublished doctoral dissertation, University of California at San Francisco. 1985.

CHAPTER TEN

Coping with Caregiving

I am in charge tonight with five nurses and 30 patients. Two of my nurses are floats who have never been on the floor; one will be an hour late, so I will have to cover her patients. Our medical-surgical patients have diagnoses [including] failure of the kidney, stroke, diabetes, cancer, sickle-cell disease, hepatitis, AIDS, pneumonia and Alzheimer's disease. The average age of our patients is seventy-nine. We have five fresh post-operative patients and one going to surgery in two hours. As I come out of report one of our stable patients who transferred from CCU (coronary care unit) yesterday is having chest pain. There is a doctor on the phone wanting to give admission orders and the anesthetist for our pre-operative patient wants the old chart, *now.* Down the hall in 4324 an elderly, confused patient has just crawled over the side rails and fallen. Two of our fresh post-op patients are vomiting as a side effect of anesthesia, [and] their families are very tense and need reassuring. One of the patients I am covering for has just pulled out his IV; another wants something for pain; another needed the bed pan and I got there too late. The lab has called with a critical low hemoglobin level on the patient who pulled out his IV; he'll be getting a few units of blood as soon as possible. This condensed version represents the first two hours of my working day. The above description of a medical-surgical floor in an acute care hospital is no fabrication. . . .

In the nine years I have been a nurse the most meaningful memories of patients and families are held in a delicate web of what I call my "love-hate" relationship with the profession of nursing. What is this dynamic, this tension, [that] is a real component in my life as a nurse? Is it a shared quality with other nurses I know? As a matter of fact, yes, it is. We share this similar yet vaguely unarticulated frustration that there is much we are unable to do because of the bureaucracy of the hospital institution [that] dictates the volume of patients to be cared for by each nurse and increasingly forces us to accomplish the minimal and more obvious aspects of our care. . . .

I must say that in dealing with the issues and conflicts in the nursing profession today I have been moved from a point of pessimistic detachment to a stance of wavering hope. I am remembering, once again, that caring is a profound act of hope and its hidden aspects may not be recognized by our health care system.   *Tracey White, RN, MA*

Coping with professional caregiving is shaped by the cultural meanings and institutional forms associated with caregiving. Nursing stands out in the literature as highly stressful (Marshall 1980). In acute care settings, nurses daily confront life-threatening situations and complicated treatment regimens that allow little margin for error. Nurses are confronted with societal failure—the breakdown in caring that is evidenced in violence, abuse, and the loss of self-care. The knowledge explosion in highly technical health care requires constant continuing education and confronts the nurse with the fear of failure. Nurses who work in hospitals must face the problems inherent in working in a complex organization. These problems are compounded by lack of authority and recognition commensurate with the life-and-death responsibility of nursing care.

Furthermore, the demands of working in complex organizations are increased by chronic nursing shortages and ill-advised reductions in nursing staff as a cost-saving measure. Salaries for nursing in hospitals are compressed. The pay increases over a clinical career in a hospital are limited to seven years' worth of increments. This compressed salary and career advancement conflicts with the current image of nursing as a career (Kalisch and Kalisch 1987). Thus, coping with caregiving cannot be addressed without addressing the meanings and context of nursing care. Here we examine why coping with caregiving presents unique stress and coping issues for nurses.

Nursing as Women's Work

Tending the sick; promoting health, growth, and development; and caring for the body have all been traditionally designated as "women's work." The similarities between the issues and dilemmas of nursing practice and what Caroline Whitbeck (1983) identifies as the core practices of women are clear:

> The practice that I consider to be the core practice is that of the (mutual) realization of people. I take this practice to have a variety of particular forms, most, if not all, of which are regarded as women's work and are therefore largely ignored by the dominant culture. Among these are the rearing of children, the education of children and adolescents, care of the

366

dying, nursing of the sick and injured, and a variety of spiritual practices related to daily life.

These practices are sometimes described as "nurturing." Although this language has the advantage of being familiar, it has often been used to evoke a sentimental picture of a woman doing a variety of mindless tasks in response to the demands of others, and for that reason I am reluctant to use it. The creativity and responsibility of all parties in the conduct of the practice in its full, liberated form is inconsistent with the sentimental picture of women's self-sacrifice (p. 65).

In the past, caring has been associated with duty and subservience. Altruism has been associated with self-immolation. As Reverby (1987) points out:

Caring is not just a subjective and material experience; it is a historically created one. Particular circumstances, ideologies, and power relations thus create the conditions under which caring can occur, the forms it will take, the consequences it will have for those who do it.

The basis for caring also shapes its effect. Nursing was organized under the expectation that its practitioners would accept a duty to care rather than demand a right to determine how they would satisfy this duty. . . .

Because nurses have been given the duty to care, they are caught in a secondary dilemma: forced to act as if altruism (assumed to be the basis for caring) and autonomy (assumed to be the basis for rights) are separate ways of being (p. 5).

Instead of altruism being the basis for caring, we maintain that caring is the basis for altruism. However, the history and implications of the word *altruism* are problematic. Although the word *altruism* implies concern for the good of others, its roots lie in an oppositional view of the self. The self is viewed as separate from and in opposition to others; therefore, any concern for others must be viewed as a separate and distinct project, set apart from "self"-interest. In this view, concern for others competes with self-concern: Concern for others must always be at the expense of the self, and therefore "altruistic." However, in a phenomenological view of the person, in which the person is viewed as related to others and defined by those relationships, concern for others is not necessarily oppositional to or competitive with self-interest. Concern for others may bring about mutual realization. Caring for others contributes to a world where one can care and expect to be cared for.

The ethics of care and responsibility may be seen as complementary but also as more basic than a strict ethic of rights and justice. For example, rights and justice are remedial in a context of caring; therefore, rights and justice, while important, are not sufficient and must be grounded in an ethic of care and responsibility (AACN Report 1987, Gilligan 1982, Sandel 1982). We maintain that autonomy is not the pinnacle of achievement in adult development. To the extent that the individual is insular and unrelated to others, it is a damaging cultural myth to view autonomy as the hallmark of maturity and health. Instead, we hold that caring and interdependence are the ultimate goals of adult development. To care and feel cared for promotes personal and societal health. Caring is the most basic human way of being in the world (Heidegger 1962, Roach 1984, 1988).

Caring is devalued and the primacy of care is culturally invisible because caring is associated with "women's work," and women's work is devalued and most often unpaid. Caring is also devalued because the extreme individualism of the American society makes caring suspect and subordinate to individual desires and needs (Bellah et al. 1985). The self is understood as private, and in keeping with the Cartesian tradition, as in opposition to others, i.e., the self is opposed to others. In the oppositional Cartesian view of the self, caring for others is a violation of, or is at the expense of, the autonomous, independent self. Thus, the association of "altruism" with caring noted above. Caring is a cultural embarrassment in this extremely individualistic view of the self because such a self should ideally engage only in "self-care." Caring and needing care point up the centrality of interdependence and our essential reliance on others.

Since we hold that stress and coping are inextricably tied to meanings, a major source of stress and a major stumbling block to effective coping in nursing lies in the societal devaluation of caring, and the lack of societal recognition and rewards accorded to caregiving. We refuse to suggest that the stresses of nursing would go away if only nurses were more effective copers. As long as the society overvalues technology's heroic promises of disemburdenment and freedom from pain and fails to recognize the care required to support such a technological self-understanding, those who provide care will feel the stress of being invisible and undervalued by the society. Also, since the status of caregiving is intimately related to the status of the ones cared for, nurses who care for the culturally devalued, such as the homeless, the poor, and the aged, may experience an even greater status inequity.

Nursing is no longer the only career path open to women, and this is a new condition. Women have increasingly gained equal access to professions and positions with greater status and economic rewards than those accorded to traditional women's work such as nursing and teaching. Rowe's (1980) definition of crisis is appropriate here:

> One world has died; another is powerless to be born. . . . The experience of it is the experience of crisis or dilemma, of being condemned to the anxious space between the no longer and the not-yet (Rowe 1980, p. 13).

The "no longer" for nursing is the large pool of women recruits who enter the field because of limited options. Nurses no longer can accept patterns of practice and organizational structures that ignore the nurse as a knowledge worker central to health care. The "not-yet" is the promise of a new recognition of the primacy of care and the resolve to create a health care system that promotes and values care.

The nursing profession is threatened with a future of chronic nursing shortages that further decrease the quality of work life. A decrease in the quality of work life decreases the opportunity for the growth of liberated caregiving—caregiving that is based on a cultural reappraisal of the value of the work and not on a duty to duty and self-sacrifice. As we discuss later, self-sacrifice and duty to duty were never a very generous basis for caregiving, anyway.

We maintain that if nurses were liberated to give the care that they want to give and were able to use their knowledge in a fully efficacious way, while being adequately rewarded, the stresses inherent in nursing would be reduced to the manageable level imposed by the legitimate demands inherent in caring. The stresses of nursing become intolerable when the demands of the situation prevent the nurse from performing with a maximum level of skill and compassion.

The illegitimate stresses (i.e., circumstances that prevent adequate caring) are the most damaging stresses and offer the fewest effective personal coping options. The "illegitimate stresses" (e.g., status inequity, staff shortages, work overload, and underpay) are damaging because they inhibit caregiving practices that are congruent with caring. Therefore, the most effective coping resources are two-pronged:

1. The uncovering of the primacy of care and a societal and personal valuing of caring
2. Societal and organizational changes that support and value nursing care with status, pay commensurate with responsibility, and more humane working conditions.

Mary Mallison's (1987) editorial "How Can You Bear to be a Nurse?" in the *American Journal of Nursing* provides an example of how to combat the cultural devaluation of nursing by acknowledging what is culturally devalued while uncovering the meanings inherent in caring:

National Nurses' Day is May 6 this year. No doubt people will ask you some of these questions. Please add to this list and send us your answers, will you?

How can you be a nurse? How can you bear the sight of blood?

Wait until you slide a catheter into a tiny vein just before it collapses. The flashback of blood you see will make you sing.

How can you be a nurse? How can you bear the sight, the embarrassment, of urine?

Wait until your new postpartum patient can't void, and her uterus is rising. Your persistent maneuvers finally work, making a catheter unnecessary. Urine then looks glorious.

How can you be a nurse? How can you bear to touch that alcoholic who hasn't had a bath in weeks?

Wait until you've repeatedly given ice lavages to that alcoholic and his esophageal varices have finally stopped bleeding. When he actually recovers enough to amble onto your unit to visit, dirt and all, you'll be happy enough to hug him.

How can you be a nurse? How can you bear to watch someone die?

Wait until you've worked for weeks helping a dying woman repair a decades-old conflict with her children, and at some point along the way you see the guilt fall from their shoulders and peace enter her eyes. Watching such a death can be an exaltation.

How can you be a nurse? How can you bear the sight and smell of feces?

Wait until you've been anxious about the diarrhea that nothing has stopped in an AIDS patient. Finally, your strategies work and you see and smell normal stool. You'll welcome that smell.

How can you be a nurse? How can you bear to watch children suffer?

Wait until you've rocked and soothed a suffering child into peaceful sleep, and you feel the child's relief washing over you like a blessing. Then you won't need to ask.

How can you be a nurse? How can you bear to look at searing trauma, at burned people?

Wait until you see healthy granulation tissue that has been given a chance because your sensitive nose detected an infection before it could take hold. That healing will look beautiful to you.

How can you be a nurse? How can you bear the stream of abusive words heaped on you by psychotic patients?

Wait until you've prodded and pulled a silent, withdrawn catatonic back over the lifeline, and she releases a string of expletives. Could Mozart sound better?

How can you be a nurse? How can you bear the sound of babies crying?

Wait until your combination of vigilance, bulldog advocacy, and gentle handling has given a preemie's lungs the time they needed to develop, and you hear his first lusty cry. You'll laugh out loud!

How can you be a nurse? How can you bear to care for frustrating, confused Alzheimer's patients?

Wait until you've devised a combination of strategies that provide exercise and permit safe wandering, and you see a lift, almost a spring, in a patient's shuffling gait. You'll feel the lightness of Baryshnikov in your own step that day.

How can you be a nurse? So many of your patients are so old, so sick, these days. How can you bear the thought that, in the end, your care may make no difference?

Wait until you've used your hands and eyes and voice to dispel terror, to show a helpless person that his life is respected, that he has dignity. Your caring helps him care about himself. His helplessness forces you to think about the brevity of your own life.

Then and there, you decide yet again to reject the pallid pastel life. No tepid sail across a protected cove for you. No easy answers.

So you keep choosing to be a nurse. You have days of frustration, nights of despair, terrible angers. Your highs and lows are peaks and chasms, not hills and valleys. The defeats come more than often enough to keep you humble: the problems you can't untangle, the lives that seep away too fast, the meanings that elude your understanding.

But you keep working at it, learning from it, knowing the next peak lies ahead.

And gradually you realize your palette is filling up with colors. You see more shades of meaning. You laugh more. You realize you are well on your way to creating a work of art, maybe even a masterpiece. So that's why you've remained a nurse. To your surprise, your greatest work of art is turning out to be your own life.

Though nursing owes much of its identity and agendas to the tradition of women's practices of "mutual realization" outlined above by Whitbeck (1983), nursing extends these agendas into the highly complex arena of caring for illness and disease and attending to the relationships between the two. During the past twenty years, science

371

and technology have become more central to nursing practice. Nurses now have the only resident knowledge of administering and monitoring a wide range of diagnostic tests and treatments (Benner 1984a, Benner and Tanner 1987).

Nurses could make their claims for increased recognition, rights, and status through the recognition of their highly specialized knowledge of science and technology related to health and illness, and they might avoid the battle to gain legitimacy and status for caring. The problem with this approach is that it ignores the essential relationship among caring, science, and technology in nursing. In the best nursing practice, science and technology are the tools for caring. Indeed, used without caring, technology becomes ominous and too frightening to be efficacious. To make science and technology the primary source of legitimacy assaults the inner logic of nursing practice even though nurses use these tools in highly skilled ways.

A second major strategy aimed at status inequity has been a deliberate attempt to decrease the sex segregation in the profession. Although efforts have been made to increase the number of men in the profession, their numbers are limited (three percent of total number registered nurses—American Nurses' Association, 1987). Also, men tend to experience the status inequities of nursing even more than women because male nurses have crossed a sexual-division-of-labor line. Women today suffer very little discrimination upon entering medicine; however, men still battle sex stereotyping upon entering nursing. The fact that entering nursing feels like a "step down" for men reveals the status problems plaguing nursing as a "women's profession." When nursing is given its proper societal recognition for the life-and-death responsibilities of nursing care, then men will not suffer the double burden of status inequity that they now experience upon entering the nursing profession.

The Modern Epidemic—Burnout

Caregiving has become an enigma for the modern person. The old meanings related to duty to duty and self-sacrifice have fallen away (see Yankelovich 1981). This is just as well, because these meanings described caring inadequately. Duty and self-sacrifice separate the notions of caring and caregiving. The separation of caregiving and caring is a good definition for the modern epidemic of burnout, which is defined as the loss of human caring (Maslach 1982). When one is burned out, things appear equally flat and meaningless. The world ceases to have meaningful distinctions. What once gave pleasure can feel like a demand.

It is a peculiarly modern mistake to think that caring is the cause of burnout and that the cure is to protect oneself from caring to prevent the "disease" called burnout. Rather, the loss of caring is the sickness, and the return of caring is the recovery. Being in the situation without caring robs one of the perspective that only caring brings and renders the resources and meanings in the situation inaccessible. Although disengagement may numb pain, one is also numbed to the resources and support of others in the situation. Recovery requires rest and respite, but it also requires the reintegration of concern and involvement (Benner 1984a).

The metaphor for burnout is that of a bank account that has been overdrawn (Selye 1974). While the metaphor captures the sense of feeling overextended and depleted, it is inadequate because it reduces the problem of caring to one of quantity of energy and ignores meanings and relationships. Burnout is a description of alienation and anomie accompanied by physical symptoms that may include stomach disorders, headaches, rashes, exacerbations of chronic illnesses, depression, fatigue, irritability, and insomnia (Maslach 1982, Smythe 1984). Besides respite and recreation, the person experiencing burnout needs to be reconnected to sustaining relationships and meanings to overcome the alienation and anomie. Norbeck (1985) found that social support from fellow nurses was the most effective way to reduce distress and burnout. Because nurses share common meanings and are subjected to similar stresses, they can provide the insights and perspectives of the insider.

Finding the Right Level and Kind of Involvement

The thesis of this book is that caring (involvement) makes things show up as stressful and dictates available coping options. Some kinds of involvement create repeated cycles of distress. Benner (unpublished research notes 1986, 1987) has found much discussion and practical wisdom among nurses about the nature and kinds of involvement. For example, many nurses talk about "overinvolvement." Overinvolvement may take the form of identification with the patient and may overwhelm the nurse with fear and anxiety. The nurse feels as if he or she knows and feels the patient's pain (see Chapter Three, p. 92). However, overidentification is less likely than overinvolvement as helper. Overinvolvement as helper may raise excessive needs to "control" and dominate the situation to ensure that one's own interests are protected. Boundaries between self and others become blurred, and the one caring may take on the role of omnipotent rescuer, overlooking the responsibility, integrity, and resources of the person and the situation. This is the kind of solicitude that "leaps in" and takes over for the person (see Chapter Two, pp. 48–49).

The stance of omnipotent rescuer may be a way to cope with the feelings of vulnerability that caring for another can engender because the one caring realizes that the one cared for may leave, bring disappointment, or die. The frantic rescuer who seeks to change another's behavior as a way of gaining control and mastery may be responding to lived meanings learned early in childhood that the world is capricious and unreliable. Such meanings can be the result of growing up in families where alcoholism or mental illness made caregiving precarious and unpredictable. The meanings learned in a chaotic or impoverished caregiving situation are that the world is a risky, chaotic place that must be pasted together by one's own efforts. Helping others becomes a way of feeling helped or cared for (see Heron 1987). Norwood (1985) describes such overinvolvement as "loving too much":

> Our own needs for love, attention, nurturing and security went unmet while we pretended to be more powerful and less fearful, more grown up and less needy, than we really felt. And having learned to deny our own yearning to be taken care of, we grew up looking for more opportunities to do what we had become so good at: being preoccupied with someone else's wants and demands rather than acknowledging our own fear and pain and unmet needs (p. 63).

Overwork and overly solicitous helping are signs of helping in order to feel that one is in control and that the world is safe. Such a helper is out of trust with the world and seeks by his or her own effort to make an unsafe, chaotic world safe. This kind of involvement does not allow the helper to see the resources in the person or the person's situation. The overinvolved caregiver takes over the patient's burdens and problems. The excessive activity of this stance is a way of warding of anxiety.

Overinvolvement with patients may also be a way of avoiding intimacy in relationships outside of nursing. Patients become intimate strangers who provide a safe sense of being close without the obligations that go with long-term relationships. Nursing becomes the person's whole life, and the nurse may withdraw from close friendships and intimate relationships outside of work. All major risks in caring occur only in the work setting, where the limits of caring are clearer.

The remedy for overinvolvement is not lack of involvement but rather the right kind of involvement. Nurse Sallie Tisdale, in her book *The Sorcerer's Apprentice* (1986), describes the narrow path to the right kind of involvement by a nurse in a burn unit:

> Somewhere in this trial is a middle way, a balance of pain and compassion. Burn nurses find it or quit. It is a narrow trail flanked by extremity. One side, the side of empathy, is filled with wrenching sorrow, anger, and despair. It is where another person's pain becomes so visible, so inarguably present, that we attempt to take it on as we might carry a burden. This fails because, though we might succeed in weighing ourselves with the burden, we cannot actually take the weight from another: the burden doubles. We have *created* pain. And when we see another's pain (this is not as easy as it may at first seem), we quickly begin to expect the person to behave in certain ways, to respond as we would respond— or are responding—to the same affliction. We make demands of the sufferer, be it patient, child, a whole population. This is the way of the martyr; it is filled first with pity and then with contempt.
>
> On the other side is a kind of total severance from the person in pain. This is more than detachment—it is actually a fissure within the person not in pain from his or her own memory and experience. Because medical science defines pain as physical, the clinician may not only fail to recognize nonphysical experience, but demand that it stop when he does recognize it. This is the World Series of artificial hearts, the unblinking preparation of the heartbeating cadaver. This is the undermedication of the patient in pain, for his own good.
>
> Along the narrow road, where the nurses scrape little Michael's nerves [she refers to a caring approach to the debridement of a burned child], is a simple acceptance. Here is now, this is happening, keep walking. To project another's experience onto one's self (how would I feel; what if this were *my* child?) is both terribly necessary and terribly dangerous. Burn nurses work here year after year, anonymously, cutting off skin and treading lightly. It is easy to slip. They must help each other up when they fall (pp. 129–130).

Tisdale (1986) captures in her prose what it is to place oneself *in* the situation without becoming enmeshed or inappropriately distanced from the situation. It is a narrow path and, as Tisdale points out, one that is best negotiated through the support of others who understand the situation (see also Norbeck 1985).

It is an art to know what one can offer in a situation without becoming overextended or assuming more responsibility for the situaion than necessary. Weisman (1981) recommends that caregivers make the "least possible contribution":

> A little goes a long way; the least possible contribution is the one with the least strain but with the best chance of making a difference, however small. Having made this contribution, which may be very insignificant against the background of need, one can make another contribution, and still another, until something quite unanticipated but substantial results. Morale in everyone seems better, care is effective, plight is less painful. Least possible contribution does not, of course, mean doing as little as possible, but doing only a little bit beyond the ordinary, something that most closely reflects the caregiver at his or her best (p. 167).

Offering the least possible contribution makes sense only in the context of a discussion of overinvolvement or being an "omnipotent rescuer." The art is to offer what you can without dictating the results and recognizing that you are not the only one to contribute. It takes courage to be involved and offer what you can, even though it may not be enough (see Michelle Marin's account in Chapter Eight, pp. 302–303).

Repeated Exposure to Breakdown and Suffering—Learning to Acknowledge the Pain

Health care workers are repeatedly exposed to breakdown, tragedy, and death. Even with the best defenses, the nurse must confront the limits of control, the inevitability of death, and in the case of violence, the very real presence of cruelty. Nurses know through their work that the worst can happen, and this infiltrates and colors one's sense of the world. Health care workers may cope with laughter, bravado, detachment, and elaborate self-protective maneuvers to feel immune to the calamity they confront, but these are temporary "Band-Aids" that can grant only fleeting immunity. In the midst of such "immunity-granting" coping, it is helpful to acknowledge to oneself and to one's coworkers the pain and threat one confronts. Margret Fenton, from Winnipeg, Canada, demonstrates the power of such an acknowledgment in a poem. She captures not only the significance, fear, and pain of confronting tragedy but also the courage required to be a nurse:

Debbie
Margret Fenton

What were you doing . . . out so late . . . and all alone?
Were you drinking? . . . Were you on drugs?
Did you even know what happened? . . .

It is now four days since you came to our unit . . . head injury, uncon-
scious, lifeless. Tonight I am your nurse . . .
You are so young, your body so lovely, so healthy . . .
your head so bruised.
You shouldn't be here, Debbie, lying so still . . . so broken . . .
You're only 19 . . .

I am so afraid . . . of the responsibility . . . of being your nurse . . .
and of being touched by the fragile thread that is your hold on
life. Can you hear me? I talk and even sing to you, in the dark as
I move around . . . checking . . . charting . . . caring . . . Can you
feel me touch you? . . . with my hands . . . with my heart . . .

Did you see your mother? . . . hear her cry . . . Her face paled, knees
buckled when she saw you. And your brother, too young to bear
such grief, circled her waist with his arm and held her up.
Watching and sensing the anguish, I felt my heart in my mouth . . .
saw one of my own daughters . . . lying . . . like you . . . myself in your
mother's place . . . and I was terrified.

You died soon after . . . I knew you would . . . and I felt helpless . . .
bitter . . . and then so very hopeless . . . Did it matter . . . what I did?
that I was there? . . . that I cared . . .

At home I cried . . . laid awake, alone at night, and wondered at the
pain I felt. I thought about quitting . . . never going back . . .
to face again the sorrow of such suffering.
Sometimes it hurts so much to care . . . to reach out . . .
I never really knew in the beginning, how much it would take . . .
to be a nurse.

Acknowledging that the pain matters sanctions the distress and
confronts the impact of the tragedy. It feels protective to rationalize or
avoid the strong feelings associated with tragedy. Depersonalizing and
objectifying the patient may serve to locate the possibility of tragedy
outside one's own life and community. However, these avoidant strategies interfere with compassionate care, and can cause an emotional
numbing that can reach all aspects of the nurse's life. The intent is not
to enhance or elaborate the pain. Acknowledgment allows one to come
to terms with feelings and move on.

In sum, avoidance of the threat inherent in being repeatedly confronted with one's own mortality, the inhumanity of others in cases of
violence, and the threat of pain and disfigurement cannot effectively be
dealt with by claiming or pretending immunity. The threat seeps
through. Therefore, acknowledging and supporting one another in confronting the threat are the most fruitful long-term coping strategies.

Acknowledging the threat and pain confronted in caring for the suffering, the dying, and those facing major disability or disfigurement opens the nurse up to the possibilities in the situation as well as the pain. Nurses learn from patients and families the unimaginable courage and resiliency of the human spirit. Nurses learn firsthand from many patients and families the situated possibility created by caring. It is here that the moral art of nursing contributes both to the one caring and to the one cared for. This is best illustrated in an essay by Susan Hager, a critical care nurse who captures the kaleidoscope of courage and wisdom she has gleaned from working with intensive care unit patients.

Courage in Intensive Care

Susan Hager, RN
Surgical Intensive Care Unit
Hermann Hospital
Houston, Texas

I'm always hearing people say that it takes a lot of "guts" to be a critical care nurse. Although I believe the statement to be absolute gospel, it is not just the nurse who needs the strength. There is often an hourly need for bravery in intensive care units that taxes everyone who becomes caught up in life's tragedies.

I have witnessed many small acts of courage demonstrated by patients, their families (I call them critical care families), and by co-workers. It is the seemingly small demonstrations of courage that return to my thoughts time and time again, for collectively they are overwhelming. It is by imitation that I am enabled to have "whatever it takes" to be a good critical care nurse.

J.B. had suffered many setbacks and complications from sub-arachnoid hemorrhage; persistent symptomatology, numerous evacuations due to re-bleeding, and permanent deficits. This woman, whom everyone had said was inconsistently visually attentive at best, eventually became my assignment. During bathing, I spoke to her course of events, including her left-sided paresis, her tracheostomy and her shaved and scarred head. I said that even though her family rarely visited, they had knowledge of her situation. It dawned on me that J.B. had been staring at me the whole time. She then began mouthing words. I told her that perhaps her family had a transportation problem, or maybe it was difficult for them to see her suffer.

Again she began mouthing words. I covered her tracheostomy with my thumb, and she said: "If they don't like me the way that I am now, then they're not going to like me any other way."

The very first words out of this neurologically crippled woman, true or not, in my opinion were words of acceptance of herself and an unalterable situation. (If life had dealt me the same blow, I have no doubt but that *my* first words would have been words of despair.)

Imitation of her attitude has become one of my favorite weapons against an occasionally wilting self-esteem.

I am learning that sometimes it takes courage to give something up, to quit. The most horrifying thing I have ever seen or known in my lifetime—AIDS—has required human beings to give up their lives, to ask that they be allowed to die without medical intervention. I cannot recall how many times I have driven home from work hoping that I might have the fortitude to make myself a "do not resuscitate" patient if ever it becomes necessary, just as so many of my patients and friends have had to do.

If critical care families are not the walking wounded, then none exist. Some of them remind me of photographs from the Holocaust that showed people wide-eyed from an overdose of constant fear, and suffering from a lack of food, water and sleep. Once I had a patient who had accidentally blown the lower aspects of his face off with a deer rifle. I had everything but his eyes covered. To look at his face had disturbed every doctor and nurse in the unit—I could feel the discomfort as co-workers passed by.

I told his new teenage wife what she could expect to see, and that even if we could "fix" him, he would still never be the same. She turned to her husband, lifted the drapes, and without even flinching, said: "I'll take him any way he comes; however you can fix him, I'll take him." What impressed me so much was that this young woman did not fall back ten yards to punt—she picked up the fumble and ran with it. Courage.

What nurse could walk away from a bedside and not be at the very least impressed, if not in some small way changed by the mother who has made her 15-year-old, an only son, the victim of a motorcycle accident, a "do not resuscitate?"

I also firmly believe that the truly compassionate nurse is in absolute awe of the significant other who sees the patient through to the end, as in the case of the AIDS patient's lover.

I hope that I will always have within me the ability to accept what is fact, as many of the critical care family members have had to do.

For those of us in the critical care trenches, life needs a steady supply of courage. My co-workers provide me with so many examples to learn from. Only one such example is the new graduate nurse who learns how to stand up effectively to the bully doctor and professionally inform him that he may not "browbeat" the nurse. It is a joy of joys to hear your orientee gently breaking the news to the rude and loud-mouthed doctor that the days of Dr. Kildare are over. As well, I will always admire those health care workers who dare to doubt the words and actions of others, e.g., the resident who believes that the fluid therapy prescribed by the attending physician will result in congestive heart failure.

And how many nurses have refused to administer a dosage that they believed to be excessive? What consistently makes my decision-making easier is not only the strength of my own convictions, but also the imitation of those experiences. I can only respect my co-workers when they act upon what they believe in their hearts to be right.

I will always remember the people in my work world who have made me a better person by teaching me little lessons about life (and death). Thinking back, I believe that I have physically touched all of them; a hug or a handshake—perhaps subconsciously hoping that their courage would rub off on me.

Nurses like myself need the strength to accept themselves, as well as take other people "as they come." Nurses must be brave enough to change priorities and to live with the decisions they make. We must have the nerve that is required to accept what is no longer an issue, but has become a fact. And, perhaps most important, we need the fortitude to learn from our failures. The application of courage for a critical care nurse means the difference between making a good choice and a bad choice. It is this sort of courage, when gained from experiences such as I have described, that manifests itself in the form of good choices.

And when it comes right down to it, good choices are the mainstay of critical care nursing.

Susan Hager has expressed directly and passionately how a notion of the good is embedded in the caring practices of ICU patients, families, nurses, and physicians. She is taught by her membership and participation. She gains wisdom and compassion. It is her answer to societal questions based on utilitarian individualism such as: How can you afford to care? How can you stand the pain and suffering? How do you manage your stress? She responds in a way that shows that she feels privileged to participate in a healing community of care and responsibility—community that has the courage to face the extremities of life. She carries with her the moral courage and self-acceptance of the woman with extreme neurological damage; she imitates it, and her patient's self-acceptance becomes a personal weapon, a coping resource. She is instructed and enriched by her caring. It is not merely a means to an end; caring is good in itself.

She does not gloss over the difficulty. She sees the suffering and yet does not try to be the omnipotent rescuer. She joins the community of care and responsibility and is strengthened. By participating in the meaning and the world of her co-workers, her patients, and her patients' families, she is able to take up new ways of being in the world. She calls this "imitation," but this is no mere mimicking of outward behavior. It is a living out of these ways of being in her own life.

It would be unrealistically optimistic to maintain that acknowledging the experience of human courage and situated possibility in the midst of suffering can eradicate the toll of repeated exposure to tragedy. Health care workers are repeatedly confronted with extreme breakdown and this cuts them off from society's general tendency to avoid the disenfranchised poor, the mentally ill, the social outcasts. Beliefs that our society is equal and just are threatened by such a confrontation, and the resultant moral outrage can be a chronic demand.

Nurses, who are most often women, are confronted with the particular societal ills that women suffer, and thus cannot help feeling the injustice. Nurses bear triple burden:

1. One's avoidance of suffering and societal injustice is rendered implausible.
2. Moral outrage follows and may be accompanied by a sense of inability to solve the "larger problems."
3. The nurse may experience an additional social stigma created by his or her association with those who are disenfranchised and suffering.

A patient who had an extreme injury that required long and extensive nursing care poignantly expresses these burdens in a letter to his nurse, Pamela Minarik:

> My Dearest Pamela,
> Hi. Hope all is well with you and the staff and that you get to see more of life than its tragedy. I know that it is sometimes hard on your head dealing with what you have to deal with, but they say that in fact women are tougher than men and can take more, so you have that on your side.

This letter stands out because in it the patient affirms the nurse's connection with tragedy—the difficult side of life—as well as his belief in the nurse's strength. The threatening realities of being confronted with extreme breakdown are best dealt with in staff support meetings, where both the threat and the courage needed to face it can be discussed. In the final analysis, there can be no magical reassurances or bravado, only the acknowledgment that the suffering is real, that it cannot be completely erased, and that we all would be imperiled if nurses were not there to care.

Affirming the Knowledge, Skill, and Responsibility in Nursing Practice

Part of the devaluation of a practice discipline lies in the Western tradition of valuing the theoretical and abstract over the practical (see Chapter Two, p. 43). For example, in intensive care nursing, it is assumed that the "real" knowledge lies in establishing the safe physiological parameters and the safe range of dosage for achieving the specified physiological parameters (the physician's domain). The knowledge and skill needed to keep particular patients safely within the established parameters are overlooked because the knowledge is informal and particular, not easily formalized or generalized. For example, titrating drugs to keep patients within prespecified physiological parameters depends on an in-depth knowledge of the pharmacological properties of the medicine (e.g., vasopressor); the possible interactions with other drugs; the effects of patient activity or agitation on blood pressure, and the judgment of whether the activity and concomitant physiological response is transient; and finally an understanding of this particular patient's responses. Martha McDermott (1987), a nurse in neonatal intensive care, who is recognized as an expert clinician by her colleagues, demonstrates the role of the particular in clinical expertise:

> It is through our repeated experience with patients that we begin to perceive the *particular* rather than the typical, care becomes *individualized* rather than standardized, and planning becomes *anticipatory* of change rather than simply responsive to change.

Martha McDermott captures the deep knowledge of the particular patient and the particular situation that the expert uses to orchestrate nursing care. Surely it is a cultural error to think that this complex, skilled knowledge is of a "lower level" than setting the physiological parameters and prescribing the range for the dosages.

Pattern recognition and configurational knowledge are also overlooked in the Greek view of knowledge. For example, Jorgenson and Crabtree (1986) quote an expert intensive care nurse describing her knowledge of Swan-Ganz wave forms:

> Sure you see them in the books, but not every wave form is the same as in the book. . . . So, the only way you learn is by doing, by experiencing. He [the physician] said, "I wish I could work as a nurse for about a month, because I need to learn these things, become comfortable with them. I may help put in a swan here and there, but I've never done it by myself.

And as far as interpreting what I see in the wave form, I understand the numbers, but the wave forms are different and you learn that more by experience" (p. 180).

The Swan-Ganz wave forms are configurational knowledge that can be attained only by direct observations of many wave forms in relation to many patient positions and arterial pressures. This configurational knowledge and the pattern-recognition ability are overlooked in the reduction of the physiological parameters to specific numbers (see Benner and Tanner 1987).

The differential status and legitimization given to formal knowledge that can be stated in laws, and preferably in mathematical equations, overlook and discredit skilled nursing knowledge by default. The same status difference can be noticed in science in the distinctions between "pure" versus "applied" and "hard" versus "soft" sciences. Giving status and legitimization to the clinical judgment inherent in skilled practice is essential to an accurate valuation of nursing care. If such status is achieved, we may come to allow sufficient teaching-learning time for teaching clinical judgment both in nursing and medicine. Certainly, status and legitimization are essential to crediting the knowledge embedded in nursing practice. When the nurse's knowledge is taken seriously, patients benefit through having the diagnostic and monitoring abilities of the nurse responded to appropriately by physicians and other health care workers.

The Intent and Challenge of Caring

Most management literature focuses on how to reengage the disenchanted and motivate the unmotivated; however, little sage advice is given on how to enable highly motivated and dedicated workers to perform at the level they want to perform. Although nurses, like other groups, have their share of the unmotivated, they also have a large share of individuals extremely committed to providing the best care possible for their patients. In a recent study of expert nurses in intensive care units, five nurses from the same unit were reported to state: "Our patients deserve the best." This shared view reflects a unit culture of excellence (Benner, unpublished research notes 1985–1987). With this zeal comes equally great frustration when the care environment does not permit the nurse to deliver the best care. Stress reduction for highly motivated nurses is not disengagement and a lowering of sights, but rather a concerted organizational effort to enable nurses to practice in the way that they want to practice.

The consequences of delivering inadequate care due to work overload erodes the nurse's self-esteem and causes real anguish. Consequently, a bad day is not experienced as just a bad day at work but a "nightmare" due to the human suffering and peril involved in inadequate care. For example, Ms Kineavy, a nurse who had been working for five months, reported in *The New York Times* a "nightmare" evening of being understaffed on a unit where with patients with AIDS, asthma, and problems related to alcoholism and drug abuse:

> "One guy admitted with lice immediately traded his clothes with another patient," she said. "A patient escaped down the back stairs, tried to jump over the fence, got a spike caught in his buttock and had to be treated in the emergency room. And then one guy punched a blind patient in the face. We had just been talking to the blind patient, and he couldn't see who hit him, so he began yelling, 'The nurse hit me, the nurse hit me.'
>
> "I closed the door and cried my eyes out." (The *New York Times,* July 7, 1987, p. 11)

This story has an undeniably sensational ring. But our direct experience and interviews with many nurses lead us to say that every experienced nurse has had a similar work experience. It is insulting to talk about individual strategies to cope with such an untenable situation. And it is hard to imagine ways to lessen the personal disappointment and turmoil created by such disastrous working conditions.

But even in the best of circumstances, with highly motivated staff, the challenge of caring remains. One's intent to care may not match the challenge of caring for patients with difficult personalities. Here one is fortunate to work with a team of nurses whose personalities and strengths are known and where assignments can be made according to the particular nurses' talents, nurse-patient relationships, and particular patient needs.

Anger is a frequent companion of illness and breakdown, and many nurses become expert at working with angry patients. However, other nurses, even those skilled in communication, may find it extremely difficult to work with angry patients. This is yet another example of why nursing cannot be reduced to mere technique. Knowledge of the dynamics of anger during illness and even communication skill training cannot ensure that the nurse will become comfortable or effective in dealing with extremely angry patients. Likewise, some patient situations may be too close to the nurse's own personal threats to allow the nurse to be effective. Although the nurse may be effective in performing the tasks of skilled nursing, she or he may not be able to be engaged in caring for the patient. These are ways in which the nurse literally may not be required or "assigned" to care.

Nursing is intimate and particular. Expert communication skills help, and understanding the illness and the disease provide unique ways of helping. But there is no way to guarantee the success of caring. Some patients are more accessible and understandable to some nurses than others are. The hallmark of the expert nurse is the recognition of her or his strengths and weaknesses and the ability to shape her or his practice toward strengths.

The Fear of Failure, and the Damage of Keeping It a Secret

Nursing care is provided in the context of highly technical medicine. Both medicine and nursing face a knowledge explosion. One response to the knowledge explosion has been increasing specialization in both medicine and nursing. Even in the most specialized nursing practice, however, nursing is by its nature more general than medical specialties. It is typical in acute care centers to care for a patient treated by several medical specialists, and it is often the nurse who plays a coordinating role, assisting with cross-specialty communication and detecting conflicting therapies and medical intents that may be at cross purposes. Nurses also typically have less control over their caseload. They are assigned patients. Although they may consult with their peers and supervisors about their assignments, in the end all patients must be taken care of, and there are limits to the nurse's choice.

The complexity of health care, the rapidly expanding knowledge base, and constant change create both qualitative and quantitative overload. That is, the demands for new knowledge and technique are qualitatively difficult to learn and perform, and the need for continued education often comes in the context of short staffing and overwork (quantitative overload).

With the knowledge explosion in medicine and nursing, it is not surprising that Larson (1987) found in a study of 495 nurses participating in professional conferences and educational programs that 20% fear making a mistake. They also fear not being able to keep up with the knowledge demands. This understandable fear is rendered more stressful, according to Larson, because nurses often keep their fear of making mistakes a secret from colleagues. Pennebaker (1985) found that "secret keeping," failure to express thoughts and feelings about a stressful event such as the divorce of parents or the death of a spouse, increases the probability both of obsessing about the event and of developing illness. This research finding seems reasonable, since one cannot receive social support (emotional, direct help, or information) as long as the fear is kept secret.

When examined, the fear of making mistakes in a health care environment where there is little margin for error is also reasonable. The fear is even adaptive if it causes the person to seek information. The fear becomes excessive if the person sees it as a personal deficit and experiences isolation and shame in relation to the demand for precise care in high-risk situations. Staff meetings need to be organized for the purpose of assessing educational needs and discussing the fear of mistakes, along with trouble-shooting and debriefing after mistakes are made. Increasingly, hospitals are organizing continuous education on the units to keep up with the knowledge demands as fast as they develop. Nurses have a right to request an immediate update or instruction on new techniques, procedures, or unfamiliar areas of care.

One-Way Giving and Too Many Demands

In the same study of nurses' fears, Larson (1987) also found five interrelated secrets:

EMOTIONAL AND PHYSICAL DISTANCING. Descriptions of wanting to or actually distancing oneself emotionally or physically from patients, families, staff, or personal family; usually accompanied by explicit expression of guilt (22% of the responses).

"I'M ANGRY." Descriptions of anger toward, frustration about, or impatience with patients, patients' family members, or other staff (20% of the responses).

"I'M IN OVER MY HEAD." Descriptions of being emotionally overinvolved with work or home situations, i.e., empathic overarousal. Can include any difficult feelings other than anger, frustration, or impatience (11% of the responses).

TOO MANY DEMANDS. Direct reference to excessive emotional and physical demands at work and in private life (5% of the responses).

ONE-WAY GIVING: "WHAT ABOUT ME?" Expressions of a desire to receive—and not just give—caring and appreciation from patients, patients' families, and other staff (3%).

All five of these categories are related to the demands for caring and the loss of reciprocity and balance. Often the imbalance is brought about by understaffing. The nurse cannot deliver the kind of care that she or he wants to deliver. Frustration spirals when patients become disgruntled about inadequate care.

Hochschild (1983) points out two unhealthy modern cultural aberrations, that of the narcissist and the altruist. The narcissist "feeds insatiably on interactions, competing desperately for love and admiration in a Hobbesian dog-eat-dog world where both are perpetually scarce" (Hochschild 1983, p. 195). The narcissist is self-absorbed. The "altruist," in contrast, is other-absorbed and is in danger of being absorbed by the demands of others to the extent that self-care is blocked and inadequate. The psychological terms *narcissist* and *altruist* denote extreme patterns of meanings, one of being needy and the other of being "subordinate to the demands" of others. Both extreme positions are inherently stressful.

The Nurse as a Knowledge Worker: Gaining Control over Professional Nursing Practice

Nurses work in complex organizations where they are the front line of defense for the patient. They are also the contact point for all other departments and services. Because nurses are there around the clock, they fill in and substitute for all other departments who do not have the same level of continuity. This structural reality in a complex organization, even under the most enlightened managerial structures, would create intermittent additional demands and pressure.

Like other professional groups made up predominantly of women, nurses have been viewed as short-term workers rather than career workers. But that view is changing. The average age of working nurses is 39, which hardly suggests a short-term worker (Registered Nurse Population, June, 1986). However, salary increases are compressed to seven years, and hospitals do not reward the nurse for a long clinical career.

Nursing administrators have not uniformly treated the nurse as a knowledge worker. To cope with high turnover rates, they often set up extensive rules, guidelines, and protocols inappropriate to the level of discretionary decision making required of the professional nurse. The organizational strategies for coping with turnover include developing extensive formal structures to provide guidance for new employees. This response inadvertently caters to the new nurse and frustrates the experienced nurse and may serve to perpetuate the turnover (Benner 1984a).

A new vision of the nurse as knowledge worker is needed. Nurses need clinical promotion programs and participatory management to increase their power to shape their own practices. Nurses must sit on governing boards and central committees in order to shape their practices. Empowering the practicing nurse is the best remedial action for the organizational stress that nurses confront in hospital settings (See National Commission on Nursing 1983).

It seems superfluous to refer to health-promotion programs in the workplace until untenable working conditions are addressed. In a time of economic retrenchment, it may seem frivolous to mention health promotion in the health industry, but it seems equally untenable to think that the health industry may be the last to adopt health-promotion programs for workers. The following charge to industry wellness programs could have come from the hospital industry; instead, it came from Roger B. Smith, Chairman of General Motors:

> American industry can't afford not to expand the wellness movement in the workplace. . . . We need to go with the prevention over the cure (Cited by Kizer 1987, p. 1).

Kizer (1987) offers concrete directions for promoting health in the workplace and for demonstrating the cost effectiveness of wellness programs in increased worker productivity, decreased absenteeism, and lower insurance costs.

The Stress of Working Around the Clock

Shift work is an unavoidable reality in caring for the sick. Productivity, accuracy, and safety can be threatened by shift work (Vidacek, Kaliterna, Radosevic-Vidacek, and Folkard 1986). Night shift work creates stress due to alterations in biological rhythms, sleep disturbance, and altered social patterns. Shiftworkers have an increased incidence of ulcers. These may be caused by the alterations in circadian rhythms and lack of adequate meals at night (Adams, Folkard, and Young 1986).

Two competing factors enter into the stress and decreased effectiveness of those working at night: (a) The effect of circadian rhythm on the performance of simple tasks is at a low point at night and workers adjust only slowly over a span of night shifts (Vidacek et al. 1986). (b) Day sleeping patterns tend to be one to four hours shorter. The night shift worker thus tends to lose sleep, accruing a cumulative sleep debt over time (Akerstedt 1985). Therefore, one's effectiveness may be expected to improve as the circadian rhythm adjusts to night work but may also be expected to deteriorate due to sleep deprivation (Vidacek et al. 1986).

For complex cognitive performance with high demands on short-term memory, performance will deteriorate over successive night shifts as circadian rhythm adjusts and sleep deprivation accumulates. For this reason, very rapidly rotating shift systems may be preferable to the long shift rotations for nurses performing complex cognitive tasks (Folkard and Monk 1979). In contrast, for simpler tasks not heavily dependent on short-term memory, the performance at night is poor when the circadian rhythm is unadjusted and improves with adjustment (Vidacek et al. 1986). Thus, as these authors point out, circadian rhythm adjustment and sleep deprivation have conflicting implications for designing the best shift rotation patterns. In light of circadian rhythms, long shift rotations are preferable because performance improves as the circadian rhythm adjusts. However, in light of cumulative sleep deprivation, short rotations are preferable.

More study is needed on actual effective coping strategies for long-term night work. Counseling is frequently recommended, but until more studies are done on effective and ineffective coping strategies, counselors will have a limited knowledge base for offering new coping options. Most of the literature focuses on strategies for sleeping during the day. For example, Felton (1975) found the following five problems associated with day sleeping:

> (1) trouble staying asleep, (2) trouble sleeping because of noise or environmental temperature, (3) fatigue, (4) difficulty switching from night to day shift, and (5) requiring a week to adjust bowel habits after night duty (p. 19).

However, day sleeping is not the only problem associated with shift work. Social isolation, altered patterns of eating, and coping with altered circadian rhythms are also troubling.

A strong commitment to working nights and a satisfaction with the night schedule, not surprisingly, make the adjustment much easier (Adams, Folkard, and Young 1986; Folkard et al. 1978; Felton 1975). Also, those who subordinate their nonwork activities to rest and recuperation fare better than those who refuse to make concessions in their social life in order to get the rest required (Adams, Folkard, and Young 1986). Structuring new patterns of eating and sleeping requires deliberate planning, since most time structures are geared to night sleeping and daytime activity. A routine such as caring for animals may help set up expectations about time for rest (Adams, Folkard, and Young 1986).

Shiftwork requires that the person develop a new habitual body as well as new social and activity patterns. The deliberate development of "timegiving" rituals, such as establishing rituals around night meals, even giving the meal a name such as "supper," helps normalize and set up signals to the body that establish new habitual body rhythms (Adams, Folkard, and Young 1986).

Distinctions Between Nurse and Family Coping with Caregiving

The distinctions between nurses, family, and significant others' coping with caregiving bear examination even though they are too numerous to discuss comprehensively. Examining even a few of these distinctions uncovers the range of meanings inherent in caring. They elucidate the cultural value and significance of investing in professional caregiving. Also, these distinctions are instructive for examining the role of the situation, the role of personal concerns, the role of temporality, and the role of embodied intelligence in coping with caregiving.

THE ROLE OF THE SITUATION

The situation for the nurse, the patient, and significant others is completely different in obvious ways that nevertheless bear review. For the loved one and for the patient, the care setting is most often foreign. Families and patients feel stripped of their familiar surroundings and their identities. By contrast, the situation is familiar to the nurse; the environment is accessible and makes sense. The tools and equipment appear functional and enabling to the nurse, whereas they may appear threatening or at least puzzling to the patient and family. The role of the nurse is to make this foreign environment feel safe and even healing to the patient.

However, the situation is far from having only one meaning for the family and patient. For trusting patients and families who have depleted their resources, the caregiving environment may give a strong symbolic message of forthcoming help. Consequently, raging symptoms may be quieted by a visit to the doctor's office, emergency room, or hospital or by the entry of a nurse. Patients and families with chronic illness may use the hospital as a source of respite, a coping resource when self-care and family caregiving resources are depleted and the patient's condition deteriorates. A major role of the nurse is to strengthen patients' and families' sense that the caregiving environment is safe and a coping resource. Nurses can make unfamiliar and threatening equipment appear enabling, if not friendly, through expert coaching and orientation.

For the nurse, the caregiving situation can become routine. She or he may experience it on a "timetable" of getting through the work day. A nurse at a conference on nursing practice directed by Benner told a story of being "unfairly" requested to admit a patient after her long and difficult night shift was over. She went to the room feeling disgruntled. She was abrupt and did not focus on the patient, who had just come from the emergency room with a possible myocardial infarction. The patient's condition deteriorated rapidly, and he became unconscious and died despite resuscitation efforts. The nurse told the story to the group of nurses as a "paradigm" case for her. It made her realize that this man's last contact before death was with a disgruntled, uninterested nurse. Her sense of the moral art of nursing was violated, and she determined never to adopt this uncaring stance again when admitting a patient. The point of her story was to remind her colleagues that what feels like routine and "one more task" may have great human significance. It is easy for the nurse to experience patient care as "routine," whereas patients and families seldom experience being sick as "routine." Thus, the experience of the situation as routine or novel is a major potential distinction for every nurse/patient-family interaction.

THE ROLE OF PERSONAL CONCERN

Caring for another in a world-defining way, as is the case for significant others, renders caregiving both threatening and necessary. This distinction is brought home by the nurse or physician who is confronted by a life-threatening illness in a family member. When the threat is extremely high, the personal concern may render those closest to the patient incapable of problem solving and providing the required action. The health care worker may not be able to perform as well for a family member as for a stranger. Memory is disrupted, and thinking processes can be chaotic due to fear and distress. Significant others may perform heroically when no other resources are available. When others are available, however, there is usually little doubt that others can cope with caregiving better in extreme circumstances.

This familiar scenario highlights how essential it is to sustain a network of care by setting up a society with paid, well-prepared, and caring caregivers to act in our stead. Such a societal arrangement is more than a business agreement, it is a moral statement. The moral injunction to provide fulltime paid caretakers is supported by the fact that every person in the society may require such assistance sometime.

Concern and a shared history with the patient, however, make significant others essential to effective nursing care. They provide the support and incentives crucial to recovery. Expert nurses talk about "knowing a patient" as a basis for assessment and intervention (Benner, Tanner, and Gordon, in progress). "Knowing a patient" for these expert nurses includes knowing his or her everyday habits, practices, and preferences as well his or her usual demeanor and self-presentation. Nurses rely on significant others to help them recognize subtle changes in the patient's behavior and mood, since such changes may be the first sign of physical or emotional distress.

TEMPORALITY

The way time is experienced by the nurse, patient, and family is widely disparate. In acute care settings, the nurse typically has an immediate timeframe that ranges from minutes to hours, depending on the acuity and degree of change the patient is experiencing. The nurse may perceive the patient's situation as stable, improving, or deteriorating in relation to the trends present in the previous minutes, hours, or days. In contrast, the patient and family may experience the illness in relation to the immediate past (weeks, months, or years) or to an uncertain projected future. Patient and family members may experience illness as interminable and without a horizon of hope within a foreseeable future. Therefore, part of the expert coaching of the nurse includes providing a perspective about the progress and recovery trajectory. Based upon prior experience with similar patients, the nurse often has a sense of the most likely immediate futures for the patient. The patient and family may experience the illness only as deficiency and discontinuity. The nurse who does not have this historical sense of the patient may more readily assess current progress and future possibility from the perspective of the current illness.

For the nurse, caregiving is timebound even though, as in the case of primary nursing, the nurse may coordinate and plan the caregiving around the clock. The structured limits to time spent in caregiving sets up obviously different possibilities for the nurse than for the patient or significant others. The intermittence or timeboundness of nursing care can be extremely functional. The time away gives perspective and renews energy for the caregiving tasks at hand. This structured time allotment is a central coping resource for nurses. The talk about time off and being off duty reflect the socially structured respites essential to effective caregiving. Failing to experience time off as a respite is a sign of fatigue and tension. Indeed this is one of the major burdens for the new nurse because much of the "time off" is spent in studying and anticipatory coping for the next shift (Benner and Benner 1979).

Although family members may have respites and even a sense of being off duty, their concerns and ongoing relatedness to the patient do not allow the same level of release available to the nurse. Nurses may think of their patients and feel concern when they are not working, but they return to an intact world outside of work. The patient's family must remain in a world altered or threatened by the illness of their loved one. Cultivating a lively world of love and leisure or even participating in one's own sets of dilemmas and projects provides an essential restorative respite from the demands of professional nursing.

From a nursing perspective, "work" and "love" are not in opposition. Work should not connote manipulative relationships governed only by efficiency. Rather, work and love are complementary sets of concerns and ways of being. Respite and restoration must be available in both spheres. The traditional view of work as competitive demands and home as the sole source of comfort does not suit any occupation, but it is untenable in nursing, where caring is central to the work. This is why health promotion and social support belong in the workplace as well as in the home.

THE ROLE OF EMBODIED INTELLIGENCE

Coping options are increased and qualitatively different when experience allows for an embodied intelligence. The body as a capacity to act has embodied orientations and expectations as a part of skilled know-how (Benner and Tanner 1987). Advanced levels of knowing

393

how are based on embodied intelligence. The body "takes over" a skill so that the task becomes easier (see Chapter Two, p. 45).

This bodily takeover of skill was described by nurses in a coronary care unit (Benner and Tanner 1987):

> And I didn't know how I would ever get to the place where I knew what I was doing. But then I learned. I knew what each drug did. I knew what the drips did. I knew what the monitors said and why. But I couldn't put it all together. But then, . . . it's almost like you visualize their arteries and veins expanding and contracting. And you know that as you turn this drip up, those veins are going to contract (she makes a gesture of contracting in the area of the leg veins). That's how you comprehend. That's how you get to be on top of something, so that you can look at any portion of this person's body and know what's expanding and contracting or what should be. And if it doesn't happen the way you visualize it, you can find that out and figure out why.
>
> During the telling of the story, the nurse became animated in describing the various bodily responses as she visualized them in her own body (p. 26).

The skilled habitual body gives the nurse access to the situation with much less effort and yet with increased sensitivity to signs and patterns. For example, the sounds from a panel of monitors recede into the background so that only the irregularities are noticed. The newcomer to a unit has to acquire a skilled habitual body in response to the patterns and actions required by the new environment. This learning period is stressful because it requires much interpretation and offers little direct effortless understanding. The skilled habitual body is a major coping resource.

Patients and families have little acclimation to the hospital situation and certainly do not have skilled habitual bodies geared to the hospital environment. Patients may experience their own bodies as awkward and strange due to the loss of skilled habitual responses. Mary Cucci, an expert critical care nurse, notices body language and reads bodily movements as a text (see pp. 247–250). In introducing patients to the unit, she points out that the "high-tech" environment looks intimidating, but she quickly reassures patients that one can continue to live here: "We eat cookies and laugh here, too," she says. Domesticating and thus normalizing the highly technical hospital environments and the strangeness brought on by illness is a central coping resource for patients, families, and nurses. Recovery for the patient means a recovery of a habitual skilled body.

Moving Beyond the Ideal and Real, Deficit View

We have presented an alternative view of the person in the situation from the Greek (and Cartesian) tradition. In the Greek view, the person has standards and ideals that are almost never actualized or lived up to in reality. Thus, a persistent view in such a tradition is that reality doesn't measure up—it is deficient. There is an expected gap between the ideal and the real, and this tension is understood as the basis for striving, goal-oriented behavior. The same picture of reality is evident in psychological testing. People are measured against an ideal norm or standard and are diagnosed in relation to that standard—how far they fall short of it or exceed it.

Although it is neither desirable nor possible to rid ourselves completely of the Greek view of reality, another cultural alternative is to view reality as a source of possibility and not only as a reflection of deficits in relation to prespecified ideals. Whereas the valuative stance is important for goal setting and guidance, the possibility stance allows one to see the actual possibilities inherent in the specific situation rather than always searching only for the "ideal" or preconceived ones. The move from viewing the situation only in relation to prespecified standards to viewing the situation as a field of opportunities and constraints is the same move made by the person moving from competent to expert levels of performance (Benner 1984a, Dreyfus and Dreyfus 1986).

The Greek-Cartesian understanding of the world in the dualities of "ideal" and "real" inevitably makes things show up as deficient. The usual therapeutic manuever for the distress created by a rift between the ideal and real is to recommend that the person let go of the importance of specific "desires" to one's happiness. For example, Borysenko (1987) offers the typical Western solution of adopting a Western version of an Oriental disengagement from desires and living in the moment:

> Wanting things is a natural part of life. Setting goals and working toward them fuel creativity and invention. The desire to change things activates progress. Wanting, per se, is not the root of difficulty; it's the pernicious attitude that we can't possibly be happy unless we satisfy a certain desire. . . . We suffer to the degree that we make our desires central to our happiness.
> . . . Deferring happiness until any condition is met—a new job, a new relationship, a new possession—leads to suffering. In clinging to

our desires, we send ourselves a strong statement that things are not okay right now. As life goes on the feeling of dissatisfaction keeps us hooked to our wants, preventing us from letting go and enjoying the present moment (pp. 117–118).

Borysenko's (1987) insight that desires (having things matter, i.e., caring) are not the problem is a good one. But then she makes the typical but incoherent therapeutic move that only specific desires are a problem and that deferring happiness to a future achievement robs us of the pleasure in the moment. Consequently, in this view, one must not make any specific desire essential, and happiness comes from living in the moment—immediacy. "Living in the now" can get the person out of endless activity, striving, planning, and preparing for the future, but it is not a coherent long-term coping solution. One's connection to the past and future, indeed experiencing continuity with past and future, is lost in this "presentism" (See Rubin, in progress).

Desires are not the problem, and loss of attachment and desires is effective only for brief periods of time. Borysenko's (1987) advice works because most people do not really lose their desires, they lose only the "ideal" forms of the desires. Ideal forms of reality that do not match up with actual situations keep the person from noticing possibilities in the situation.

Making all specific desires unimportant creates detachment at the expense of involvement. Presentism is an alternative to the Western temporality error of experiencing meaning only in future achievements. One can neither afford to arrive (reach the goals) nor can one focus adequately on the pleasures of the journey. (See Benner 1984b for an explication of goal-oriented, progress-oriented meanings.) Presentism or devaluing the importance of the specific goals creates a detachment that may cut one off from the things that matter to one. It is better to shift one's perspective from the "ideal" strategy (trying to stamp one's own version of reality on the situation) to a more flexible strategy (looking for one's possibilities inherent in the situation while at the same time looking for the coherence and possibility inherent in the situation itself). This is a shift from the technological understanding of the situation as chaotic raw material that must be wholly shaped by the self to one of expecting coherence and possibility in the situation.

Shifting one's perspective from that of a deficit view of the situation (i.e., assessing how deficient the real is compared to the ideal standard) to one of discovering the possibilities inherent in the situation opens up new coping options. Seeing only the deficits can block perceptions of the possible, but the deficit view may also paralyze action if the emotional response is one of moral outrage or disappointment. If one reacts with moral outrage, one may not see alternative lines of action that would help in this situation. Disappointment may breed disillusionment, and the person may cope by giving up the ideals altogether. Therefore, a shift in perspective to what is possible in this particular situation may open up new avenues for action, decreasing the sense of disappointment and powerlessness. Questions that open up possibility are: "What can be done now, in the meantime (before the ideal can be realized)?" "Is there another way to achieve the same end?" "Is the end in sight the most worthy?" Looking for the possibility inherent in the situation still requires a notion of the good one is trying to achieve. However, decreasing the preconceived notions about how that good ought to be achieved or even the nature of the particular good can offer a new point of departure.

Learning to look for the possible is a good antidote for the paralysis of reality shock (Kramer 1974), defined as the surprise and shock encountered when real practice does not meet the ideal expectations generated in school. Reality shock is reframed in the phenomenological perspective to be a description of learning by experience. Experience, according to Gadamer (1975), is a turning around of preconceptions that allows one to learn something new or add nuance to prior views.

Instead of expecting theoretical accounts to be precise (true to the situation), Heidegger (1962) offers the corrective that theory is derived from practice and that any practical situation is more complicated than any skeletal model or theoretical prediction. Theory derives power from leaving out detail. This is why the expert practitioner who has opportunities to test theories directly in practice has knowledge that goes beyond any theoretical account. Human expertise is based on the ability to compare current whole situations with past whole situations complete with the nuances (Benner 1984a, Dreyfus and Dreyfus 1986). In Heidegger's view, all practice becomes a dialogue with theory. Theory is confirmed, not confirmed, or extended in practice. This, too, is a departure from the deficit view of reality. One no longer expects to find a precise one-to-one relationship between theories of human action and the actual situation. The situation contains new possibilities. The practitioner develops clinical knowledge by subjecting the theory to practice and then using the practice to confirm, disconfirm, or extend the practice.

Effective Caring—A Basic Mode of Being

We have argued that caring is a basic way of being in the world and that caring creates both self and world. When nurses are permitted to care for patients and families to the best of their knowledge and ability, the "stresses" in nursing are reduced to those legitimate to the realm of caring. We do not seek to trivialize or sentimentalize the difficulty and pain inherent in liberated caring. We only want to point out the power, challenge, and stunning human victory when the difficulties are met with a caring intent.

In the best of nursing practice, we experience a common humanity. Nurses find it important to convey to patients that they consider it possible to experience the same fate as patients or family. A television reporter once commented that technology had given more power and liberation to nurses than feminism. Her reporting was more intelligent than her commentary, however, because she also taped a nurse giving care to a cancer patient. It was obviously less than heroic care, and it was obviously care. Seeming to be truly puzzled, the reporter asked, "Don't you have a problem with burnout? Why do you do this?" The nurse gave a profound response from the ethics of care and responsibility. She said, "I would like to think that someone would be here for me if I had cancer." This sense of membership in a common humanity that not only loves, competes, aspires, wins, consumes, and gets promoted but also suffers and gets sick is illustrated when an expert nurse gives a patient an exquisite coaching session on what to expect from surgery. (See Chapter One, p. 13.)

We believe that we have much to learn from the best and worst of nursing practice. In the best practice, we discover selves of membership related to a common humanity and given over or defined by specific concrete concerns and human relationships. By being experts in caring, nurses must take over and transform the notions of expertise. Expert caring has nothing to do with possessing privileged information that increases one's control and domination of another. Rather, expert caring unleashes the possibilities inherent in the self and the situation. Expert caring liberates and facilitates in such a way that the one caring is enriched in the process. Instrumentalism, contract language, cost-benefit analysis, social exchange, enlightened self-interest, and all the language of the autonomous self of possession misses the relationship of the person constituted by concerns and human relationships.

The self of membership and participation requires a language of commitment, meanings, skills, concerns, and aspirations. The systematic study of such human beings requires narrative and interpretation. Human capacities are best described in terms of possibilities and skilled practice, and not just in terms of how well the person measures up to predetermined, context-free criteria of performance.

Managerial language and practices that seek to objectify, quantify, and decontextualize conflict with the nature of caring practices. Patients feel cared for when they are not treated as merely customers, consumers, or resources. When we are ill we want to feel cared for. Even the most autonomous, modern person wants to feel confident that humane, sensitive care will be available if she or he were incapacitated and unable to be assertive or demand rights. The notions of the self in opposition to others and an ethic limited to rights and justice cannot account for caring for another who is without full powers, except in "paternalistic" terms. An ethic of relatedness, care, and responsibility is needed to account for the mutual trust required for caring for the incapacitated. Caring practices in the context of familial and community membership need not be paternalistic. A culture that emphasizes independence and individualism cannot survive without a safety net of care and caring practices.

The rational-technical model of management has no language or strategies for determining what are worthy goals (MacIntyre 1981, March 1976). The rational-technical model is limited to the assumption that we know what are the appropriate ends and that the only problem is how to be more efficient in reaching them. To go beyond the rational-technical model we need to develop a discourse on worthy ends. We need to examine our caring practices and augment the rational-technical model of management with narrative forms about what is required to support and facilitate excellence in caring practices. This narrative can develop by examining practice actually considered excellent. Such an approach allows the manager to move beyond deficit management, where practice is always compared to standards or pre-specified managerial goals and found deficient or merely adequate, to develop a positive project based on worthy ends already demonstrated in the best of practice. Such an approach demands respect for the practicing nurse and an expectation that new standards of excellence are being developed daily in practice.

TAKING OVER WORK LIFE

If nurses are to liberate caring practices, organizations will have to be redesigned to facilitate and sponsor caring practices. The nurse is both a knowledge worker and one who cares. The thesis of this book is that knowledge is dangerous if it is divorced from caring, and that human existence requires care and caring practices. Furthermore, human expertise is based on care—having things and people matter. Caring and caring practices must set the health care agenda, and managerial strategies must be shaped to serve caring. In a health care environment that has switched from non-profit to profit-based, from community-based organizations with volunteerism and planned charity to corporate-based ownership and accidental charity, the time is ripe for creating radically new approaches to both community and hospital-based care.

The hospice movement and birthing centers, along with the change in caring practices in childbirth, are examples of shaping organizations to fit the nature of caring (Corless 1985). For example, labor-and-delivery nurses and childbirth educators have provided the rest of nursing, and indeed the rest of society, with an important cultural dialogue—and even cultural victory—over a completely totalizing, technological self-understanding of birthing. Approximately twenty-five years ago, nurses began to raise consciousness with the suggestion to their patients that the birth of a baby need not be experienced as a disease. Nurses contended that women need not be separated from other family members, drugged, operated upon, and alienated from the birthing of their family; that babies need not arrive drugged, bruised from forceps, and incapable of a lusty cry. In twenty-five years the cultural practices surrounding childbirth have become a public dialogue, and sweeping changes have occurred in birthing practices. Many have participated in this change. But this cultural revolution would have been much slower, and may not have occurred at all, without many nurses beginning childbirth education classes, often in a hostile medical climate. Also, nurses working in labor and delivery actively coached women into new birthing alternatives. Nurses were very clever and cloaked this revolutionary change in the guise of consumer demand, but it was primarily the nurses who taught the consumer to make new demands. Of course these changes in birthing practices were helped along by an emerging identity of women as active determiners of their bodies and experience instead of passive victims.

Though many nurses resisted this new vision of birthing a family, in schools of nursing and in the majority of labor-and-delivery suites, nurses coached women into new alternatives. In this one area, technological practices that had run rampant were turned back—an amazing accomplishment, and nurses deserve credit for this.

That victory is tenuous. Each day newly developing technology threatens to convince us that birthing is a dangerous, chaotic process. Technology should be shaped by necessity, not by its mere existence. Unnecessary technical procedures and practices convey to us that our bodies are unreliable and passive. They imply that participation and skilled know-how are unrelated to birth. This is a technological self-understanding, i.e., bodies are understood as machines or chaotic raw material that must be controlled and dominated by technology. Means are separated from ends and means are considered relatively unimportant.

Lisa Chickadonz, a nurse-midwife, describes in an interview how cultural statements are embedded in the way the work of labor and delivery is carried out. She sees the lithotomy position as a cultural statement, an embodiment of the technical-expert model:

First of all, sitting at the foot of the bed when somebody's delivering can be a total power feeling. For some it's a big rush to sit there, but I don't like to do births from the foot of the bed, partly because of that. It is as if you are enthroned and everything is there for *your* convenience. You as the expert become the center of the process. Literally, the configuration centers around you.

Interviewer: So how do you deliver if you aren't at the foot of the bed?

I like the sidelying position a lot. Those are my favorite births. You don't give the mother any particular position; it is just the position most women labor in. And then, when they push, sidelying is the best position for circulation for the fetus. At the time of delivery you just have [her partner] hold her knee up a little bit. Stabilize the top leg, and the baby slides right out. It's almost anticlimactic! Part of the mystique about the lithotomy position is that it is so dramatic compared to having these little babies just go "plunk" and slip out into the bed.

I watched a movie once, a twin birth in Appalachia, and this woman is just lying in the bed having some pains, and pretty soon this little baby comes squirting out, and the midwife picks it up and wraps it and puts it next to her, and pretty soon the mother's had a few more pains and another baby squirts out, and the midwife puts it next to her, makes the bed up, and goes home. Compared to the kind of production we make for the birth of twins in the hospital, it was unbelievable. I am not convinced that our way is warranted. It seems to be about the glorification of the expert rather than the safe delivery of the baby. There are a lot of advantages to sidelying deliveries also, in that the babies tend to fit better and do better in delivery. It is just a very nice way for women to deliver. A lot of patients I've delivered that way have said that it is very comfortable and that it felt really good to them.

Lisa Chickadonz gives a strong sense of a notion of good in her practice. She tries to empower, coach, and facilitate. She is aware that her practice is laden with meanings. It is this kind of critique based on the caring practices of mutual realization and empowerment that must shape the organizational life of health care and guide managerial practice.

TAKING OVER OUR EDUCATION AND SCIENCE

Nursing education has been too enmeshed with the rational-technical model and needs reform that will enable nurses to critique organizational life based upon expert caring practice. Practice must not be viewed as a deficient imprint of ideal theoretical propositions. Instead, practice must be viewed as coherent and more complex than can be captured by any formal theoretical statement (Benner 1984a). The practicing nurse is on the forefront of knowledge development, and educational practices need to prepare the nurse to engage in a dialogue with practice. As Donald Schon (1987) states:

> The question of the relationship between practice competence and professional knowledge needs to be turned upside down. We should start not by asking how to make better use of research-based knowledge but by asking what we can learn from a careful examination of artistry, that is, the competence by which practitioners actually handle indeterminate zones of practice—however that competence may relate to technical rationality (p. 13).

Such an examination of expert practice can uncover new areas of knowledge not yet described or accounted for in the research literature (Benner 1984a). An enhanced respect for the knowledge embedded in expert practice will set up new agendas for nursing education.

How do we take over our science and education so that it can do justice to our practice? This is a central question in this scientistic age. Since science is our major authority and source of legitimization, how can we transform our science so that the definition of what it means to be a person is not always construed in advance to be an unrelated, autonomous agent, gripped in a homeostatic presentism, seeking strategic ends based only on self-interest, enlightened or otherwise.

A revision of our understanding of the person will give us a new science and new therapies. These therapies already exist in the best of our caring practices, but we require a language and science that captures the nature and intent of these practices as they are carried out in real contexts and real relationships. Such a science will give us a new respect for the concrete and specific, the courageous and meaningful over time. We will come to understand heroic action not only in terms of technological breakthroughs but also in terms of skillful comportment and excellence in the current situation.

Dorothy Merner, a nurse from Toronto, Canada, gives such an account of the power of caring:[1]

PARADIGM
A Pot of Coffee
Dorothy Merner

A sixty-seven-year-old man was admitted to the psychogeriatric assessment unit from his own apartment. He was divorced and lived alone. His presenting diagnosis was acute behavioral problems. His other diagnoses were COPD (chronic obstructive pulmonary disease) and terminal cancer with metastasis to the lungs and brain. He was grossly obese, due in part to fluid retention. He had stopped bathing and caring for himself physically, and so he had skin breakdown and a strong body odor. He was loud, exhibiting obnoxious physical and verbal behavior. He seemed to be saying: Here I am, what can you do for me that hasn't been tried? He was showing his anger over his increased dependency and loss of power. His admission was like an invasion of the unit.

The patient's history showed that he was a very sociable retired newspaperman. He exhibited a fiery intelligence and a fierce independence. Soon after his admission, dissension was created between himself and the staff. He felt he should have access to the staff coffee supply when thirsty just as the staff did. Suffering from periodic bouts of nausea, he didn't always eat his meals when they were available. The staff denied him access to the coffee pot. He solved the problem by escaping from the hospital. He returned the next day with his own identical coffee pot plus coffee. The coffee machine became the focus of his attempt at independence as well as something tangible toward which to direct his

---

1. Dorothy Merner was selected by her peers as an outstanding clinician, Sunnybrook Medical Centre, Department of Extended Care. She presented this exemplar from her practice at a conference entitled "From Novice to Expert: Recognizing and Rewarding Excellence in Practice," sponsored by the Ontario Registered Nurses Association, October 23, 1986.

anger and frustration. The opportunity to have and to offer people coffee was an integral part of his lifestyle.

This incident precipitated considerable discussion among the nursing staff. I intervened, getting permission and special safety clearance from the hospital biomedical engineering department. The nurses agreed that he would have to be monitored closely to prevent him from burning himself or leaving the pot on while empty. I interpreted this preparation of coffee to my colleagues as a nursing measure to restore his sense of control and provide an access to his more sociable side. Planned outings to the mall to purchase his own supplies would prevent further hospital disappearances. The coffee would provide an avenue for interaction with the rest of the multidisciplinary team. He was a Jewish agnostic but gained great comfort from serving coffee and talking to the chaplain about how he did not believe in God. He also did not believe in psychiatry but became much less agitated when the psychiatrist chatted over coffee about his recent emotional upheavals.

He was estranged from his family, and we were able to encourage them to come in for coffee and a visit. The alienated family members eventually "stopped by" for coffee and to say hello. As his condition deteriorated, he still enjoyed the opportunity of offering coffee to others. It served as a solace and relieved visitors' discomfort, allowing the emphasis to be on the coffee pot instead of the illness.

We could analyze the stress incurred in caring for such an angry, alienated, unkempt man, but like Dorothy Merner we celebrate the opportunity to participate in the restoration of caring for this man, his family, and the nurses. The "objective threats" are turned into challenges and triumphs and that exemplifies the best in human coping and caring. As Tracey White states, "Caring is a profound act of hope."

REFERENCES

Akerstedt T: Adjustment of physiological circadian rhythms and the sleep-wake cycle to shiftwork. In Folkard S, Monk TH (eds): *Hours of Work: Temporal Factors in Work Scheduling,* Chichester, England: John Wiley and Sons, 1985.

Adams J, Folkard S, Young, M: Coping strategies used by nurses on night duty. Ergonomics 29(2):185, 1986.

American Association of Colleges of Nursing. Final Report, Pew Foundation Study: Essentials of College and University Education for Professional Nursing. Washington, D.C.: The Association, 1986.

American Nurses' Association: *Facts About Nursing, 86–87.* New York: The Association, 1987, p. 10.

Bellah RN, Madsen R, Sullivan WM, Swidler A, Tipton SM: *Habits of the Heart.* Berkeley: University of California Press, 1985.

Benner P: *From Novice to Expert: Excellence and Power in Clinical Nursing Practice.* Menlo Park, Calif.: Addison-Wesley, 1984a.

Benner P: *Stress and Satisfaction on the Job: Work Meanings and Coping of Mid-Career Men.* New York: Praeger Scientific Press, 1984b.

Benner P, Benner RV: *The New Nurse's Work Entry: A Troubled Sponsorship.* New York: Tiresias Press, 1979.

Benner P, Tanner C: Clinical judgment: How expert nurses use intuition. Am J Nurs 87:23, 1987.

Benner P, Tanner C, Gordon DG: The phenomenology of knowing a patient (forthcoming).

Borysenko J: *Minding the Body, Mending the Mind.* Reading, Mass.: Addison-Wesley, 1987.

Corless IB: Implications of the new hospice legislation and the accompanying regulations. Nurs Clin N Amer 20:281, 1985.

Dreyfus HL: *Being-in-the-World: A Commentary on Heidegger's Being and Time, Division I.* Cambridge, England: Cambridge University Press, in press.

Dreyfus HL, Dreyfus SE, with Athanasiou T: *Mind over Machine: The Power of Human Intuition and Expertise in the Era of the Computer.* New York: The Free Press, 1986.

Felton G: Body rhythm effects on rotating work shifts. J Nurs Admin 5(3):16, 1975.

Folkard S, Monk TH: Shiftwork and performance. Human Factors 21:483, 1979.

Folkard S, Monk TH, Lobban MC: Short- and long-term adjustment of circadian rhythms in "permanent" night nurses. Ergonomics 21:785, 1978.

Gadamer H: *Truth and Method.* New York: Seabury, 1960, 1975.

Gadow S: Existential advocacy: Philosophical foundation of nursing. In Spiker SF, Gadow S (eds): *Nursing, Images and Ideals,* pp. 79–101. New York: Springer, 1983.

Gilligan C: *In a Different Voice: Psychological Theory and Women's Development.* Cambridge, Mass.: Harvard University Press, 1982.

Heidegger M: *The Basic Problems of Phenomenology.* Hofstadter A (trans). Bloomington: Indiana University Press, 1982.

Heidegger M: *Being and Time.* Macquarrie J, Robinson E (trans). New York: Harper and Row, 1962.

Heron E: *The Story of a Nurse: Intensive Care.* New York: Atheneum, 1987.

Hochschild AR: *The Managed Heart: Commercialization of Human Feeling.* University of California Press, 1983.

Jorgenson MJ, Crabtree AS: Exploring the practical knowledge in expert critical care nursing practice. Unpublished master's thesis, University of Wisconsin-Madison, School of Nursing, 1986.

Kalisch PA, Kalisch BJ: *The Changing Image of the Nurse.* Menlo Park, Calif.: Addison-Wesley, 1987.

Kizer WM: *The Healthy Workplace: A Bluebook for Corporate Action.* New York: Wiley, 1987.

Kramer M: *Reality Shock: Why Nurses Leave Nursing.* St. Louis: C. V. Mosby, 1974.

Larson DG: Internal stressors in nursing: Helper secrets. J Psychosocial Nurs 27(4):20, 1987.

Mallison M: How can you bear to be a nurse? Amer J Nurs 87:419, 1987.

MacIntyre A: *After Virtue.* Notre Dame, Indiana: University of Notre Dame Press, 1981.

McDermott MJ: The nature of advanced clinical practice. Unpublished paper presented at conference entitled: Career Development in Nursing, Developing Programs of Clinical Promotion, Berkeley, California, September 19, 1987.

March JG: The technology of foolishness. In *Ambiguity and Choice in Organizations,* pp. 69–81. Universitetsforlaget, 1976.

Marshall J: Stress amongst nurses. In *White Collar and Professional Stress,* Cooper CL, Marshall J (eds.). pp.19–59. New York: John Wiley & Sons, 1980.

Maslach C: *Burnout—The Costs of Caring.* Englewood Cliffs, N.J.: Prentice-Hall, 1982.

National Commission on Nursing. Summary Report and Recommendations. Chicago: The Hospital Research and Educational Trust, 1983.

Norbeck J: Coping with stress in critical care nursing: Research findings. Focus on Critical Care 12:36, 1985.

Norwood R: *Women Who Love Too Much.* Los Angeles: Jeremy P. Tarcher. Distributed by St. Martin's Press, New York, 1985.

Pennebacker JW: Traumatic experience and psychosomatic disease: Exploring the roles of behavioral inhibition, obsession, and confiding. Can Psychol 26:82, 1985.

Registered Nurse Population, June 1986. U.S. Department of Health and Human Services, Public Health Services, Health Resources and Administrative Services, p. 5, 1986.

Reverby S: A caring dilemma: Womanhood and nursing in historical perspective. Nurs Res 36:5, 1987.

Roach S: *Caring: The Human Mode of Being: Implications for Nursing. Perspectives in Caring.* Monograph 1. Toronto: Faculty of Nursing, University of Toronto, 1984.

Roach S: *The Human Act of Caring.* Ottawa: Canadian Hospital Association, 1988.

Rowe SC (ed): *Living beyond Crisis.* New York: Pilgrim Press, 1980.

Rubin J: *Too Much of Nothing: Modern Culture and the Self in Kierkegaard's Thought* (forthcoming).

Sandel M: *Liberalism and the Limits of Justice.* London: Cambridge University Press, 1982.

Schon DA: *Educating the Reflective Practitioner.* San Francisco: Jossey-Bass, 1987.

Selye H: *Stress without Distress.* Philadelphia: Lippincott, 1974.

Smythe EM: *Surviving Nursing.* Menlo Park, Calif.: Addison-Wesley, 1984.

Stein LL: The doctor-nurse game. Am J Nurs 68:101, 1968.

Tisdale S: *The Sorcerer's Apprentice: Tales of the Modern Hospital.* New York: McGraw Hill, 1986.

Vidacek S, Kaliterna L, Radosevic-Vidacek, B, Folkard S: Productivity on a weekly rotating shift system: Circadian adjustment and sleep deprivation effects. Ergonomics 29(12):1583, 1986.

Weisman AD: Understanding the cancer patient: The syndrome of caregiver's plight. Psychiatry 44:161, 1981.

Whitbeck C: A different reality: Feminist ontology. In Gould CC (ed): *Beyond Domination: New Perspectives on Women and Philosophy,* pp. 64–88. Totowa, N.J.: Rowman & Allenheld, 1983.

White T: On nursing. Unpublished academic paper, New College, Berkeley, 1986.

Yankelovich D: *New Rules in American life: Searching for Self-Fulfillment in a World Turned Upside Down.* New York: Random House, 1981.

Glossary

Actual Projected Body   The way the body is set to act at any particular moment. In carrying out skilled activity in any particular situation, the body responds as the situation requires by drawing on past history and skilled know-how that are relevant and needed.

Background Meaning   What a culture, subculture, family and personal life experience give a person beginning from birth. It determines what counts as real for the person. It is a shared, public understanding of what is. Background meaning is not itself a thing, like formal, explicit knowledge. It is rather what allows for the perception of the factual world.

Being (*Dasein*)   Heidegger chose the word *Dasein* to describe the ongoing activity and practical coping of everyday life. In German, the word *Dasein* means everyday existence, but it also means "being there." Dasein is the beginning point of human experience and existence for Heidegger. He saw *Dasein* as an alternative to private, separate subjects and objects. *Dasein* can refer to the ways of being of individuals, cultures, organizations, historical eras, or other collective activity. (See footnote, page 104.)

Being-in-the-World   A Heideggerian term that describes how people are involved in situations through their concerns, skills, and practical activity. (See *Concern.*)

Bodily Intentionality   Refers to the person at home in the body in such a way that the body has a capacity to respond to and act in meaningful situations without conscious reflection.

Body (Bodily) To be distinguished from features of the body such as cellular changes and hormonal changes. The body as a whole is a knower, an actor, and an experiencer of situations. There is an impoverishment in the English language to describe bodily ways of being in the world. Possibly because of the transparancy of bodily ways of being and because of a cultural emphasis on cognition as the source of all action, *body* does not show up in daily discourse as an expression of being, of action, or of an organized level of functioning.

Caring Practices   Organized, specific practices related to caring for and about others. Caring practices are lived out in this culture primarily in parenting, child care, nursing, education, counseling, and various forms of community life. An ethic, a way of knowing, and practical knowledge are lived out in specific caring practices so that it is possible to recognize and discuss what counts as caring—or not caring, in specific instances.

Cartesian   Refers to the thinking of Descartes.

Cognitivism   Refers to the approach that views each individual person's knowledge, understanding, intentions, and actions as originating only in the mind.

Concern   A way of being involved in one's own world in which people and things matter to one. It describes a phenomenological relationship in which the world is apprehended directly in terms of its meaning for the self. Concern is the reason why people act. It is necessary for life.

Constitutive   Descriptive of the way people become involved in situations so that what they experience in those situations changes them and their personal meanings. A situation or a concern is constitutive when it gives actual content or style to one's self-understanding or one's way of being in the world.

Coping   What people do when personal meanings are disrupted and smooth functioning breaks down. Since the goal of coping is the restoration of meaning, coping is not a series of strategies that people choose from a list of unlimited options. Coping is always bounded by the meanings and issues inherent in what counts as stressful. (See *Stress.*)

Descartes, René   French philosopher and mathematician (1596–1650). We trace to Descartes' philosophy the origins of the representational model of the mind and the mind-body split, both of which have currency in contemporary thought. (See *Representational Model of the Mind* and *Mind-Body Split.*)

Embodied Intelligence   Refers to the fact that the body itself is a knower and an interpreter. It includes capacities that range from innate proprioception to habitual, cultural knowledge, to complex skills. (See *Embodiment, Bodily Intentionality,* and *Body (Bodily).*)

Embodiment   The ways meanings, expectations, styles, and habits are expressed and experienced in the body.

Epistemology   Concerns how and what people know.

Existential   A way of being in the situation.

Formal Theory   The version of theory handed down by Greek philosophers, particularly Plato and Socrates. To count as formal theory, knowledge must be propositional, context-free, formalizable through mathematical relationships, general, and ahistorical.

Habitual, Skilled Body   This aspect of embodiment includes all culturally and socially learned postures, gestures, and customs, as well as the capacity to acquire and use bodily skills.

Heidegger, Martin   German phillsopher and writer (1889–1976). Heidegger was a student of Husserl. He critiqued Husserl as being the last of the Cartesians because of his cognitivist project. (See *Phenomenology* and *Husserl.*)

Husserl, Edmund   German philosopher (1859–1938). Founder of phenomenology and a teacher of Heidegger. Husserlian phenomenology is not followed in this book because it is based on a representational model. Husserl's notion of the *noema* is that it is an internal, mental organizer that assigns meanings to perceptions. Husserl is the culmination of the Cartesian tradition that understands the world in terms of conscious subjects knowing objects. (See *Phenomenology.*)

Inborn Complex   The pre-cultural body that the baby is born with.

Interpretive Theory   Interpretive theory refers to an explanation in meaning terms. In contrast to formal theory, interpretive theory can attend to the local, particular, and specific as it relates to similarities and differences in content, meanings, and qualitative distinctions.

Lived Experience   The way people encounter situations in terms of their own personal concerns, background meanings, temporality, habitual, cultural bodies, emotions, and reflective thoughts.

Lived Meaning   The way personal meanings arise from and exist in the situation as the person experiences it. Lived meanings are part of the person's precognitive understanding. They are not explicit and cannot be made explicit—nor are they propositional, but they are part of the person's understanding of what is real.

Mechanism or Mechanistic Model   The view, based on physics and mathematics, that something can be broken down into components and understood by the analysis of separate elements.

Mind-Body Split   The idea, which originated with Descartes, that the mind and body are separate and distinct entities. Although many people have attempted in various ways to dispute the notion, it is a necessary corollary to the representational model of the mind. As long as the mind is the only source of meaning and interpretation, the body cannot be understood as a knower but only as a means of bringing information to the mind. (See *Representational Model of the Mind.*)

Ontology   Concerns how people are or exist.

Phenomenal Body   The phenomenal body is the body aware of itself. This is the ability to imagine the body. Body image, as it is typically described, is the same as the phenomenal body.

Phenomenology   A philosophical approach based on the study of the thing(s) perceived. Heideggerian phenomenology, the approach used in this book, differs from other approaches in that it posits that the very act of perception is a grasp of meaning, an interpretation.

Positivism (Logical Positivism)   Positivism has its roots in the work of the nineteenth-century French philosopher Auguste Comte, who believed that the same scientific methods used for the natural sciences could be applied to morals and the study of human affairs. Logical positivism is an extension of Comte's thesis and was developed in Austria and Germany in the 1920s. The most influential of this group of scientists were known as the Vienna Circle. Their goal was to eliminate metaphysics from science and to develop a scientific discourse in the human sciences that relied on interpretation-free data, or observation statements that were "direct and indubitable" descriptions of sense experience. The verifiability principle of this school limited meaning to what things could point to, represent, or stand for; meaning that referred to human experiences of feelings or significance had to be excluded from this account.

Practical Knowledge   Know-how or knowing how. It is the opposite of theoretical knowledge. It depends in large part on bodily intentionality and the habitual, skilled body.

Precognitive   Refers to awarenesses and interpretations and any resulting actions that do not rely on deliberate and intentional cognitive reflection.

Presencing   To be with someone in a way that acknowledges or participates in the person's experience. To presence oneself means that the person is available and accessible to another so that the other feels that he or she is understood and supported.

Present-at-Hand   Refers to equipment described as an object and not as part of the way the person is in or experiences the situation.

Projective Body   The way the body is set to act in normal skilled comportment.

Radical Freedom   A term coined by French philosopher Jean-Paul Sartre that refers to the ability to choose any meaning consciously and deliberately and to live by it. In this view, the person is free to choose any course of action and interpret the meaning of any situation through conscious, explicit choice. (See *Situated Possibility.*)

411

Ready-to-Hand   Refers to equipment that is transparent, unnoticed, and experienced as an extension of the body because of the way the person is actively involved in the situation.

Representational Model of the Mind   The notion that people perceive and understand experience by representing their experiences mentally and then interpreting or assigning meanings to them. This assumption of how the mind works is the basis for all analogies of the mind to a computer. (See *Mind-Body Split.*)

Set to Action   The bodily anticipation of action and the embodied preparedness to respond.

Significance   Meaning as it is lived, and the world as it is experienced in a qualitatively differentiated way. Significance allows some things to show up as relatively important or relatively unimportant.

Situated Freedom   The freedom that is available when people are involved in a network of social relations, meanings, concerns, and equipment. Certain actions and experiences show up as possibilities or as choices against the background of this network or situation. The person's situatedness makes some choices more relevant and appealing than others. (See *Radical Freedom* and *Situated Possibility.*)

Situated Possibility   The possibilities people have when they are engaged through concern with their current situation. (See *Situated Freedom* and *Radical Freedom.*)

Situation   The relevant concerns, issues, information, constraints, and resources at a given span of time or place as experienced by particular person(s).

Stress   The disruption of meanings, understanding, and smooth functioning so that harm, loss, or challenge are experienced, and sorrow, interpretation, or new skill acquisition is required. (See *Coping.*)

Temporality   The way the person simultaneously lives in the present, is influenced by the past, and is projected into the future. It does not refer to the linear passage of time, but to the way the person is

412

anchored in a present that is made meaningful by past experience and by the person's anticipated future.

Unready-to-Hand Refers to equipment that is noticed because of breakdown. Breakdown occurs either because the equipment itself does not work smoothly or because the person has cause to notice it, perhaps through loss of maximum grasp or self-consciousness.

World A collective term used by Heidegger to refer to the fusion of temporality, concerns, and the situation.

PERMISSIONS

AUTHOR INDEX

SUBJECT INDEX

Winner of American Journal of Nursing *Book of the Year Awards in Nursing Education and Nursing Research!*

FROM NOVICE TO EXPERT

Excellence and Power in Clinical Nursing Practice

Patricia Benner, RN, PhD, FAAN

After reading this book, one appreciates the richness of knowledge, skill, and sensitivity in nursing practice.

Roberta Ann Smith
Women and Health

A "must" for all nurses at any stage of their professional development.

Martha D. Clark Balser
MCN

Must reading for all who bemoan present-day nursing practice . . . clearly describes the scope and depth of nursing practice.

Barbara A. Munjas
Journal of Psychosocial Nursing

It may just help you see your career in a whole new way.

Mary Mallison
Editorial *AJN*

Anyone involved in nursing today could profit from this book, but it is especially relevant for practicing nurses and nursing faculty.

Mitzi L. Duxbury
AJN

Captures the nature of nursing practice in exquisite narrative relying on the cases of practicing nurses.

Judith Krauss
The Yale Nurse

To all members of the profession it fosters a sense of pride in saying "I'm a nurse."

Linda Hodges
Journal of Neurosurgical Nursing

A testimonial to the importance of nursing, this landmark book includes many clear, colorful examples from actual nursing practice, presented in nurses' own words. A special epilogue describes how the findings of this study have been applied in five major hospitals.

Book Code #00299. 335 pp, soft cover. $26.95.
For fastest service in ordering, call Toll Free (800)447-2226 or write:

Addison-Wesley Health Sciences
390 Bridge Parkway
Redwood City, CA 94065

ISBN 0-201-12002-X